The New Politics of Old Age Policy

The New Politics of Old Age Policy

Edited by Robert B. Hudson

The Johns Hopkins University Press
Baltimore

The Johns Hopkins University Press
2715 North Charles Street
Baltimore, Maryland 21218-4363
www.press.jhu.edu

Library of Congress Cataloging-in-Publication Data

The new politics of old age policy / edited by Robert B. Hudson.
    p. ;   cm.
  Includes bibliographical references and index.
  ISBN 0-8018-8074-2 (hardcover : alk. paper) — ISBN 0-8018-8075-0
(pbk. : alk. paper)
  1. Older people—Government policy—United States. 2. Older people—
Services for—United States. 3. Old age pensions—United States.
4. Medicaid. 5. Social security—United States. 6. Old age—United States.
  [DNLM: 1. Public Policy—Aged—United States. 2. Medicaid.
3. Pensions—United States. 4. Social Security—United States.
HQ 1064.U5 N532 2005] I. Hudson, Robert B., 1944–
  HV1461.N76 2005
  362.6'0973—dc22   2004015975

A catalog record for this book is available from the British Library.

To Perry and Tim—
the lights of my life

Contents

Contributors

Robert Applebaum, Ph.D., Professor, Scripps Gerontology Center, Miami University, Oxford, Ohio

Robert H. Binstock, Ph.D., Professor of Aging, Health, and Society, Case Western Reserve University, Cleveland, Ohio

Alan Burnett, M.A., Director, Area Agency on Aging, Ohio Region 9

Chenoa A. Flippen, Ph.D., Research Scientist, Center for Demographic Studies, Duke University, Durham, North Carolina

Judith G. Gonyea, Ph.D., Associate Professor of Social Research, Boston University School of Social Work, Boston, Massachusetts

Colleen M. Grogan, Ph.D., Associate Professor, School of Social Service Administration, University of Chicago, Chicago, Illinois

Madonna Harrington Meyer, Ph.D., Associate Professor of Sociology, Director of the University Gerontology Center, and CPR Senior Research Associate, Syracuse University, Syracuse, New York

Pamela Herd, Ph.D., Assistant Professor, LBJ School of Public Affairs, University of Texas at Austin, Austin, Texas

Martha B. Holstein, Ph.D., consultant in ethics and aging research, Chicago, Illinois

Robert B. Hudson, Ph.D., Professor and Chair, Department of Social Policy, School of Social Work, Boston University

Eric R. Kingson, Ph.D., Professor of Social Work and Public Administration, and CPR Senior Research Associate, Syracuse University, Syracuse, New York

Marc Molea, M.H.A., Director of Planning and Evaluation, Ohio Department of Aging

Marilyn Moon, Ph.D., Vice-President and Director, Health Programs, American Institutes for Research, Silver Spring, Maryland

John Myles, Ph.D., Professor of Sociology and Canada Research Chair, University of Toronto, Toronto, Ontario, Canada

Christy M. Nishita, doctoral candidate, Andrus Gerontology Center, University of Southern California, Los Angeles, California

Angela M. O'Rand, Ph.D., Professor, Department of Sociology, Duke University, Durham, North Carolina

Jon Pynoos, Ph.D., United Parcel Service Professor of Gerontology, Leonard Davis School of Gerontology, and Professor of Urban Planning, University of Southern California, Los Angeles, California

Sarah Poff Roman, M.G.S., Research Associate, Scripps Gerontology Center, Miami University, Oxford, Ohio

Steven M. Teles, Ph.D., Assistant Professor, Department of Politics, Brandeis University, Waltham, Massachusetts

Preface

The New Politics of Old Age Policy addresses the policy issues posed by a series of demographic, economic, and political trends now well under way in the United States. The aging of the U.S. population, growing disparities in economic well-being among older Americans, and the reemergence of a political agenda questioning the federal role in social policy have transformed traditional understandings of the status of older people in public policy. In the early years of the American welfare state, the politics surrounding age-based policy were relatively benign because the programs' direct costs were modest and the opportunity costs were few. In subsequent decades, the politics became more highly contested as program costs escalated, the needs of the aged population became more variable, and other social issues emerged. Most recently, the politics have become even more heated as a resurgent political conservatism, raising fundamental questions about the relative responsibilities of the public and private sectors, has emerged in conjunction with dire budgetary forecasts tied to expected demographic and economic developments.

This volume explores the policy issues and options resulting from this convergence of population, economic, and political forces. The book's opening section provides theoretical perspectives on aging policy. Martha Holstein makes the normative case for maintaining today's age-based policies, arguing that their reduction or elimination would result, not in greater equity across populations, but in major retrenchment of universalism in American social policy. John Myles reviews alternative steps that might be taken to heighten the fairness of age-related policies, invoking the standards of both intergenerational and intragenerational justice. Madonna Harrington Meyer argues that today's emergent conservatism would shift longstanding public responsibilities toward individuals and their families in a manner that would have serious ramifications, especially for the very old, for women, and for family caregivers. Taking a far different view, Steven Teles reconstructs the political meaning of Social Security as the cornerstone of a new "welfare state conservatism" so entrenched that meaningful reform has essentially become impossible and allied opportunity costs have grown very large.

The book's second section focuses on the changing makeup of the older population, with a principal emphasis on increasing differentials in well-being now being found among different segments of this population. Angela O'Rand, in exploring the question of when old age begins, emphasizes how variable life-course trajectories make any old-age marker empirically problematic and, in turn, how policy shifts toward increased individual responsibility leave selected older subpopulations very much at risk. Chenoa Flippen concentrates on one of those at-risk populations—older workers of color—documenting high levels of involuntary job loss besetting middle-aged and older African Americans and Hispanics. Judith Gonyea turns attention to the oldest old, seeing both collective vulnerability and surprising diversity within this population. She concludes that our public policies continue to lag in recognizing the growing and multiple needs of many very old people.

The book's third section investigates the workings of our principal age-based and age-related policies. Pamela Herd and Eric Kingson tackle the debate centered on the future of Social Security, arguing that proposals to privatize and "individualize" the program, rather than being necessary to assure its future, are in fact a direct assault on the core principles of a program highly valued by the American public.

Marilyn Moon believes that Medicare still "makes sense" as an age-based program (although the eligibility age of 65 may ultimately need to be raised), concluding that in the current environment any major alternative would likely be in the direction of eliminating the program rather than expanding it. Colleen Grogan argues that even though Medicaid is a residual or public-assistance program, the political standing of at least its older beneficiaries may nonetheless make possible expansion of eligibility through a process she labels "universalism within targeting." In the case of housing for elderly persons, Jon Pynoos and Christy Nishita find pressing issues around program costs and beneficiary deservingness, but they juxtapose this set of concerns against the indisputable need for more and new types of senior housing.

The book's concluding section looks to national, state, and local politics associated with age-based policy in the United States. Robert Binstock reviews how demographic and ideological developments have transformed aging politics in recent years and have abetted the development of major new policy options that—depending on one's perspective—would either save or eviscerate longstanding aging programs. Finally, Robert Applebaum and his colleagues review the dynamics that have led Ohio's taxpayers to support local tax levies on behalf of older people in need of community-based long-term care services, asking in particular if what appears to be good politics also constitutes good policy.

The editor and several authors involved in the preparation of *The New Politics of Old Age Policy* were also associated with an earlier volume published by the Johns Hopkins University Press (in cooperation with the American Society on Aging) entitled *The Future of Age-Based Public Policy*. By virtue of the participation of additional contributors and the preparation of new chapters by earlier authors, *The New Politics of Old Age Policy* stands as an entirely new work. For their assistance in the preparation of this volume, I would like to thank Wendy Harris, medical editor of the Johns Hopkins University Press, Bob Binstock, consulting editor in gerontology to the Press, and Judith Gonyea, my colleague, friend, and unceasing source of innovative thinking.

The New Politics of Old Age Policy

1. Contemporary Challenges to Age-Based Public Policy

Robert B. Hudson

Provisions benefiting older people have long been a hallmark of social policy in the United States. Given their life circumstances, it is perhaps not surprising that aged persons receive a far greater volume of public benefits than do younger populations. Nonetheless, social policy in the United States is distinctive because it allocates a higher proportion of social welfare expenditures to elderly people than do other industrial nations; it employs age as an eligibility criterion more than is the case elsewhere; and, in using chronological age, it puts greater emphasis on the needs of the old than those of the young.

Old Age as a Policy Variable

There are compelling reasons, both historical and current, for recognizing advanced age as a major variable in social policy. The most obvious is that age has long stood as a formidable proxy for demonstrable need and, in turn, the receipt of support from the larger society. Indeed, old age has long been understood—in addition to illness, disability, and unemployment—to be one of the "bad things" (Rubinow 1934) that can happen to people in industrial society.

In the United States, greater recognition has been given to old age as a bad thing than has been given to other risks or contingencies associated with modern life. Outliving one's income was long considered the most dire prospect facing older persons. That prospect was far from remote, given that as recently as seventy years ago at least half of older people are estimated to have been poor and that some three-quarters of elders' income in that period, it is estimated, came from their adult children (Upp 1982). Few would have argued with Franklin Roosevelt's contention, made while governor of New York, that "poverty in old age should not be regarded either as a disgrace or necessarily as a result of lack of thrift or energy. . . . It is a mere by-product of modern industrial life" (Rimlinger 1971, p. 212). Or, as noted by Carole Haber (1983), from an early time in American history, aged persons were consciously omitted from "the redeemable" (i.e., those who should be expected to earn their own support).

Historically, chronological age has served as a central proxy for need, as an important marker of an inability to work, and as an essentially inevitable predictor of illness and disability. Separately and in combination, these traits have given the old a uniquely legitimate claim to policy benefits in the U.S. context. If one cannot work due to age (or if employers choose not to employ older people for real or alleged work-related limitations), provision should be made for income transfers in old age. If older people are understandably more ill than younger ones and if the private insurance market will not serve them, provision should be made for publicly sponsored health insurance. And in those cases where advanced age creates especially desperate situations, means-tested supplements to existing income and health provisions may come into play. A "positive political construction" of the aged (Schneider and Ingram 1993) has long held sway in the United States, and this construction goes a long way toward explaining the historic generosity public policy has shown toward older Americans.

An important contextual factor contributing to the old's positive political standing has been the nation's more ambivalent attitudes toward other population groups and social problems. In such prominent social policy arenas as public welfare, national health care, unemployment relief, mental health care provision, family supports, or child care, the U.S. policy effort has been relatively limited and restrictive. The widely analyzed reasons for this distinctive U.S. profile extend to historical patterns of immigration (Hartz 1955), a consensual political culture (Huntington 1966), national devotion to individualism (Rimlinger 1971), divided governmental institutions (Skocpol 1985), and "the failure of socialism" (Esping-Andersen 1985). Whatever the reasons (and justifications), the comparative level of benefits and the basis for benefit receipt in the United States have historically been more generous in the case of the age-based policies than in the other social policy arenas.

Until the late 1970s, a comparatively benign economic and political environment, coupled with the widely accepted deservingness of the aged, allowed for and fostered the growth of age-based public policy in the United States. In more recent years, of course, that environment has changed fundamentally as the scope of conflict around aging policy has broadened and sharpened. The singular legitimacy long enjoyed by the aged—albeit largely based on a negative stereotype—has more recently morphed into an imposing institutional standing generated by a monumental policy presence and a new-found political identity. Yet this development itself has generated fiscal, generational, and ideological concerns, which in turn have created the highly charged political atmosphere in which aging-based policy today finds itself.

The Development of Age-Based Policies

In both absolute and relative terms, the development of policies on aging in the United States has been impressive. The country's first national social policy took the form of Civil War pensions for Northern soldiers. Unprecedented in scale, these pensions were subject to large-scale fraud and abuse throughout the late nineteenth century, to the point that their policy legacy largely died with the passing of the veterans themselves (Skocpol 1991). In the twentieth century, the dire needs of many elderly or widowed Americans were first recognized in modest state-level "mothers pensions"; and, in the 1930s, these needs were given federal recognition through Old Age Assistance, the Title I public assistance program for the destitute aged under the original Social Security Act.

The broader economic issue facing the aged centered on the transition from work to retirement and was addressed in the Act's Old Age Insurance (OAI) title, the cornerstone for today's Social Security program. Roosevelt and his brain trust were able to overcome opposition to OAI by designing an insurance program that would reward only those who had contributed to Social Security during their working years and who would receive benefits based on those earnings only at the advanced age of 65, an age beyond which work was not to be expected. In 1939 benefits were made available to the survivors of deceased workers—a matter of some controversy at the time because, unlike the retiree's benefit, the survivor benefit was independent of work history. In the 1950s, Disability Insurance—originally covering only individuals over the age of 50—was enacted, providing an important transitional benefit to older disabled individuals whose inability to work often turned them into "younger retirees."

The high-water mark of aging-based public policy came in the decade from the mid-1960s to the mid-1970s. While much social legislation associated with Lyndon Johnson's Great Society was enacted during the period, policy for older Americans continued to stand out. Most notable was the passage of Medicare, a program that represented—in addition to economic need and inability to work—the illness element of elderly Americans' deservingness triad. In Marmor's well-known words, the elderly were "one of the few population groupings about whom one could not say the members should take care of their financial-medical problems by earning or saving more money" (1970, p. 17). The Medicaid program, also enacted in 1965, addressed both need and illness among the old. Medicaid broadened an earlier federal-state grant program by paying for the long-term care health costs of low-income frail elders. Primarily supporting nursing home care, Medicaid filled an important gap by recognizing the chronic care needs of many poor elders that were expressly omitted from Medicare coverage. Today Medicaid is the nation's largest payer of long-term care health benefits for the old and for the disabled.

Growing recognition of the needs of the growing elderly population led to additional enactments during this ten-year period. The Older Americans Act, a non-means-tested program that served in part as symbolic recognition of the growing policy place of the old in Washington was also enacted in 1965. The OAA grew dramatically throughout the 1960s and 70s and became the focal point of the so-called aging network, an array of planning and service agencies in both the public and private sector that now blanket the nation (Hudson 1994).

Major civil rights legislation for the old was enacted in 1967 through the Age Discrimination in Employment Act. The ADEA initially outlawed workplace bias against workers aged 40–65; in 1978, the upper age was raised to 70, and in 1987, the upper age was eliminated altogether, resulting in the effective elimination of mandatory retirement for the vast majority of older workers. ADEA is also important for giving legislative acknowledgment to the contemporary reality that not all older individuals wish to cease working and that not all older individuals are beyond employment. In the years since, whether the old can or should work has become a matter of prominent policy debate, raising important questions about age-based employment and retirement policy.

The need for private pension protection for retired workers was recognized through passage of the Employee Retirement Income Security Act (ERISA) in 1974. Under ERISA, workers in traditional or defined benefit retirement plans were vested after five years service, and the federal Pension Benefit Guarantee Corporation was established to insure employer pension plans in the case of bankruptcy or forfeiture. Finally, the National Institute on Aging was created within the National Institutes of Health in 1974. Creation of NIA represented a victory for researchers in geriatrics, who argued that the health needs and the particular health profiles of older people were not adequately recognized in disease-specific institutes directed to heart disease, cancer, and other illnesses.

Emerging Pressures on Age-Based Public Policy

By the late 1970s, known and anticipated age-based expenditure and program growth began garnering focused attention: Estes (1979) spoke of the "aging enterprise"; Hudson (1978), of "the graying of the federal budget"; and Samuelson (1978), of "shouldering the growing burden." Short-term economic pressures, emergent concerns about the aging of the U.S. population, and a new conservative presence in Washington led to a halt in the enactment of additional age-based programs after the long expansionary period.

Nonetheless, expenditures under existing programs were continuing to grow "automatically" (Weaver 1988), "unsustainably" (Concord Coalition 2003), or even "understandably" (Ball 2000). In the case of Social Security, retirement benefits had been increased more than 60 percent between 1967 and 1972, and future benefits were now tied to cost-of-living increases. These liberalizations and growing numbers of beneficiaries resulted in OASDI expenditures for those aged 65 and above increasing from $29 billion in 1971 to $85 billion in 1980, and to $307 billion by 2000. Medicare costs began spiraling shortly after the program's enactment, with doctors' historical cry against the government promoting "socialized medicine" being replaced by their recognition that they were beneficiaries of a massive new health care funding stream. Indeed, critics suggested that Medicare had succeeded in "socializing" the costs of health care to the elderly while "privatizing" the benefits to physicians and other health care providers. Due to higher payments to providers, growing numbers of beneficiaries, and new technological developments, Medicare expenditures for the old rose from $8 billion in 1971 to $29 billion in 1980, and to $189 billion by 2000 (U.S. CBO 2001, p. 200). Finally, nursing home and other long-term care costs were rising as well, even as concerns about the quality of long-term care for the elderly and disabled escalated (Walker, Bradley, and Wetle 1998). Table 1.1 presents information on the growth and size of federal expenditures on behalf people aged 65 and above from 1971 to 2000 and projected to 2010.

Program developments in the 1980s and 1990s centered on concerns about expenditure growth. Social Security legislation enacted in 1983—drawn from a commission headed by Alan Greenspan—incorporated both cuts in benefits—notably, the gradual raise in the normal retirement age to 67—and increases in payroll taxes. Also in the early 1980s, expenditure growth in the Medicare program led to the institution of a prospective payment system limiting how much Medicare would reimburse providers for particular medical procedures. Additional measures to curb Medicare spending, directed at physicians and at escalating home health care costs, were later imposed. In the late 1980s, the Medicare Catastrophic Coverage Act, a seemingly expansionary piece of legislation incorporating new hospital and drug benefits, was enacted. However, invoking concern about the aging of the population and data about the new-found well-being among the old, the Reagan administration insisted that these new benefits be paid through income tax surcharges on older people themselves rather than by current workers through the payroll tax. The outcry by older voters in response to this provision was so heated that Congress was forced to repeal the law two years after passage (Himmelfarb 1995).

The 1990s saw a major effort by Republicans in Congress to cut Medicare and Medicaid benefits—the stalemate leading to a government shutdown for several days—but legislation passed in 1997 imposed cuts that were less sweeping (Smith 2002). During the late 1990s several proposals to partially "privatize" Social Security were put forth, two of them being contained in the official Report of the Social Security Advisory Council. Proponents of privatization pointed to the need to rein in what they saw as unsustainable growth in program costs that would accompany retirement of the baby boom generation. Critics of these proposals, however, saw a different agenda at work, namely, to curtail the responsibility of the federal government to honor its obligations to these future old-age cohorts.

Table 1.1 Estimated federal spending for elderly persons under selected programs, 1971–2010 (by fiscal year, in billions of dollars)

	1971	1980	1990	2000	Projected 2010
Mandatory programs					
Social Security	29	85	196	307	471
Federal civilian retirement	2	8	21	33	50
Military retirement	1	2	7	14	21
Annuitants' health benefits	*	1	2	4	9
Benefits for coal miners/black lung	*	1	1	1	1
Supplemental Security Income	1	2	4	6	10
Veterans' compensation and pensions	1	7	4	9	14
Medicare	8	29	96	189	377
Medicaid	2	5	14	33	77
Food stamps	*	1	1	1	1
Total	44	137	349	597	1,026
Discretionary programs					
Housing	*	2	4	7	10
Veterans' medical care	1	3	6	9	13
Administration on Aging programs	*	1	1	1	1
Low-income energy assistance	n.a.	*	*	*	1
Total	1	6	11	17	24
Total, all federal spending on people age 65 and older	46	144	360	615	1,050
Federal spending on people 65 and older					
As percentage of budget	21.7	24.3	28.7	34.8	42.8
As percentage of GDP	4.2	5.3	6.3	6.4	7.1
Per elderly person (in 2000 $$)	8,896	11,839	15,192	17,688	21,122

Source: U.S. Congressional Budget Office 2002
* = less than $500 million; n.a. = not applicable

In what now seems a *fin de siècle* fiscal mirage, the booming economy and stock market of the late 1990s led Clinton administration and other officials to predict that the entire federal budget debt could be retired by 2015, a development that would have dramatically eased long-term pressures on Social Security. The more recent return of annual budget deficits well in the hundreds of billions of dollars and long-term debt projections of many trillions of dollars have, however, reinforced notions of Social Security as the "third rail of American politics" and Medicare reform as an even dicier prospect.

Age-Based Policy Today

The shift in political and economic climate, coupled with the remark-
able success of public policy in improving the overall well-being of the
old, has generated policy debates that would have been hard to imagine thirty years ago. Have policy accomplishments (and expenditures)
on behalf of the old gone beyond being a notable policy success to a
form of policy excess? Do growing disparities in well-being among the
aged call for a more targeted and less universal approach to age-based
benefits? Are longstanding policy assumptions around the reciprocity
of relations between the generations now dated and unfair to emerging generations? And, most fundamentally, has government come to
play too large a role on behalf of the aged, and should steps be taken
in order that individuals, their families, and the private sector shoulder greater responsibility for well-being in old age?

Varieties in Well-being among the Old

Much contemporary debate about age-based public policy lies in re-
markable improvements in well-being among the old, many of which
can be laid to the benefits of public policy, notably Social Security and
Medicare. By no means can it any longer be said that old people are
universally needy or, as was historically nearly the case, singularly
needy. Poverty among the old has declined from nearly 40 percent in
the 1950s to 10.4 percent in 2002 (U.S. Bureau of the Census 2003).
The broader aging population has also made notable economic
progress in recent decades, its median income having risen (in constant
2002 dollars) from $19,900 in 1970 to $33,800 in 2001 (U.S. Bureau
of the Census 2002). In comparison, the incomes of those under 65 increased only 26 percent from 1967 to 1992 (Radner 1996). The role
of Social Security in these developments is seen in a study by the U.S.
Bureau of the Census (1988), which concluded that social insurance
programs, principally Social Security, have done more to alleviate
poverty and inequality among the old than either the tax system or
other social programs, including welfare.

There is also a new twist on the matter of older Americans' ability
to work. While it was long common knowledge that older people
"couldn't work," in fact, they did. As recently as 1950, the labor force
participation rate among older men was 46 percent, a figure that fell

steadily into the early 1990s—to the point at which only about 16 percent of older men were working—before leveling off and rising slightly since (Quinn 1997). The pattern for older women has been largely unchanged over recent decades due to "the combined effects of increased participation by women and decreased participation by the elderly" (Quinn and Burkhauser 1990). Social Security, which had historically been designed not only to support older people who were not in the workforce but also to encourage them to leave the workforce, has been a major factor in this trend. Thus, labor force participation falls off precipitously at age 62, the age at which workers are eligible for early retirement benefits under Social Security.

Most recently, however, the growing presence of relatively well-off elders and policy enactments predicated on their emergence are modifying historical patterns of work and retirement. The 1990s have seen a gradual increase in the labor force participation rate of men and also an increase in older workers turning to so-called bridge jobs (Ruhm 1995) (i.e., different from their principal occupation but representing a clear substitute to retirement). For members of these emerging cohorts of older workers, improved health and job opportunities make work a more rewarding option than was once the case. For growing numbers of workers, whether and when to retire is now more of a choice than a decision forced by illness or unemployment.

Contributing to the trend toward greater labor force participation are new work-related opportunities and incentives that have been introduced into public policy in recent years. Originating in concerns over population "graying," these moves build as well on assumptions about improved age-specific health status among the old. The most obvious provision is the rise in the normal retirement age (eligibility for full benefits) from 65 to 67 currently being phased in for workers born after 1938. Elimination of mandatory retirement under the ADEA is also making it possible for more workers, principally white collar middle-class workers, to remain in the labor force at their choosing. More important yet has been elimination of the so-called earnings test under Social Security. Historically, workers aged 65 to 69 forfeited up to one-third of their Social Security benefits if they continued to work and earn relatively modest amounts. After several years of liberalizing the test, the reduction in benefits has now been entirely eliminated, no matter what the level of earnings are.

Improvements in well-being among many contemporary elders have led to the development of new constructs capturing the phenomenon, such as "productive aging" (Bass, Caro, and Chen 1993), "the young-old" (Neugarten 1974), and the "third age" (Laslett 1987). In place of the traditional monolithic view of the old as poor, frail, and unemployable, these categorizations center on the strengths and abilities to be found among many contemporary older people. Policy is moving to discourage retirement among a population now argued to be increasingly in good health and around which old age policy can now be notably "reconstructed."

Yet, lurking just beneath the aggregate improvements in elders' well-being are enormous disparities and imbedded levels of need. In addition to differences by race and gender, there are differences within the overall older population. Poverty among older African Americans stands at 27 percent and among older Hispanics at 21 percent in comparison to 9 percent among white older Americans. At 13 percent, the poverty rate among older women is nearly double that among older men. Among people aged 65–69, the median income is $20,893, compared to $11,251 among people aged 80 and older (Crown 2001). The multiple jeopardy associated with these otherwise discrete attributes paints yet a starker picture as seen in the poverty rate among "young-old" white men (aged 65–69) standing at 5.7 percent in comparison to the rate among "old-old" African American women at 28.3 percent (U.S. Bureau of the Census 2001). And were it not for Social Security, these figures would be much more pronounced, because Social Security constitutes 82 percent of income among the poorest 20 percent of the elderly and only 19 percent among the most well-off 20 percent (U.S. Bureau of the Census 2002).

Major vulnerabilities face members of the young-old as well as the old-old populations. For all of the talk in policy circles about the "productive old" and the "able old," millions of older workers struggle, frequently caught in an economic black hole where they are neither able to work (due to illness and unemployment) nor to retire (due to nonexistent or inadequate pension protection and savings). Involuntary job loss and forced retirement remains an enormous problem for low-income and minority workers (Hayward, Friedman, and Chen 1996). Concern about these younger vulnerable workers helped preserve the age-62 early retirement benefit under Social Security when the normal retirement age increases were phased in. However, that age and benefit will be on the table again when, as seems likely, moves are made to increase the normal retirement age beyond age 67.

At the other end of the old-age spectrum, the plight of the very old has become more rather than less pronounced. The old-old are disproportionately women, living alone, often physically or mentally frail, unable to work, and in possession of only meager savings and modest policy benefits. When widowed, women's Social Security benefits decline by one-third. When incapacitated by long-term illness or disability, their needs extend beyond the protections offered by Social Security and Medicare, forcing them to rely on Medicaid's means-tested benefit. And while evidence is growing that age-specific disability levels are declining modestly, individual and aggregate-level long-term care needs are certain to remain among the most pressing problems of the old.

Overall, we left with a clear pattern of "structured diversity" among the old. Aggregate improvements in well-being, many of them policy induced, are notable, even historic. Yet in the face of these overall improvements, clearly identified groups of the old find themselves at social and economic risk. In a time of governmental retrenchment, this diversity poses major questions for public and policy and especially for age-based public policy.

Future Costs and Responsibilities

Coloring all discussions of the status of the aged is the question of growing costs of age-based programs and how those costs should be distributed. In the late 1980s and early 1990s, this discussion largely took place in terms of intergenerational transfers. The demographic bulge represented by the baby boom cohort brought into question a historic assumption that successive generations of workers would be able and willing to support earlier generations in their old age. Sustaining these programs largely unchecked, critics argued, would be unfair to future workers and would place onerous burdens on the U.S. economy. While acknowledging that the contributions of Social Security and Medicare "deserve our respect," Lamm and Lamm (1996) contended that if these programs continue to go untouched "with taxes as high as 60 percent of each paycheck, the next generation will have little incentive to work." Devising a "generational accounting" construct, Kotlikoff (1996) pointed to a dire future for the young and unborn. For generations born throughout the twentieth century, he argues, lifetime net tax burdens have risen only moderately, from 24 percent for those born in 1900 to 34 percent for those born in 1993. He estimates, however, that the comparable rate for future generations may run as high as 84 percent. To right this generational imbalance, he contends, we would have to either cut income taxes by 69 percent or cut Social Security and Medicare benefits 45 percent beginning today (Kotlikoff and Burns 2004), this being an increase in his 1996 estimates requiring a 41 percent income tax hike or a 30 percent cut in program spending. Several recent analyses see estimates of future unfunded liabilities for Social Security and Medicare easily running into the trillions of dollars. The Bush administration estimates an $18 trillion shortfall over a 75-year period, but economists Kent Smetters and Jagadesh Gokhale (2004) project a long-term deficit of no less than $44 trillion. A different but parallel calculation derived by Howe and Jackson (1999) forecasts, under intermediate assumptions, that the percentage of the gross domestic product devoted to governmental benefits (of which Social Security and Medicare are the largest items) will jump from 13 percent in 1998 to 22 percent in 2040. Finally, the 2004 Report of the Medicare Trustees forecasts that the Medicare Part A hospital trust fund will be exhausted by 2019, seven years sooner than was predicted in the 2003 report.

In joining this debate, proponents of the current programs argued that modifications were required but could be undertaken within present framework, the critical elements of that framework being universal coverage, single insurance pool, defined benefits, and a progressive benefit formula. With these bedrock provisions remaining in place, reforms put forth by program defenders have included extending coverage to additional state and local workers, reducing benefits slightly by computing them over 38 rather than 35 years, taxing benefits in a manner similar to private sector defined contribution plans, raising the earnings ceiling, and investing part of the trust fund in equities (Jones 1996). To bring long-term liabilities under control, Diamond (2004) suggests steps such as eliminating the "legacy debt" (i.e., benefits received by early participants well in excess of their contributions plus interest) by imposing a 3 percent tax on earnings above the maximum earnings base.

These are certainly modest reforms compared to the proposals by

Kotlikoff and Smetters and Gokhale calling for massive tax increases and benefit cuts and fundamental restructuring of both Social Security and Medicare (Kotlikoff and Burns 2004). But if one remembers that there was a time when the very thought of taxing Social Security benefits was considered political suicide (Stockman 1975), it becomes clear how the debate over the future of these programs has changed. Or, as Moon says in this volume, there was a time when shifting Medicare from an age-based policy meant expanding it to cover other populations and conceivably approximating national health insurance; today, a discussion of moving Medicare away from age-based eligibility would probably mean its elimination.

Moon's comment speaks to a critical broadening of the public policy debate that has taken place over the past decade in which age-based policy has been centrally featured. In short, the contemporary social policy debate is more about political ideology than it is about population dynamics. The interrelated cost and generational issues are still important, but these concerns are taking a back seat to deeply rooted convictions among different parties about what the appropriate role of the federal government should be in addressing individual and social problems. Quadagno (1989) picked up on this shift earlier than many observers, noting that the so-called entitlement crisis proclaimed by intergenerational equity critics of aging-based programs was centered more on the responsibilities and expectations of the federal government than it was on expenditures and deficits.

In the case of Medicare, White (2003) argued that Republican efforts to "save Medicare" were of such magnitude that they would have ended the program as we know it. More recently, the battle over the Medicare legislation signed in December 2003 has been as much about creating, restructuring, and subsidizing a private sector delivery system and limiting the government's future exposure to cost increases as it has been about adding a prescription drug benefit to the program. Proposals to partially privatize Social Security, once couched in language tied to fiscal solvency, are now discussed more openly as shifting responsibility for well-being in retirement from government to individuals. In the case of Medicaid, tax incentives to promote sale of private long-term care insurance policies have the same objective. Structural reforms proposed by Kotlikoff are very much along these lines, including eliminating the OASI payroll tax, imposing a national sales tax to pay transitional Social Security benefits, eliminating the

Medicare fee-for-service program ("traditional Medicare"), issuing "participant-specific" vouchers, and limiting the voucher amounts to the future growth of real wages (Kotlikoff and Burns 2004).

The overt introduction of ideological bases and rationales for program restructuring is an important and, arguably, a welcome addition to the age-based policy debate. Arguments and reforms based on age and generation have often contained a subtext that was both mean-spirited ("greedy geezers") and flew in the face of much public opinion and social science understanding of the positive and reciprocal relations that exist between members of different age groups and generations (Cook and Barrett 1992; Campbell 2003). There will indeed need to be equitable trade-offs among different generations that involve benefits for the old and taxes on current workers (see Myles in this volume), but this debate is now openly addressing "the locus of responsibility" question, that is, what should be the balance between public sector, private sector, and individual responsibility for assuring population well-being among young and old alike.

Age-Based Policy: Politics and Prospects

For the foreseeable future, it is increasingly certain that the politics of age-based policy will run along the contentious lines of "immovable object meets irresistible pressure." The magnitude of old-age policy and the salience of older people in the political process represent an imposing institutional presence. Yet impinging on aging policy's continued standing are economic and political constraints on the growing need for massive infusions of new funds to honor pending program commitments.

These developments place arguments about the merits and dangers of age-based public policy in sharp relief. On the one hand, it is clear that old age—certainly where age 65 continues to be invoked as the threshold year—is an increasingly imperfect proxy for singular physical, economic, and social vulnerability. Heterogeneity among the older population is great and growing, and the characteristics of many older people are becoming less distinct from the young than may have once been the case. Moreover, recent sociological research (see O'Rand in this volume) makes clear that patterns of divergence marking people in old age emerge many years before individuals attain age 65. Whatever its historical contributions, the unique case for age-based public policy is weakened by trends pointing to greater heterogeneity among the old and growing levels of similarity and connectedness between the old and the young.

As a political matter, however, the growth and acceptance of age-based policy in the United States results in large part from the nation's unwillingness to entertain other populations or population character-istics as legitimate bases for receipt of public benefits. There has been an enduring reluctance for policy to embrace vulnerabilities defined by poverty, class, race, health, and employment status. As a result, age-based policy has assumed something of a default-drive character in the context of U.S. social policy. The reason for the U.S. welfare state's not having developed universal health insurance or children's allowance programs, perhaps the two most pressing policy gaps, is not that we have devoted substantial resources to those who are old. Rather, our age-based programs assume a special place—certainly when compared to other industrial nations—because we have chosen to pay little heed to an array of risks and vulnerabilities facing many middle-aged and younger people.

We must be mindful of these patterns and realities in addressing the future of age-based public policy. Specifically, there must be clarity about what the problem is that we might choose to address. The ear-lier debate centering on "old versus young" has receded in part be-cause the underlying argument that public policy does so little for young because we do so much for the old has lost much of its credi-bility. No one believes that cutting expenditures in Social Security or Medicare would result in new policy benefits for young families—in-deed, the welfare reform embodied in the Temporary Assistance to Needy Families program moves in a dramatically different direction.

A more legitimate question is whether today's older people require all of the benefits now being made available to them. For many, that is clearly not the case. But "need" has a very particular meaning in so-cial policy terms, invoking means-testing, exclusion, and residualism. Americans have tried to spare the old many of the indignities associ-ated with such systems, but the newfound well-being of many old people gives rise to this option again. Means-tested options in age-based programs have gained little ground in recent years, although there has been a notable increase in the targeting of benefits toward low-income and functionally impaired elders in recent years (Binstock forthcoming). More clearly, "affluence-testing" among well-off elders in the financing of Social Security and Medicare benefits is gaining ground, a step that alarms many liberal adherents of social insurance programs (Hacker and Marmor 2003). In the newly contested arena of old-age policy, upward adjustments in contributions and fee schedules are certainly on the table, as are further weighting of benefits toward the economically and functionally vulnerable old.

Beyond these types of adjustments, the overriding question today comes back to sector responsibility. In the case of the old, the inexorable growth in program expenditures has led to loud and growing calls for major structural reform. The earlier argument centered on intergenerational inequity has more recently evolved into one centering on the income and tax burdens resulting from massive levels of increased spending on the old that will fall on future workers. No one knows with precision how great that burden will be, with that very unknown quality constituting a major reservation among liberals about too aggressively tackling the problem today (Marmor, Mashaw, and Harvey 1990; Aaron 2002).

Yet these burdens, whatever their size, will need be tackled somewhere. If it is not provided through the public sector, it will need to be provided by individuals, families, and, perhaps, private entities. These alternatives will satisfy concerns about excessive taxation, but they cannot hide age and generational issues that will arise even if the units in question are families and communities rather than governments. Filial obligation—significantly relieved by Social Security, notably so by Medicare, and to a lesser extent by Medicaid—might move back closer to center stage if pending political choices result in a retreat from the overall twentieth century pattern of building "institutionalized solutions to individual risks" (O'Rand 2003).

References

Aaron, H. 2002. Budget estimates: What we know, what we can't know, and why it matters. In S. H. Altman and D. I. Shactman, eds., *Policies for an Aging Society*. Baltimore: Johns Hopkins University Press.

Ball, R. 2000. *Insuring the Essentials*. New York: Century Foundation.

Bass, S., F. Caro, and Y.-P. Chen, eds. 1993. *Achieving a Productive Aging Society*. Westport, Conn.: Auburn House.

Binstock, R. H. Forthcoming. What changes will be needed in social policy, and who will determine them? Commentary. In M. Smyer and R. Pruchno, eds., *Policy and Responsibility across the Generations*. Baltimore: Johns Hopkins University Press.

Concord Coalition. 2003. Seniors still come first in the budget. *Facing Facts Alert* 9(2) (March 19).

Campbell, A. L. 2003. *How Policies Make Citizens: Senior Political Activism and the American Welfare State.* Princeton, N.J.: Princeton University Press.

Cook, F. L., and E. J. Barrett. 1992. *Support for the American Welfare State: The Views of Congress and the Public.* New York: Columbia University Press.

Crown, W. 2001. Economic status of the elderly. In R. H. Binstock and L. K. George, eds., *Handbook of Aging and the Social Sciences,* fifth ed. San Diego: Academic Press.

Diamond, P. 2004. What Are the Best Alternatives for Meeting the Impending Crisis in Social Security Financing? Presentation to Conference on Public Policy and Responsibility across the Generations. Boston College, Newton, Mass.

Esping-Andersen, G. 1985. *Politics Against Markets.* Princeton, N.J.: Princeton University Press.

Estes, C. 1979. *The Aging Enterprise.* San Francisco: Jossey-Bass.

Haber, C. 1983. *Beyond 65: The Dilemmas of Old Age in America's Past.* New York: Cambridge University Press.

Hacker, J., and T. R. Marmor. 2003. Medicare reform: Fact, fiction, and foolishness. *Public Policy and Aging Report* 13(4):1, 20–23.

Hartz, L. 1955. *The Liberal Tradition in America.* Cambridge, Mass.: Harvard University Press.

Hayward, M. D., S. Friedman, and H. Chen. 1996. Race inequities in men's retirement. *Journal of Gerontology: Social Sciences* 51B:S1–10.

Himmelfarb, R. 1995. *Catastrophic Politics: The Rise and Fall of the Medicare Catastrophic Care Coverage Act of 1988.* University Park: Pennsylvania State University Press.

Howe, N., and R. Jackson. 1999. *The Graying of the Welfare State* (Policy Paper No. 117). Washington, D.C.: National Taxpayers Union.

Hudson, R. B. 1978. The "graying" of the federal budget and its consequences for old-age policy. *Gerontologist* 18(4):428–40.

Hudson, R. B. 1994. The Older Americans Act and the defederalization of community-based care. In P. Kim, ed., *Services to the Aged: Public Policies and Programs.* New York: Garland.

Huntington, S. 1966. Political modernization: America vs. Europe. *World Politics* 18:378–414.

Jones, T. 1996. Strengthening the current Social Security system. *Public Policy and Aging Report* 7(3):1, 3–7.

Kotlikoff, L. 1996. Generational accounting. *Public Policy and Aging Report* 7(4):4–6, 17.

Kotlikoff, L., and S. Burns. 2004. The perfect demographic storm: Entitlements imperil America's future. *Chronicle of Higher Education,* March 19, B6–10.

Lamm, R., and H. Lamm. 1996. *The Challenge of an Aging Society.* Denver: Denver Center for Public Policy and Contemporary Issues, University of Denver.

Laslett, P. 1987. The emergence of the third age. *Ageing and Society* 7:133–66.

Marmor, T. R. 1970. *The Politics of Medicare.* Chicago: Aldine.

Marmor, T. R., J. Mashaw, and P. Harvey. 1990. *America's Misunderstood Welfare State.* New York: Basic Books.

Neugarten, B. 1974. Age groups in American society and the rise of the young-old. *Annals of the American Academy of Political and Social Science* 415:187–98.

O'Rand, A. 2003. The future of the life course: Late modernity and life course risks. In J. T. Mortimer and M. J. Shanahan, eds., *Handbook of the Life Course.* New York: Plenum.

Quadagno, J. 1989. Generational equity and the politics of the welfare state. *Politics and Society* 17:253–76.

Quinn, J. 1997. Retirement trends and patterns in the 1990s: End of an era? *Public Policy and Aging Report* 8(3):10–14.

Quinn, J., and R. Burkhauser. 1990. Work and retirement. In R. H. Binstock and L. K. George, eds., *Handbook of Aging and the Social Sciences,* third edition. San Diego: Academic Press.

Radner, D. 1996. Incomes of the elderly and non-elderly. *Social Security Bulletin* 58:82–97.

Rimlinger, G. 1971. *Welfare Policy and Industrialization in Europe, America, and Russia.* New York: Wiley.

Rubinow, A. 1934. *The Quest for Security.* New York: Holt.

Ruhm, C. 1995. Secular changes in the work and retirement patterns of older men. *Journal of Human Resources* 30:362–95.

Samuelson, R. J. 1978. Aging America: Who will shoulder the growing burden? *National Journal* 10:1712–17.

Schneider, A., and H. Ingram. 1993. Social construction of target populations. *American Political Science Review* 87(2):253–77.

Skocpol, T. 1985. Bringing the state back in: Strategies of analysis in current research. In P. Evans, D. Rueschemeyer, and T. Skocpol, eds., *Bringing the State Back In.* New York: Cambridge University Press.

Skocpol, T. 1991. *Protecting Soldiers and Mothers.* Cambridge, Mass.: Harvard University Press.

Smetters, K., and J. Gokhale. 2004. *Fiscal and Generational Imbalances: New Budget Measures for New Budget Priorities.* Washington, D.C.: AEI Press.

Smith, D. 2002. *Entitlement Politics: Medicare and Medicaid, 1995–2001*. New York: Aldine de Gruyter.

Stockman, D. 1975. The social pork barrel. *Public Interest* 39:3–30.

U.S. Bureau of the Census. 1988. *Measuring the Effect of Benefits and Taxes on Income and Poverty, 1986*. Washington, D.C.

U.S. Bureau of the Census. 2003. *Consumer Income Series, P60-222*. Washington, D.C.

U.S. Bureau of the Census. 2002. *Current Population Survey, Annual Social and Economic Supplement*. Washington, D.C.

U.S. Bureau of the Census 2001. *Current Population Series. Annual Demographic Survey* March 2001 Supplement. Table 1.

U.S. Congressional Budget Office. 2001. *An Analysis of the President's Budgetary Proposals for Fiscal Year 2002*. Washington, D.C.

U.S. Congressional Budget Office. 2002. www.cbo.gov/showdoc.cfm?index =2300&sequence=0 (accessed 4/23/04).

Upp, M. 1982. A look at the economic status of the aged then and now. *Social Security Bulletin* 45:16–20.

Walker, L. C., E. H. Bradley, and T. Wetle, eds. 1998. *Public and Private Responsibilities in Long-term Care*. Baltimore: Johns Hopkins University Press.

Weaver, R. K. 1988. *Automatic Government: The Politics of Indexation*. Washington, D.C.: Brookings Institution.

White, J. 2003. The Social Security and Medicare debate three years after the 2000 election. *Public Policy and Aging Report* 13(4):15–19.

I. Perspectives on Age-Based Policy

2. A Normative Defense of Universal Age-Based Public Policy

Martha B. Holstein

Advanced age plays a significant role in the development and growth of U.S. social policy, perhaps more than in any other industrial nation. The Old Age Insurance (OAI) program under Social Security and the Medicare program are the principal policies in which age is the determining factor for eligibility. In other policy arenas, such as housing and transportation, age is also an important, but not necessarily the primary, factor in determining eligibility.

Social insurance and public assistance are fundamental and distinct program types; age is a critical contributing factor in the workings of each. Thus, older Americans are rendered eligible under OAI—this country's major social insurance program—based on prior contributions made through employment and independent of their current economic need. Medicare is similarly based on age and not need. In contrast, an older person becomes eligible for benefits through such public assistance programs as Supplemental Security Income or Medicaid on determination of current pressing economic need; benefits are paid from general government revenues.

In recent years, attacks on the prominent role advanced age has played in the workings of U.S. social policy have become familiar and recurrent. One argument has centered on the cost of such programs both now and in the predicted apocalyptic future. These critics, if not alarmists, point to the programs' current size, their large constituency of beneficiaries, and the anticipated future growth of the older population. Another argument has centered more on the real or presumed opportunity costs associated with these programs. What else might we be doing if we devoted fewer resources to older people? In some cases, these arguments center on the well-being of children; in other cases, they are more economic in nature. These critics argue that entitlement expenditures on behalf of old persons negatively affect the national savings rate. Few critics, however, have moved beyond theoretical and rhetorical claims about redistribution.

I will argue in support of the role age plays in these programs. These programs do not represent my ideal for public sector social allocation, but I believe that universal, age-based, minimally fragmented programs are the best practical way to translate the values I support under the present political and economic circumstances found in the United States. I will thus make a case for preserving the fundamentals of both Social Security and Medicare. While far from perfect, these programs protect key values better than the alternatives critics have offered in recent years. In particular, I continue to value the importance of a "common stake" (Kingson et al. 1986) among Americans of different ages and generations.

To be clear, I am profoundly concerned about poverty, ill health, and inadequate housing facing Americans of all ages. Given the poor odds that new government initiatives addressing those concerns are in the offing, it seems critically important to preserve—and, it is to be hoped, to improve—the two age-based programs that have succeeded in moving many Americans out of poverty and in providing widespread access to health care services. We need only remember that in the absence of Social Security, 41.7 percent of white men and 53.2 percent of white women would fall below the poverty line (Calasanti and Slevin 2001). For its part, Medicare has assured that almost all older Americans have acute health care insurance coverage, more than doubling the pre-Medicare proportion of older people so covered.

Much as I would like to see benefits found through Social Security and Medicare extended to middle-aged and younger populations, current political and ideological debates around these programs focus on preservation rather than extension or expansion. Thus, while rightist critics speak of "saving Social Security and Medicare," their proposals actually would transform, if not essentially destroy them.

Creating individual retirement accounts tied to returns on investments under Social Security introduces elements of high risk and reward not found in the current pooled system. It also eliminates the ability, found in the current system, to modestly redistribute benefits in the direction of lower-income beneficiaries. Instead, it would continue, and likely exacerbate, current income differentials between low and high earners. This result would be experienced particularly by older women. In short, steps to individualize and privatize Social Security threaten many current beneficiaries rather than extend the provisions of the current system to yet new populations. In the case of Medicare, the seeming liberalization of the program found in the recent prescription drug legislation includes more fundamental structural changes. Inducing elders to join managed care plans may ultimately limit rather than expand their choices. Similarly, capping payments or tying them to various benchmarks would transform the program from one assuring defined benefits to one guaranteeing only defined contributions.

These current proposals to curtail laudable features of both Social Security and Medicare allow me to speak to the empirical wisdom of maintaining these age-based programs. Age-based features have allowed these and selected other social policies in the United States to do much material good and to bind us together at least nominally as a caring society. They support the values—dignity, social solidarity and justice, particularly gender and racial justice—that are often lost in our individualistic, consumer-oriented society. Normative values such as these reflect our common humanity, our vulnerability to pain and suffering, and the need that most of us have to believe that we are persons worthy of respect. They also remind us that because being old is different than being young in ways that can imminently threaten integrity, we must make extra certain that public programs do not reinforce the physical, psychological, and social vulnerabilities that create those threats.

Following a brief glance at history, I will turn to a more expansive discussion of the values that make these programs highly defensible even in the absence of their expansion to other populations.

Social Security and Medicare: Value Assumptions

By convention, U.S. welfare policy consists of those public programs providing money, goods in kind, or services that are designed to offset regularly occurring events that are generally beyond individual control. Collective responses at least partially funded and managed by government have responded to losses of income associated with old age, disability, unsupported motherhood, and fluctuations in the business cycle. When government also assumed some responsibility for older people's health care, it did so in part because retired people were excluded from employer-supported health insurance and, being overwhelmingly of low income, were unwanted by the private insurance market. Social Security and Medicare were, from the beginning, universal and age-based. This strategy, as contrasted to Old Age Assistance and Medicaid—and similar to Workman's Compensation, Railroad Retirement, and Veterans Benefits—avoided stigma and secured "buy-in" from all groups. These programs also responded specifically to a critical condition that set older people apart from other age groups (i.e., their exclusion from the labor market, by choice or by necessity, which for most older people meant sharp declines in income and elimination of any health care coverage they may have had).

Most historians of social welfare consider the Social Security Act of 1935 the initial cornerstone of the modern U.S. welfare state. However, the act contained both social insurance and public assistance titles, ones that sharply bifurcated social provision. Based on a social insurance model, Old Age Insurance was distinguished by clearly established contractual benefits for older workers. Old Age Assistance and Aid to Dependent Families was of the latter type and as such was stigmatized as "the dole" or "welfare" (charity) made grudgingly available for those who had not worked or were not currently working. Not coincidentally, there was clear gender bias in this division of benefits, reflecting familiar ideas about deservingness and nondeservingness, on which American responses to poverty and vulnerability had long rested (Achenbaum 1978; Holstein and Cole 1996).

Medicare was a response not only to the economic and physical vulnerabilities of old age but also to private market failure. In 1965 as now, the private health insurance market was closely tied to employment. Employers are the primary providers of health insurance to their workers. As a result, except for the few retirees covered by retirement health benefits, older people were effectively excluded from the private health care market. Private insurers had no interest in insuring them because of anticipated high use of medical care and their documented inability to pay the requisite premiums. Hence, older people had no fallback but their own or their children's resources, or the beneficence of kindly physicians should they need high-cost medical care. Though not without intense advocacy efforts, Medicare resulted from this situation, tapping both payroll and general revenue to bring older people into the mainstream health care system. Implicitly, Medicare affirmed several important values—that health care was an important social as well as a personal good and that older people "deserved" access to mainstream medicine without having to prove need because they had clearly been cut off from it through no fault of their own. The prevailing belief that sickness and ill health were unavoidable conditions of old age lay centrally behind the sense of age-based deservingness that has underpinned Medicare politically.

Achieving Core Values: Dignity

How, then, do these two programs reflect the values that I have proposed as the foundation for public policies that serve older people? Central to philosophical thinking and infusing personal concerns is dignity, a morally significant concept relating to the sense that we are people of worth, respected by those whom we respect. A dignified life—and a dignified death—are profound human wants. As a core value, dignity trumps virtually all others. When California Health Decisions asked recipients of MediCal (California's Medicaid system) about the most troubling features of their health care, they overwhelmingly reported "not being treated with dignity." Once providers learned that they were "on MediCal," these individuals felt rushed, silenced, and not heard (California Health Decisions 1993). While dignity is putatively universal and egalitarian as an abstract quality owed to all human beings, society and its members can easily withhold it. "Withholding [dignity] can be a blow to a person's identity, because a society *shapes* the identity of its people by mirroring back to them an image of themselves. If that image is distorted—if it is not an image that accords a person a measure of dignity, and thus cannot serve as the basis of self-respect—then it can be crippling" (Elliott 2003, p. 41).

In *A Theory of Justice*, philosopher John Rawls emphasized the need to secure self-respect or self-esteem. People, he argues, "would wish to avoid at almost any cost the social conditions that undermine their self-respect," which is "perhaps the most important of all the primary goods" (1972, pp. 440, 396). For political philosopher Charles Taylor, dignity shapes—and therefore is prior to—our choices, desires, and interests and gives them a strong evaluative component. What we consider to be our autonomous choices actually rest on some moral vision that is "uncommonly deep, powerful, and universal" (Taylor 1989, p. 4) and helps define who we are. To avoid anomie, we must be able to live according to these deeply held values and know that others recognize and respect who we are. Our dignity requires this recognition.

Political philosopher Robert Goodin (1982), identifies what he calls moral primitives for which no further justification is needed, and he finds dignity to be central. This moral concern is not secondary to "either rational articulations of what an unencumbered human would choose or what utility calculations [e.g., cost-benefit analysis] suggest" (Taylor 1989, p. 8). Dignity demands a minimum standard of decent treatment for every individual "not to be sacrificed for any less weighty considerations" (Goodin 1982, p. 85). We are obliged, then, to shape the "right kind of respect" (Moody 1998, p. 20).

While dignity is important at all ages, it becomes particularly important in old age because in old age illness, ageism, and accumulated losses threaten identity and erode dignity. "Dignity in old age matters," Moody points out "because everyone of us carries this sense of vulnerability and because we fear becoming less of ourselves in the last stages of life" (1998, p. 14). This condition of old age makes it particularly essential that public policies reinforce, rather than reduce, self-respect.

In recent years many commentators on aging have come to emphasize the "productive" capacities of older people. This heralding of "successful" aging, though well-intentioned, can also serve to threaten the self-esteem of people who cannot or do not choose to live up to those new norms. It can also challenge the underlying sense of deservingness that has been the hallmark of policy addressing the situation of the old. Gerontology's enthusiastic embrace of the positive features of old age can easily lead to unintended and troubling consequences (see Holstein and Minkler 2003). These consequences (e.g., devaluing one's own condition and status, judging others by external appearances, presuming that old age does not present unique and complex needs) threaten dignity and self-respect.

Despite these positive admonitions attached to the "productive aging" construct, older people very much retain a sense of being the "other" (de Beauvoir 1972). Appearance, disability, or advanced age itself may be powerful estranging factors, ones that, among other consequences, erode one's sense of dignity. Very important in this context is the largely unspoken role that age-based public policy has assumed in supporting dignity. It provides this support in several ways. By helping to assure a modicum of medical and financial security on the basis of age alone, policy affirms the unique situation of old age. It acknowledges that age often is a marker of decremental changes, ones that in policy terms may constitute "contingent events" (Hudson 1993). No matter how much exercise, nutrition, and engagement elders bring to their lives, major economic, social, and physical barriers may impair self-reliance. A good society recognizes that acknowledging such contingencies and anticipated life events is not a derogation of old age but is rather a sign of respect. Because American society provides few recognizable norms for old age against which individuals can measure themselves, and because our new global society can further erode customary anchors to identity, Social Security and Medicare indirectly affirm that becoming and being old requires social acknowledgment.

British social gerontologist Chris Phillipson observes that for many older people, who are unable or unwilling to create new, flexible biographies in old age, "the negative features of ageing may actually increase" as the period of disorganized capitalism fragments and abandons what had been relative secure institutions (1998, p. 48). For all the changes in the status of the old in our society, including what may be the growing irrelevance of age as a "predictor of lifestyle or need" (Binstock 1994, p. 726), many, if not most, older people will find age a profound reality that threatens dignity and self-respect. While old age may be discursively created, the not-unfamiliar aches, pains, silent invisibility, and fears about "making it" are real. The state and society cannot give an individual his or her dignity or self-respect, but they can provide conditions that may either support or discourage its recognition and achievement (Walzer 1983).

Achieving and maintaining dignity is a serious matter for which a commitment of some financial security is essential. While there may be a number of arguments about the virtues of charity and the dangers of entitlement, the conditions for dignity are best supported through simple entitlements, comparable to earning one's salary and receiving benefits by virtue of doing one's job. While not usually phrased this way in the policy debate, it is this notion of dignity that is at the heart of the distinction between Social Security and Supplemental Security Income or Temporary Aid to Needy Families (TANF). Stigma cannot coexist with dignity. Dignity cannot survive alongside humiliation (see Margalit 1996 for a powerful discussion of humiliation). At no time in our history have means-tested programs recognized the elemental importance of dignity. Through contributory and universal financing, Social Security has supported the dignity of its recipients. And because of its contractual features, Social Security is not subject to the annual downward pressures of means-tested programs.

For all their limitations, Social Security and Medicare offer older people a rightful place in society. They could, of course, do much better, but the current elements of the program are solid starting places, especially in a country that has a limited view of social citizenship or social rights. This more generous approach, taken for granted by many European countries, guarantees certain benefits, not on the basis of charity or a particular work history or even age, but simply by belonging to a state or country (Myles 1995). Viewed along a continuum, citizenship rights affirm dignity most strongly, while means-tested or charity least affirm it. Along that continuum, contract, which is the implicit model on which Social Security rests, is closer to the citizenship end. Because benefits that derive from an implicit contract are considered earned, and because older people have been among the deserving, at least until recently, contract supports at least a minimalist conception of dignity.

Unlike the situation in the mid-1990s, means-testing of benefits is not today a central threat to either Social Security or Medicare. However, changes favored by conservatives and neoliberals do pose a challenge to elder dignity as I have constructed it. Thus, while partially privatizing Social Security will not alter the fundamental idea that this benefit is an earned one, it could erode the ability of the system to mildly redistribute benefits to lower-income individuals. Were the annuity feature abandoned (not currently being proposed) some elders, notably women, might outlive their income. As well, lower-wage earners could be harmed by the vagaries of the equity market. When one has few opportunities to recoup losses, and worry becomes a fact of everyday life, dignity inevitably suffers. Losses among low-income beneficiaries could also have the effect of forcing more older people back to the vagaries of means-tested benefits, the very end that Social Security's design and workings have largely eliminated. The much-touted emphasis on autonomy counts for little if income constraints leave us with few options that support our deeply held values. Privatization would most likely harm women and the least well off, a topic to which I now turn.

Gender, the Least Well Off, and Justice

The fullest expression of dignity takes place in a just system of benefits. While Social Security does not go nearly far enough, its mildly redistributive features (an equity-based conception of justice with some consideration of adequacy)—assuming a basically unchanged system—also mitigate, at least partially, the economic effects of lifetime differences in work histories. In essence, these redistributive features are essential for older women, whom society tends to marginalize, who describe themselves as invisible, and who pay the price of a work history that rarely conforms to male norms. It also matters for African Americans and other historically low-wage workers who rely on Social Security as the mainstay of their income.

Even without privatization, these programs, because of the way they are currently structured, contribute to the continued—indeed, expanding—inequality among the aged. Some elderly persons have contributed little to Social Security and so receive minimal benefits; their work in low-wage occupations provided them with no pensions and little opportunity to save. Similarly, Medicare does not provide much support for their chronic health problems, and they have no retiree health benefits. Any change in either Medicare or Social Security that makes those programs less universal or less comprehensive would hurt these people the most.

These prominent features of the system mean that it falls short of protecting *all* older people. The system's link to employment limited deservingness to those people who worked for pay outside of the home. Women homemakers, farm workers, and domestic laborers were some of those originally omitted from coverage. Homemakers still receive no benefits in their own name; caregiving—of the home, children, spouses, or other relatives—is granted no economic valuation and, in practice, constitutes a net economic loss for women. The system presumes that our society is "an association of free and independent equals" (Kittay 1999, p. 4), an assumption that does not hold for women involved in dependency relationships and thus is a threat to important justice-based values. In the same way, medicine also fails older women in ways that it does not fail men.

The normative life course that Social Security helped establish did not reflect women's experiences then and does it less so now. Not only could they not "retire" from the domestic responsibilities in which they had engaged for much of their lives, but their responsibilities for the health and well-being of children, grandchildren, elderly parents, and their spouses also continued. Women can rarely retire from the many and often unchosen obligations that govern their lives. They have fewer "excuses" than men for not providing care, for example, to elderly relatives. Even women who are employed do not have the excuse of work as readily accepted as do men as reasons justifying limiting their caregiving responsibilities (for an extended discussion of these themes in connection with caring for elderly relatives at home, see Holstein 1998; Parks 2003). While women may treasure these responsibilities (and may also resent them or feel a combination of pride in accomplishment and resentment simultaneously), they are essentially unchosen. These duties are expected at the same time as they are unrecognized and uncompensated.

The connection with Social Security is direct. Even women with careers or at least regular employment rarely have the same continuous work histories as men. They often drop out of the workforce to have children and may drop out again to care for elderly relatives. Both anticipated and unanticipated interruptions of work affect Social Security benefit levels. Any program that is tied to the labor market will inevitably have the effect of rewarding those people who conform to certain, but not other, socially valued behaviors.

The philosopher Martha Nussbaum and the economist Amartya Sen (1993) argue persuasively that societies ought to support basic capacities that give individuals maximum agency and choice. Such support, I suggest, includes provisions to compensate for non-work-related activities that are central to women's lives. By "choosing" to provide care or to assume certain obligations, women make sacrifices in the present that simultaneously benefit others but can negatively affect their future well-being. Without assurance that such chosen or unchosen responses to people in need will be supported, neither dignity nor justice is possible. Nussbaum asked, "What activities characteristically performed by human beings are so central that they seem definitive of a life that is truly human?" (1999, p. 39). Humans, she says, need a life in which their dignity is not violated by "hunger or fear or the absence of opportunity" (p. 40). This requirement places a claim on government to respond. Only programs that do not require us to "prove" that we lack the capabilities to achieve these important ends will serve both dignity and justice. Politics, she notes, "has an important role to play in giving citizens the tools they need, both to choose at all and to have a realistic option of exercising the most valuable functions" (p. 46). People need the resources and conditions to exercise their capabilities. Women and many other low-wage workers do not now have the support needed to give them the agency and choice to so exercise their capacities.

If Social Security is to remedy its blind spots so that it sustains the care of dependents no matter their age, it cannot opt for partial or complete privatization or means-testing, which pose the greatest risk to people who take on the care of dependents. A society preoccupied by rights and by the individualistic orientation that rights rest on often has a difficult time recognizing the essential fact of dependency, which places often unchosen demands on others to respond. Yet our lives are built around unchosen obligations. I would thus argue that the values I have proposed as grounding for public policy for the aged remain critical for this time and place, even if they do not go far enough in respecting the needs for care that are ineliminable.

Similarly, Medicare, as now structured, does not adequately support the ends of gender justice, but neither will privatization or fragmentation. Women suffer from more chronic illnesses than do men, and because they tend to outlive their spouses, they do not have a readily available caregiver in the home. Because Medicare inadequately covers the costs of chronic illness, women frequently must turn to children, most often daughters and daughters-in-law, who must then take time out from work and other responsibilities to provide care. This action, in time, penalizes them in terms of future benefits while often making older women feel like a burden. Only a radically re-envisioned Medicare system that no longer relies on the donated services of women will serve the ends of gender justice. Current efforts to move more people into Medicare HMOs can theoretically partially address this problem if they offer adequate home care benefits. But recent history suggests that HMOs do least well with chronic care. There is little to make us sanguine that this problem will be remedied.

A more just system, one that takes dependency seriously, would contain a principle such as the following: "To each according to his or her need for care, from each according to his or her capacity for care, and such support from social institutions as to make available resources and opportunities to those providing care, so that all will be adequately attended in relations that are sustaining" (Kittay 1999, p. 113).

Social Solidarity and Human Interdependence

Universal entitlements, particularly Social Security, also invoke muted values of social solidarity and human interdependence. In an era that focuses almost exclusively on protecting individual autonomy, Social Security reminds us, in the language of many folk beliefs, that "I am because we are." Each of us owes a debt to past generations; we would, quite literally, not exist "had not someone and some society taken responsibility for our welfare. . . . If we value our own life at all, then we must value and feel some obligation toward those who made that life possible" (Callahan 1981, p. 77). Such ties are a "matter of moral intuition, social common sense, and obligatory notions of reciprocity, part of what once was called civil society" (Wolfe 1989, p. 101). Social Security thus recognizes that we are, throughout our lives, inevitably and importantly connected to others (Wolfe 1989).

Social solidarity is a "necessary condition for the flourishing of the subjective life." A human being understood holistically is more socially committed, socially shaped, and socially nourished than much recent ethical thinking would have us believe (Anjos 1994, p. 139). It reminds us that we share a common human identity. In the terms of Western religious traditions, humans are made in the image of God; even metaphorically understood, that image suggests we have responsibilities for others as we have for them.

Over the course of a life, ties of social obligation and reciprocity are ways to assure that, for example, we raise the next generation of children to understand the meaning of justice or to know what a promise means (Baier 1994). As we do with organ transplantation and other acts of spontaneous generosity, we need to retain the gift relationship among generations (Johnson 1995). Social Security—because of its contractually constructed pay-as-you-go features—more accurately embodies deeply held notions of reciprocity. While relations of social obligation and reciprocity are not always freely chosen, they are required for the continuity of a just society (Baier 1994). The fact that each of us pays in to the Social Security system and then anticipates receiving benefits through a legally based relationship with generations to follow reinforces the important moral value of reciprocity. This aspect of what the system's proponents often refer to as the "Social Security compact" deserves more attention than it has received. Such bonds are not merely incidental; they are morally honorable and necessary. Recent suggestions to privatize Social Security, while subject to criticism on many grounds, would fundamentally challenge the intergenerational compact that the existing system embodies. Furthermore, by elevating the self and denying social obligations, privatization reinforces those American values most likely to sharpen divisions along class, race, and gender lines.

Instead of deliberately creating the situation for these untoward consequences, a refurbished notion of generational solidarity "will ease political uncertainty that rests on short term worries about the 'burdens' of an aging population with broad risk sharing, the bonds of generation's can be protected" (Johnson 1995, p. 252). Social Security permits sharing of risks at a time in life when risk is potentially imminent. By providing some help to younger generations in terms of financing their parents' retirement, Social Security also helps to assure the stability of generations over time. One need only recall the "family economies" of the late nineteenth and early twentieth centuries (Haber and Gratton 1994) to understand the potentially bruising results that future generations would experience from heightened economic responsibility for family elders.

The Depression dramatically re-emphasized what most middle- and working-class families already knew—the family economy could not withstand endless pressures. In the years since, as age groups increasingly segmented, it became clear that the middle generation needed assistance in caring for its parents. For the older generation, Social Security lessens fears about being a burden on its children and, for some, facilitates continued contributions to successor generations. In this way, it encourages the ongoing recognition and practice of reciprocal and interdependent relationships while mitigating the troubling aspects of asymmetrical relationships that develop as parents need more from their children.

Second, age-based policy honors social solidarity and the interdependent features of being human. As the Social Security system evolved and it became clear that individuals were not, in actuality, saving for their own retirement, the program's intergenerational features emerged more sharply. While cloaked in individualistic language, Social Security represented a collective effort, what Martin Kohli described as "morally bounded claims and expectations" (1991, p. 276), that joins one generation to another in a formally enacted system of transfer. In this way, Social Security also created what Kohli labeled a "social citizen." By virtue of having met certain criteria in the past, one has claims on common social resources. Each subsequent generation has similar claims. An intergenerational compact, tacit or otherwise, must exist for this claim to be practically realized.

This social citizen had "legitimate claims to continuity throughout the life course" (Kohli 1991, p. 286). The operative word here is continuity. Such claims, when combined with Social Security provisions that support adequacy (in addition to equity), illuminate efforts to incorporate two conceptions of justice: the meritarian or "just deserts" notion and protection of the most vulnerable among the aged population. Indirectly, by giving the individual the wherewithal to live his or her life in rough continuity with the past, the system nurtured individual autonomy. In this way, the response of the United States to the perceived situation of its older members has blended different—and conflictive—normative assumptions. How the tension between these conceptions of justice will change during the conservative ascendancy in the United States is a critical question.

In contemporary American society, with its prevailing emphasis on atomistic individualism, there are few public expressions of social solidarity and interdependence. Yet many of our deepest moral sentiments, supported by research in moral psychology and other domains, reinforce the importance of the social. Without visible expressions of community, we lack the social glue that binds individuals into a society. Yet we rarely acknowledge the social goals of Social Security and therefore do not stimulate informed discussion about the losses that might occur if those goals withered. We need reminding that the promise of the contract is that adequate income and care of the old is an "enduring right" (Johnson 1995, p. 261).

Social Security can also make a practical contribution to maintaining ties of interdependency and solidarity. The normative life course, which Social Security helped to create and sustain, frees up a number of individuals, often in relatively good health, to contribute to society in ways often unavailable to younger working people, especially parents in families. We might, of course, achieve the same ends if benefits were needs-based, but doing so would be less likely for two reasons. First, the sense of security that comes with age-based entitlements is liberating and can encourage the person to pursue socially constructive interests. Second, there is always the risk that means testing can, for example, insist on work requirements for the healthy without concern for the number or quality of jobs available. In this way, the possibilities of contributing to the social good through alternative activities would be reduced.

By maintaining its current structure, Social Security does not place the elderly in a position of subordination to the legislators and bureaucrats who make decisions about other social welfare policies. It signals a strong, visible, and public commitment to the well-being of the elderly as a group rather than to their well-being as individuals. Perhaps older people are not a group in any conventional meaning of that term, but they are, I believe, a group in their common vulnerabilities to disease, death, and society's ageist responses. While some are better able to isolate themselves from the worst ramifications of these features of old age, none, I would suggest, can be immune from them. The next section will briefly examine the reasons I make this particular claim.

The "Condition" of Old Persons in the United States

As noted above, in recent years the language of productive and successful aging, and nontraditional or postmodern aging have all moved toward deconstructing the very category of old age. If we don't need to be old—except in terms of years since birth—then it is also possible to undermine the very need for universal age-based programs. Yet freedom is a chimera for people without resources, in poor health, or responsible for the well-being of others. Old age is not merely middle age with a few added years. Most older people no longer work. Whether by choice, because of ill health, or because of job downsizing, this situation means the loss of a steady income and the health insurance that comes with most jobs. Pension income has become more volatile, as defined benefit plans increasingly disappear and holdings in 401(k) defined contribution plans erode. Long periods of unemployment sustained by many workers in this economic downturn are also eroding savings. These trends make clear that income insecurity is still a looming concern of old age, despite the notable progress the United States made in earlier decades. Freedom to live the self-created life, so touted by postmodern or post-traditional views of old age (Gergen and Gergen 2000), is possible only with a reliable income floor. It is hard to be self-creating when every expenditure represents a potential threat to security. Nor do endless projects of self-creation and the radical pluralism about which our society is so proud foster care and responsibility for others. If we are forever free to chose to give or not give care, what will happen to people of any age whose physical or mental condition demands care provision?

While Social Security and Medicare have secured for many a more stable income and access to health care, there are still significant problems of poverty or near poverty among the old. Reduce Social Security and those numbers will climb. In the mid-1980s, groups such as Americans for Generational Equity (AGE) contrasted poor children with affluent older people as if children set up households and had a hard time putting food on the table, while elders dined on caviar and champagne. But kids were poor then as now because they have poor parents or, more likely, poor mothers, and this country prefers to see their poverty as an individual rather than a social failing. Similarly, while elders at the turn of the twenty-first century have more income and a more comfortable lifestyle than previous generations, many older people have incomes under 200 percent of the poverty line. In particular, those commentators who focus on affluent elders erase—or give mere lip service to—distinctions based on race and gender. AGE has faded into oblivion, but its central agenda—reconstituting Social Security and Medicare—has not disappeared with it.

Conclusion

It is true that neither Social Security nor Medicare is today threatened with repeal, however closely some proposals to save them would come to transforming them beyond easy recognition. However, the changes proposed will certainly not move them closer to already illusive gender and racial equity, and they will undermine political support and a common stake. These threats are political and ideological rather than actuarial. A political agenda to delegitimize Social Security by urgently insisting that unless major changes are made the whole system is in jeopardy can do more to cancel popular support than would any threat to its fiscal solvency. The need for a "bold" response to a looming crisis becomes the justification for potentially undermining the program's guaranteed benefits. Similarly, in the name of choice and cost savings, to transform Medicare into what may well ultimately become a voucher plan will pit those with resources against those without and make access to comparable health benefits for comparable conditions unlikely. Shopping for health plans with no guarantee that the costs will not climb or that benefits will stay the same is a strenuous task, one bordering on the impossible for people burdened by chronic health conditions. Such fragmentation may both politically and actuarially divide people on the basis of health condition and income and, in turn, impose new risks at a time when risk has become a daily fact of life.

In our rights-oriented society, where freedom and independence are our nation's prevailing narrative, it is particularly difficult to uphold values that reflect community, intergenerational solidarity, and obligations. It is also difficult to recognize that dignity is a social and not an individual value. Dignity emerges in and through relationships and can be very fragile. Without a foundation of security vested in justice, rendered visible through public policies, our society's repeated commitment to autonomy becomes a hollow promise for many people. Autonomy demands real choices that are meaningful to people.

While not doing the job well enough, Social Security and Medicare, as they are now structured, support the values of dignity, social solidarity, and gender and racial justice better than any proposed alternatives. If Robert Putnam (2000) is correct and Americans increasingly "bowl alone," then more than ever we need public policies that remind us of our obligations, interdependencies, and connectedness to one another.

References

Achenbaum, W. A. 1978. *Old Age in the New Land: The American Experience since 1790*. Baltimore: Johns Hopkins University Press.

Anjos, M. 1994. Bioethics in a liberationist key. In *A Matter of Principles: Ferment in U.S. Bioethics,* ed. E. Dubose, R. Hamel, and L. O'Connell. Valley Forge, Pa.: Trinity Press International.

Baier, A. 1994. *Moral Prejudices: Essays on Ethics*. Cambridge, Mass.: Harvard University Press.

Beauvoir, de, S. 1972. *The Coming of Age*. New York: Putnam.

Binstock, R. 1994. Changing criteria in old age programs: The introduction of economic status and need for services. *Gerontologist* 34:726–30.

Calasanti, T., and K. F. Slevin. 2001. *Gender, Social Inequalities, and Aging*. Walnut Creek, Calif.: AltaMira Press.

California Health Decisions. 1993. *California Health Care Divide: Involving the Public in Health Care Choices*. CPN On-Line.

Callahan, D. 1981. What obligations do we have to future generations? In *Responsibilities to Future Generations: Environmental Ethics,* ed. E. Partridge. Buffalo, N.Y.: Prometheus.

Elliott, C. 2003. *Better Than Well: American Medicine Meets the American Dream.* New York: Norton.

Gergen, K., and M. Gergen. 2000. The new aging: Self construction and social values. In *The Evolution of the Aging Self: The Societal Impact of the Aging Process,* ed. K. W. Schaie and J. Hendricks. New York: Springer.

Goodin, R. 1982. *Political Theory and Public Policy.* Chicago: University of Chicago Press.

Haber, C., and B. Gratton. 1994. *Old Age and the Search for Security: An American Social History.* Bloomington: Indiana University Press.

Holstein, M. 1998. Home care, women, and aging: A case study of injustice. In *Mother Time: Women, Aging and Ethics,* ed. M. U. Walker. Lanham, Md.: Rowman and Littlefield.

Holstein, M., and T. Cole. 1996. The history of long-term care in America. In *The Future of Long-term Care,* ed. R. Binstock, L. Cluff, and O. von Mering. Baltimore: Johns Hopkins University Press.

Holstein, M., and M. Minkler. 2003. Self, society, and the new gerontology. *Gerontologist* 43(6):789–96.

Hudson, R. 1993. Social contingencies, the aged, and public policy. *Milbank Quarterly* 71(2):253–77.

Johnson, M. 1995. Interdependency and the generational compact. *Ageing and Society* 15(2):243–66.

Kingson, E., B. Hirshorn, and J. Cornman. 1986. *Ties That Bind: The Interdependency of Generations.* Cabin John, Md.: Seven Locks.

Kittay, E. 1999. *Love's Labor: Essays on Women, Equality, and Dependency.* New York: Routledge.

Kohli, M. 1986. "The World We Forgot: A Historical Review of the Life Course." Pp. 271–303 in *Later Life: The Social Psychology of Aging.* Beverly Hills, Calif.: Sage.

Margalit, A. 1996. *The Decent Society.* Cambridge, Mass.: Harvard University Press.

Moody, H. R. 1998. Why dignity in old age matters. *Journal of Gerontological Social Work* 29(2/3):13–38.

Myles, J. 1995. Neither rights nor contracts: The new means-testing in U.S. aging policy. *Generations* 19(3): on-line, 7 pp.

Nussbaum, M. 1999. *Sex and Social Justice.* New York: Oxford University Press.

Nussbaum, M., and A. Sen. 1993. *The Quality of Life.* New York: Oxford University Press.

Parks, J. 2003. *No Place Like Home? Feminist Ethics and Home Health Care.* Bloomington: Indiana University Press.

Phillipson, C. 1998. *Reconstructing Old Age: New Agendas in Social Theory and Practice.* London: Sage Publications.

Putnam, R. 2000. *Bowling Alone: The Collapse and Revival of American Community.* New York: Simon and Schuster.

Rawls, J. 1972. *A Theory of Justice.* Cambridge, Mass.: Harvard University Press.

Taylor, C. 1989. *Sources of the Self.* Cambridge, Mass.: Harvard University Press.

Walzer, M. 1983. *Spheres of Justice: A Defense of Pluralism and Equality.* Cambridge: Cambridge University Press.

Wolfe, A. 1989. *Whose Keeper? Social Science and Moral Obligation.* Berkeley: University of California Press.

3. What Justice Requires
A Normative Foundation for U.S. Pension Reform
John Myles

It is hardly surprising that retirement systems designed under conditions of high fertility and sustained labor force growth might require some serious tweaking once those conditions have disappeared. Prudence suggests we do something about the social policy legacy we leave to our children now that we are having so few of them. But because there is much uncertainty about the imputed second-order effects of population aging on both the economy (what will happen to wages, prices, and capital markets?) and the polity (will retirees really control the political agenda?), even the most socially responsible reformer risks doing too much as well as too little. So what is to be done?

Schokkaert and Van Parijs (2003) propose a noncontroversial starting point: a minimal requirement of intergenerational justice is that we leave future generations a stock of physical, human, and environmental capital at least as valuable as the one at our disposal. But our legacy to future generations also includes the real welfare gains embedded in the social institutions inherited from the past. As Schokkaert and Van Parijs highlight, our income security systems for both the old and the young are among these institutions: the traditional family structure in which parents care for children when they are too young to work and children support their parents when they are too old and frail to work is an important characteristic of the human species, probably with deep biological roots. Contemporary historiography confirms that the emergence of mandatory public pensions were as important for the children of elderly Americans as for the elderly themselves, a form of risk sharing not only against the risk of one's *own* longevity but also against the risk of one's *parents'* longevity and the imperative of supporting parents financially through an extended old age (Haber and Gratton 1994). For a species motivated by "filial piety," old age insurance is also insurance for the young. Rising Social Security costs may lead our children to complain about high taxes or to ask us to retire later. It is unlikely, however, that they will be grateful if we expose them to the risk of supporting us directly to the age of 95. Just as intergenerational justice requires us to leave them with a sustainable environment, it also requires us to leave them with sustainable pension systems at least as good as those we have had to care for our parents in their old age.

My goal in this chapter is to identify reform strategies that satisfy standards of both intergenerational equity *between* workers and retirees, and intragenerational justice *among* workers and retirees. To deal with intergenerational equity, I advocate an expanded variant of the "Musgrave rule" elaborated by Richard Musgrave at the beginning of the 1980s (Musgrave 1986). The idea is simple: "fair" or "proportional" sharing *between* workers and retirees of the *additional* retirement costs that result from demographic change. Unlike Musgrave, however, whose main concern was the political viability of public pay-as-you-go pension schemes, I conclude that satisfying the principle of "intergenerational equity" requires application of the rule to both sides of the retirement income ledger: to private as well as to public pensions. With respect to intragenerational justice, I begin from a normative position that is broadly Rawlsian in inspiration—changes to the status quo should be of most advantage to the least advantaged—and propose two complementary strategies inside public sector schemes: greater reliance on interpersonal transfers, on the one hand, and, on the other, a shift from payroll taxes toward greater reliance on general revenue financing in public sector plans.

The origins of this discussion lie in earlier work written mainly for a European audience.[1] Unlike the situation in the United States, large-scale pension reforms have been commonplace in Europe since the 1980s, and these comments were written in part as a reflection on these reforms. I do not pretend to have worked out all of the implications of the very different institutional environment of the U.S. retirement system for these proposals. Lest they appear "utopian" (normatively desirable but practically unfeasible) within the U.S. context, however, I hasten to add that the strategies advocated here are presented, not as proposals for an instantaneous "grand redesign" of existing institutions, but as guidelines or "litmus tests" against which *particular* reforms introduced incrementally can be evaluated. Pension reform in the United States, though hotly contested now for several decades, still gives no clear indication of its likely destination. My purpose here is to highlight some of the normative implications—what justice requires—of alternative pathways toward that destination. Some of the flaws I perceive on both sides of the U.S. debate are taken up in the conclusion.

The Economics of Population Aging: Three Dilemmas in Search of Solutions

Following Thompson (1998), we can highlight the problems facing societies with aging populations with a simple accounting identity. The economic cost of supporting the retired population is simply the fraction of each year's economic activity given over to supplying the goods and services the retired consume, or:

$$\text{Cost of supporting the retired} = \frac{\text{Consumption of the retired}}{\text{Total national production}}$$

which in turn, following Hicks, can be written as:[2]

$$\text{Cost of supporting the retired} = \frac{\text{Number of retirees}}{\text{Number of employees}} \times \frac{\text{Average consumption of retirees}}{\text{Average production per employee}}$$

Assuming that all else remains fixed, population aging raises total retirement costs. A 10 percent increase in the ratio of retirees to workers results in a 10 percent increase in the cost of supporting retired persons. Higher retirement costs are not a problem per se. In a stable population (with no population aging), we might expect future generations to behave much like earlier ones and take some of the gains that result from higher productivity (the "wealth effect") in the form of more retirement. Population aging, however, acts as a "multiplier," raising the cost for the same amount of leisure over each person's life course.

Cost shifting to the private sector does not per se change this scenario.[3] Public and private pensions are simply alternative ways for working-age individuals to register a claim on future production (Barr 2001). The share of total consumption of the retired rises irrespective of whether it is financed with state pensions or with investment returns from bonds and equities. Indeed, as Thompson (1998, p. 44) observes, proposals to shift toward group or personal advanced funded accounts are often made on the grounds that retirees will receive higher returns from their contributions. If this turns out to be true, the effect of change will be to *raise* future retirement costs.

The most obvious strategy is an extension of the working life. Simulations for a "stylized" Organization for Economic Cooperation and Development (OECD) country indicate that the impact of a *5 percent reduction* in the number of beneficiaries—equivalent to an effective increase in the average retirement age of 10 months—is equivalent to a *10 percent reduction* in average retirement benefits (OECD 2001). The reason for the difference can be understood by referring to the equation introduced above. An increase in the retirement age changes both the numerator and the denominator of the retiree/employee ratio. A reduction in benefits affects only the numerator of the ratio between the average consumption of the retired and average productivity per worker. The combination of more work among young and old alike would, in abstract, also conform to a basic standard of *intergenerational* equity according to Musgrave's fixed proportional shares' principle (see below). Finally, on average, the potential "welfare loss" that might otherwise result from a longer working life will be offset by increased longevity. Because people are (and will be) living longer, more working years does not mean fewer retirement years.

Policymakers, however, face a formidable political obstacle to implementing later retirement ages. Most workers in most countries look forward to retirement, and raising the age of eligibility for retirement benefits is among the least popular reform options. Because the relevant policy lever is not the "normal retirement age" (age 65 or 67) but the age at which retirement benefits can first be accessed (62 for Social Security), such a strategy raises difficult equity issues (discussed below) and regulation of the age at which private as well as public retirement wealth can be accessed (Myles 2002). Later retirement is likely to be part of the solution, especially given anticipated increases in labor demand, but it is unlikely to be the whole solution.

Another strategy is to leave the problem of cost allocation to markets and families.[4] In a totally privatized system based on advance funding and other personal assets, the business cycle and changes in demand for labor and capital that are uniquely attributable to population aging would solve the problem of cost allocation by producing lucky and less lucky generations (Thompson 1998). Some cohorts and individuals would benefit from favorable wage histories and returns to their capital and so be in a position to retire early in relative comfort. Other cohorts and individuals would be less fortunate and be required to work longer to avoid an impoverished retirement. Families would decide about the intergenerational transmission of wealth so that (perversely), *within* generations, children from wealthy families and with few siblings would be the winners.

For most nations, however, relinquishing the problem of cost allocation to markets and families is not a feasible option for both political and economic reasons. Even if one believes such a choice to be desirable, it is simply not on the menu of feasible options available to most countries because they are not starting from a tabula rasa.[5] The possible choices available today are, in the jargon of political economy, *path dependent,* that is, constrained by choices made in the past. For example, because of the high transition costs associated with moving from a mature pay-as-you-go to a private advanced funded design, the public pension systems now in place will endure well into the future so that policymakers have no option but to make choices about cost allocation. Even in the absence of this economic constraint, however, the past decade has shown that popular support for established retirement income programs is both broad and deep, so that truly "radical" reform of this sort faces an equally daunting political constraint (Myles and Pierson 2001).

There are also sound normative reasons for a public role in allocating the transition costs arising from changes in population structure. The rising retirement costs produced by the baby dearth and increased longevity is a collective risk like other exogenous "shocks" (natural disasters, recessions) and hence an appropriate target for intercohort risk sharing. Sinn (2000) raises an alternative possibility: cohorts that have reduced their fertility, and hence are the "cause" of the problem, should be held accountable for their fertility behavior and have their pensions reduced accordingly. In philosophy, the logical form of this argument is known as the problem of the *any* and the *all* (Hernes 1976, p. 516). Fertility rates, like prices, are "aggregative outcomes" that depend on decisions made by *all* individuals but not on the decision of *any* particular individual.[6] Because only individuals, not collectivities (e.g., cohorts or generations), are moral agents, it is difficult ex post to sustain Sinn's claim and others that take this form.

To throw into relief the core issues facing policymakers, it is helpful to begin from an imaginary starting point—a "useful fiction"—in which all of the consumption of the retired (including health care and other service costs) comes from pensions financed from payroll taxes on the wages of the nonretired, assumptions that can be relaxed once the main elements of the story are in place.

Intergenerational Equity and the Musgrave Rule

Following Musgrave (1986), the challenge facing policymakers in pay-as-you-go systems is in the first instance a dilemma of intergenerational equity[7] that can be illustrated by contrasting two ideal-typical pay-as-you-go designs. In the standard defined benefit model with a fixed replacement rate (FRR) common to the majority of developed countries, retirees are entitled to a given fraction of their earnings in the form of benefits plus an adjustment factor to reflect productivity gains and higher wages in the subsequent generation. When the ratio of retirees to workers changes, workers must adjust their contribution rates accordingly. In effect, benefits drive taxes (so that taxes are the dependent variable) and *all of the costs associated with demographic change fall on contributors and their dependants.*

An alternative to a fixed replacement rate is a pay-as-you-go design based on a fixed contribution rate (FCR).[8] The working population is required to contribute a fixed fraction of its income for the support of retirees. In this design, taxes drive benefits so that benefits are the dependent variable. As the ratio of retirees to workers rises, benefits must decline and *all of the costs associated with demographic change fall on retirees.* Traditionally, U.S. Social Security has been based on the FRR design. A decision to freeze current contribution rates and allow benefits to fall proportionately would produce a de facto shift to the FRR model.

How might a three-generation household faced with the prospect of demographic aging but committed to intergenerational risk sharing resolve this dilemma? Assuming they are satisfied with the status quo (current consumption levels of the generations relative to one another are neither too high or too low), the solution would undoubtedly approximate the fixed ratio or fixed relative position (FRP) model advocated by Musgrave (1986, chap. 7).[9] Contributions and benefits are set so as to hold *constant* the ratio of per capita earnings of those in the working population (net of contributions) to the per capita benefits (net of taxes) of retirees. Once the ratio is fixed, the tax rate is adjusted periodically to reflect both population and productivity changes. Along with the fixed contribution method, it obviates the need for projections but allows, in addition, for proportional sharing of risk. As the population ages, the tax rate rises, but benefits also fall, so that both parties "lose" at the same rate (i.e., both net earnings and benefits rise more slowly than they would in the absence of population aging).[10]

The FRP principle says nothing about what the relative position of retirees to workers and their dependants *should* be. It simply provides a rule for allocating the *additional* costs of demographic change between generations once an acceptable ratio is established.[11] From the perspective of multigenerational household facing the prospect of fewer workers and more retirees in the near future, it reflects a joint commitment to maintaining the status quo in relative terms. In the same way that pension benefits are usually indexed so that wages and benefits will rise together with increases in productivity, so too the Musgrave rule "indexes" *both* contributions *and* benefits to population aging.[12]

Our hypothetical three-generational household faces a *point-in-time* decision concerning the allocation of costs between generations already alive. Such a situation is very close to the real life political choices facing policymakers both now and in the future: should they raise payroll taxes on younger workers, reduce benefits for retired workers (or those about to retire), or some combination of the two? This perspective is useful because all politics is, in an important sense, "point-in-time" politics (i.e., in the hands of those currently alive). If payroll taxes rise significantly relative to pension benefits for retirees (the FRR solution), policymakers can anticipate the displeasure of workers and their employers. If, alternatively, real benefits are falling year after year relative to national living standards (the FCR solution), retirees and those near retirement will be unhappy.

If we shift our perspective from a "point-in-time" to a life course framework, however, the case for the Musgrave rule is even more persuasive. What are the implications of the three designs from the point of view of the *entire* life course of cohorts born in the future, the legacy that we will leave to our children and grandchildren?

Under FCR, the living standards of future generations would be preserved during childhood and over their working years, but they would experience a sharp decline in living standards in retirement. Under FRR, in contrast, successive cohorts would experience declining living standards in childhood and during the working years but a relatively affluent old age. FRP, in contrast, effectively smoothes the change across the entire life course and maintains the status quo with respect to the lifetime distribution of income. In this respect, FRP is a conservative strategy based on the assumption that, on average, the lifetime distribution of income available to current generations should be preserved more or less intact into the future. Future generations may, of course, disagree with our judgments and conclude that they want a different allocation of income over the life course. It would seem presumptuous, however, for the current generation to "lock in" future generations in advance by adopting either the FCR or the FRR design.[13]

The core of Musgrave's life course argument, however, rests on practical, political, grounds. His main rationale for the FRP model is based on the assumption that neither of the alternatives, FRR or FCR, are *politically* sustainable under conditions of population aging. They are based, in his terms (1986, p. 109), on an intergenerational contract that cannot be kept or at least generates great uncertainty about its future. As the opinion polls make clear, under the prevailing FRR model, young, working-age contributors are skeptical that future generations will continue to support a system in which the active population bears all of the retirement costs associated with population aging. The result is a sense of "injustice" and cynicism rampant among many young adults as a result of being required to contribute to a system that "won't be there for me."

Under FRP, taxes/contributions will undoubtedly increase as a result of demographic aging, though less quickly than under the FRR design. Thus, the FRP principle runs counter to the notion that a "hard budget line" should be established for contribution levels or that there is an upper ("acceptable") limit to tax levels associated with "sound public finance." Implicitly, the assumption of an "upper limit" implies a level of taxation that will automatically trigger a general application of the FCR model ("no new taxes") in response to changes in the retirement dependency ratio. Thus far, empirical evidence and historical experience makes us skeptical or at least agnostic concerning claims that there are "natural" limits to taxation levels that can be known a priori. Consequently, we see no sound reason for "locking in" specific upper limits as long-term policy targets and should leave such a determination to future generations. As taken up below, however, we do think there is good reason for reconsidering the *mix* of taxes used to finance pay-as-you-go pension schemes.

In a dynamic context of change, "fixed replacement" (FRR), "fixed contribution" (FCR), and "fixed relative position" (FRP) can be thought of as alternative principles for the intergenerational allocation of the *change* in retirement costs attributable to changes in the retiree dependency ratio. Moreover, the choice of which principle is applied is a matter of degree. The choice is a normative one that will be determined via "politics," and it is conceivable, perhaps even desirable, that the mix of choices might change over time in response to changing circumstances.[14] One reason for expecting future departures from the FRP principle, as Frank Vandenbroucke (2002) highlights, is that *proportional* sharing measured in income terms does not guarantee *fair* sharing measured in terms of consumption. To use his example, proportional sharing may be unfair if there are large changes in the relative prices for essential goods and services (e.g., long-term care versus education and training) consumed by the old and the young. Hence, we advocate the Musgrave rule as a "litmus test," not as an "iron law." That is, we propose the FRP principle as a litmus test for intergenerational equity in the sense that the burden of proof falls on the would-be reformer who would allocate the costs that result from demographic change in ways that depart from FRP.

Although application of the Musgrave rule is relatively straightforward in nations where all or most of the consumption of retired persons comes from pensions financed with payroll taxes on the wages of nonretired persons, it is decidedly messier in "mixed" systems like that in the United States, where occupational plans and personal retirement accounts provide a large share of retirement income. As noted above, to satisfy requirements of intergenerational equity and to bequeath a sustainable pension regime to the next generation, the Musgrave rule must be applied to the entire retirement budget, to the "private" as well as to the "public" (= *total social*) costs that result from demographic change. The important implication of this conclusion is that in mixed pension regimes where both public and private sources provide a large share of retirement income, the future share of public pensions in the retirement budget is indeterminate. Application of a Musgrave-like strategy means that whether or not total *public* expenditures should be allowed to rise or fall is contingent on future levels of retirement income from private retirement savings. Applying the Musgrave rule or any other standard of intergenerational equity to the increase in retirement costs that result from demographic change by reference to the public budget alone (e.g., for Social Security and SSI) would, justifiably, erode any public trust in the policy process. Moreover, the favorable tax regime available to occupational plans and to personal retirement accounts clearly warrants that they too be charged with social goals.

Analytically, the major difficulty is to provide the appropriate accounting frameworks so that the intergenerational allocation of costs associated with any *specific* reform to either side of the public/private ledger (and their interaction) is transparent to the political process. A full accounting scheme of the allocation of retirement costs among the working and retired populations also requires estimates of likely second-order "behavioral response" to policy changes. Thus, when policy changes intended to induce greater personal saving for retirement are made, the intended (or probable) effects of such changes on the intergenerational allocation of retirement costs (including the possibility that retirement costs could rise) need to be established.

Intragenerational Justice

As Wolfson et al. (1998) have shown, the enormous heterogeneity *within* generations (or cohorts) "swamps" differences between generations with respect to the distribution of "winners" and "losers" that result from population aging. The upshot is that the *intergenerational* dilemma is compounded by at least two *intragenerational* dilemmas, one among retirees (beneficiaries), a second among the working-age population (contributors). The notion of "justice" adopted here is broadly Rawlsian in inspiration: changes to the status quo should be of most advantage to the least advantaged.

When Pension Systems Contract:
Intragenerational Justice among the Retired

The problem on the benefit side (i.e., among retired persons) can be highlighted by comparing a pension system that is expanding with one that is contracting. Expansion/contraction can take two forms: (a) an increase or decrease in the number of years of retirement; and (b) an increase or decrease in the benefits received during retirement. When retirement ages are falling, the social welfare "gains" in additional leisure and free time tend to go disproportionately to the least well off. An additional year of retirement, for example, represents a larger proportional gain for someone with a seven-year life expectancy than for someone with a twelve-year life expectancy. But the reverse is also true: an additional year of employment represents a proportionately greater loss for those with shorter life expectancies. Raising the retirement age for public sector benefits has the largest effect on those without sufficient means to finance early retirement on their own, and the least impact on those who do. Because health (life expectancy, disability) and wealth tend to be correlated, the equity problem is compounded.

As with changes in the retirement age, more disadvantaged persons tend to gain most when public pension benefits are expanding because they are less able or likely to provide income security for themselves. But conversely, they stand to lose the most when income security systems are contracting. The standard result from studies of savings behavior is that the savings to permanent income ratio rises with permanent income and does so in a sharply nonlinear fashion (Diamond and Hausman 1984). The implication is that behavioral response to lower mandatory pensions will be a function of income level: low-income families are less likely to compensate with more savings than high-income families. If a proportional share of the costs of population aging is to be transferred to retirees, how can this be done so that they do not fall disproportionately on the least advantaged among them?

Financing Pensions: Intragenerational Justice
among the Working Population

On the contribution side, pay-as-you-go pensions are financed with a tax on wage income—the payroll tax—while income from capital and transfers are exempt.[15] The payroll tax is a flat tax, often with a wage ceiling that makes it regressive. Unlike income taxes, there are no exemptions and no allowances for family size. Low-wage workers and especially younger families with children typically bear a disproportionate share of the cost as a result. These effects are compounded to the extent that high payroll taxes discourage employment, especially at the lower end of the labor market, where the social safety net, minimum wages, or industrial relations systems make it difficult for employers to pass such costs on to employees.

Application of the Musgrave rule, however, implies that a proportional share of the increased retirement costs that result from population aging will fall on the working-age population (i.e., that contributions will rise). Clearly, however, allocating these costs based on a flat-rate tax without deductions for children or other circumstances (i.e., flat-rate payroll taxes) is inconsistent with the notion that these costs should be of greatest advantage (or the least disadvantage) to the least well off within the working-age population. In effect, charging the costs of the transition to the working-age population via a payroll tax creates a huge problem of intragenerational justice among the working-age population because the distribution of the additional costs in no way reflects ability to pay. Not surprisingly, the main target of European pension reform in the 1990s was to slow or freeze the rate of growth in payroll contribution rates, an objective embraced not only by employers and governments but also by labor organizations.

Redesigning Benefits: Intragenerational Justice for the Retired

If a proportional share of the costs of population aging is to be transferred to retirees, how can this be done so that they do not fall disproportionately on the least advantaged among them? Clearly, reforms that simply cut all pensioner benefits by a proportional amount (e.g., by reducing all pensions by 5 percent) do not satisfy this standard. Moreover, behavioral response to such reductions can be expected to increase inequality among the retired. The standard result from studies of savings behavior is that the savings to permanent income ratio rises with permanent income and does so in a sharply nonlinear fashion (Diamond and Hausman 1984). The implication, then, is that behavioral response to reduced *mandatory* pensions will be a function of income level: lower income families are less likely to compensate with more *voluntary* retirement savings than higher income families.

The notion that the costs of restructuring should be borne by those most able to afford it and the weakest members of society should be protected is hardly novel. But how to implement it? We propose two forms of "targeting" public sector benefits to meet this challenge drawn from the real world experience of contemporary affluent democracies.

Eliminating Old Age Poverty

Building or enhancing generous basic security schemes with a minimum guarantee above the poverty line goes a long way toward addressing the Rawlsian problem identified above. It establishes a floor beyond which the most disadvantaged pensioners bear *none* of the additional costs of population aging and thus meets at least a minimal requirement of intragenerational justice for the retired.

Declining poverty rates among elderly persons have been a distinguishing feature of all OECD countries since the 1960s. Old age poverty rates below 10 percent are now common, and a number of countries have achieved rates of 5 percent or less (Hauser 1997; Smeeding and Sullivan 1998; Table 3.1). The major flaw in the U.S. design is that it lacks such a plan, and hence old poverty rates remain high by international standards (Table 3.1).

The most effective antipoverty systems are not necessarily the most costly. Both high-spending Sweden and low-spending Canada achieve poverty rates of less than 5 percent (see also Smeeding and Sullivan 1998) because both provide guaranteed minimum benefits that raise the vast majority above standard "poverty lines." Canada provides a guaranteed annual income to elderly persons, and Sweden, a guaranteed minimum pension. Both make benefits conditional on the presence or absence of other economic resources (i.e., they are "targeted") but in a way that departs significantly from traditional *means-tested* programs such as SSI. To distinguish traditional means-testing from these modern variants, it is useful to draw some distinctions.

- *Means-testing.* Individuals qualify for benefits on the basis of a test for both *income* and *assets,* requiring individuals to "spend" their way into poverty to qualify. Tax-back rates (the rate at which benefits are cut as other income rises) are typically high and can be in excess of 100 percent. Supplemental Security

Table 3.1. Poverty rates among the population aged 65+, 1990s

<5%	5–9%	10–14%	15–19%	>20%
Canada	Finland	Austria		Australia
Sweden	France	Belgium		United States
	Germay	Denmark		
	Luxembourg	Italy		
	Netherlands	Norway		
	Switzerland	Spain		
		United		
		Kingdom		

Source: Data from LIS Key Figures, Luxembourg Income Study, 2001.

Income (SSI) in the United States is an example. Usually the aim is to restrict benefits to a small fraction of the population (the "poor"), and benefits are modest. Because of the intrusiveness of the means test, there is often considerable stigma attached to accepting benefits so that take-up rates tend to be low. Poverty rates among seniors remain high as a result.

- *Income-testing.* As the term suggests, income-testing is based on a test of income but not of assets, so there is no requirement to spend oneself into poverty to qualify. Interest or dividends from investments are included in the test, but not the underlying capital that generates the income. Tax-back rates are always *much* less than 100 percent, so benefits are not "for the poor alone" but often extend well into middle-income groups, albeit at declining rates. The implicit model is closer to Milton Friedman's design for a negative income tax (NIT) or a guaranteed annual income (GAI) than traditional means-tests for the "poor" (see Myles and Pierson 1997). Canada's *Guaranteed Income Supplement* for seniors is the exemplar.[16] Because such plans are administered through the tax system, stigma is minimal and take-up rates are high. In the United States, the Earned Income Tax Credit (EITC) provides one model for such a strategy.

- *Pension-testing.* As practiced in Sweden and Finland, pension-testing is a yet more restricted type of test, including only income that comes from the *public* pension program in those countries. Unlike a Guaranteed Annual Income scheme, it functions to provide a Guaranteed Annual Pension. Individuals with

earnings histories and contributions below the minimum are
provided with pension supplements on a sliding scale. Where all
or most of the income of retirees comes from the public pension
system, of course, the distinction between income-testing and
pension-testing is merely a formal one.

Providing all elderly citizens with a minimum guarantee above a
poverty line indexed to national living standards is well within the
reach of most rich democracies because the poverty gap—the difference between family income and the poverty line—of the poor elderly is typically modest compared to that of working-age families
(Table 3.2).

Providing retirees with a high guaranteed annual income or minimum pension is less problematic than providing such benefits to
working-age families, because the issue of work incentives does not
arise.[17] Over some range of the earnings distribution, a high guarantee level may have an impact on savings behavior, but this is likely to
occur over a short time period, relatively late in the work career, when
the impact of more or less savings on retirement income is known.

Building or enhancing generous basic security schemes with a minimum guarantee above the poverty line goes a long way toward addressing the Rawlsian problem identified above. It establishes a floor
beyond which the most disadvantaged pensioners bear *none* of the additional costs of population aging and thus meets at least a minimal
requirement of intragenerational justice among retirees. Because a
guaranteed annual income or minimum pension involves interpersonal
redistribution, there is a strong case for general revenue (from income,
consumption, and other taxes) rather than payroll taxes as the source
of financing. Payroll taxes impose all of the cost on the working-age
population with perverse distributional effects within that population.
A large or rising share of general revenue financing provides a powerful tool for reallocating the costs of population aging based on ability
to pay among the retired as well as the working-age population because, like the young, the old are also subject to income and consumption taxes.

The cost of eliminating poverty among elderly persons will be higher
in nations like the United States with higher earnings inequality over
the working life because there will be more retirees who are eligible
for such benefits. One might think of these additional costs as an "in-

Table 3.2 Cost of eliminating old age poverty, National Accounts Estimate, 1990s

Country (Year)	Number of Poor Households with Old People (thousands)	Poverty Gap (local currency)	Extra Cost (as percentage of GDP)
Canada (1994)	118	1,591	0.025
United States (1997)	5,565.9	2,931	0.201
Finland (1995)	21.7	3,708	0.015
Norway (1995)	60.6	6,612	0.043
Sweden (1995)	27.2	10,524	0.017
Netherlands (1991)	36.9	5,312	0.036
Germany (1989)	633.8	3,617	0.080
France (1994)	664.1	8,083	0.073

Source: Data from LIS Databases and OECD National Accounts.
Note: Extra cost as percentage of GDP = (number of poor households x poverty gap)/GDP. Estimates are based on the objective of bringing families containing persons 65+ above 50 percent of the median adjusted disposable income line. This exercise ignores the fact that this, in itself, will alter the overall distribution and, thus, also the median.

equality tax," the cost of which must be evaluated on the basis of one's prior assumptions concerning the effects of wage inequality during the working life on employment and labor market flexibility.

Rationalizing Redistribution in Earnings-Related Schemes

The modern institution of retirement rests on much more than a promise that retirees will not fall into "poverty." Postwar retirement patterns reflect the development of institutions that promised much more, namely, that the majority would be able to maintain living standards not unlike those reached during their working years. All of this suggests that the main challenge raised, once an adequate basic security scheme is in place, is the probable impact of reform on workers with average and below average earnings who, under current provisions, would have retirement incomes well above the guaranteed minimum. The challenge, moreover, is not gender neutral. The distribution of income security "losses" that can result from lower public pensions will have a greater impact on women because they typically have lower lifetime earnings and longer life expectancies than men.

Although earnings-related pension schemes ostensibly reflect individual work histories and contributions, all systems have traditionally incorporated design features that produce significant interpersonal transfers and cross-subsidies. Eliminating transfers and cross-subsidies that could be identified as "inequitable," "perverse," or "outdated" (such as special privileges for public employees) provided many European countries with an effective means of cost reduction during the 1990s. At the same time, some of the savings were used to provide new cross-subsidies considered to be socially desirable, such as pension credits for child and elder care. This "rationalization" of the redistributive design features to achieve equity or to more clearly realize socially desirable distributive outcomes offers policymakers a potent tool for solving the Rawlsian problem among the non-poor.

The 1995 Swiss reform is especially striking (and relevant for the United States) because the reform was about introducing gender equality and was subject to a national referendum (Bonoli 1997). As in the United States, a married man with a dependent spouse was eligible for a "couple pension" corresponding to 150 percent of his own pension entitlement, a practice that disproportionately benefits higher-income families (Meyer 1996). Women's organizations successfully took the lead in demanding the end of the couple pension. In the new design, all contributions paid by the two spouses while married are added together, divided by 2, and counted half each. Strikingly, however, couples with children below the age of 16 now receive additional credit equal to the amount of contributions payable on a salary three times the minimum pension (56 percent of the average wage). Compensation is provided for years spent in child rearing but, unlike the previous formula, not for providing housekeeping services to a spouse. The result is a cross-subsidy to families with children from those who remain childless.

An Appropriate Role for General Revenue Financing

A rising share of general revenue financing in the retirement budget provides a powerful tool for reallocating the costs of population aging based on ability to pay not only among the working-age population but also among retired persons. While retirees are not subject to payroll taxes, they do pay income and consumption taxes.[18] Assuming the more affluent among both retirees and the active population pay higher taxes, their share of the additional costs associated with demographic change rises proportionately with increases in the share of retirement costs financed from general revenue.

General revenue is the appropriate financing mechanism for all retirement benefits that involve interpersonal transfers whether inside Social Security (the spousal benefit, benefit formulas that favor lower-income workers) or outside of it (SSI). Changes to the financing mechanism of this sort have been a common strategy in the European reforms of the 1990s, and Bonoli's (1996) interviews with party officials and labor leaders in France and Germany provide striking evidence for the self-conscious character of this strategy. In the words of a French trade unionist: "The financing of contributory benefits . . . must be done through contributions based on salaries. In contrast, non-contributory benefits must be financed by the public purse." Tuchs-zirer and Vincent (1997) highlight a similar logic underlying the 1995 Toledo pact, an all-party agreement on the framework for reforming the Spanish social security system.

If pursued aggressively, if only incrementally, the criteria for reform outlined above imply a strategy that potentially alters the traditional social insurance model of old age security, at least in the long term. On the benefit side, any reductions required by the Musgrave rule are offset by new or expanded interpersonal transfers for less advantaged retirees. On the contribution side, these additional costs are met, not through higher payroll taxes, but with general revenue financing raised among both the retired and the nonretired, based on ability to pay. The implication on the benefit side is that with time the earnings replacement function of public sector insurance scheme diminishes somewhat for higher income families (which may be taken up by second and third tier savings).[19] And with time, the share of general revenue financing for the income security system as a whole rises. The exact mix at the "end" of the process will vary from country to country because we assume that there is a wide variety of initial starting points and that the strategy is applied incrementally only to the allocation of the *change* in retirement costs that results from population aging.

Conclusion

In the U.S. context, critics of the status quo often appeal to intergenerational equity to justify reforms, but only within the context of addressing the public finance (i.e., Social Security) implications of population aging. Concerns over intergenerational equity can be mostly resolved in such a framework in pension regimes where all or most retirement income is from publicly financed sources but not in mixed systems such as that in the United States. Supporters of the status quo, in contrast, often highlight the fact that reducing Social Security benefits has the largest impact on the least advantaged among the retired, but they have largely overlooked the implications of rising payroll taxes for the least advantaged among the working population. Allowing payroll taxes to rise solves the public finance problem, but financing the transition to an older society on the backs of lower-income and especially younger workers does not satisfy the principle of intragenerational justice. The one-sided focus on long-term public finance issues posed by Social Security has also distracted attention from the equally pressing *point-in-time* challenge of constructing an adequate basic security system for retirees. By international standards, Social Security and SSI perform poorly in protecting the least advantaged, despite their redistributive features.

Notes

1. Specifically, this chapter draws on material from Myles (2002) originally written as part of a larger report on welfare state reform for the European Union and a subsequent exchange (Myles in press) with Erik Schokkaert and Philippe Van Parijs (2003) in the *European Journal of Social Policy*. For reasons of space, I only briefly allude to the discussions of gender equality and later retirement contained in these papers.

2. Peter Hicks, personal communication, December 2001.

3. Advocates for privatization typically argue that the result would be higher investment and hence larger gains in productivity under a privatized system, but as discussed later, this is a result over which there is considerable skepticism.

4. On this, see the exchange between Richard Epstein and David Braybrooke in Laslett and Fishkin (1992).

5. The important distinction between tabula rasa choices and transformation choices is developed by Orszag and Stiglitz (1999). As they note (p. 7), the social effects of *transforming* a mature pension system into a system of individual accounts may be substantially different from the social effects of the initial choice between a public defined benefit system and individual accounts.

6. Aggregative outcomes such as prices or fertility rates, writes Hernes (1976, p. 516), "are partly under human control and partly the result of

chance processes; in part they can be affected by conscious action but to a considerable extent they are unintended."

7. In the context of the issues addressed in this chapter, the principle of *equity* should be understood as referring to "fair burden sharing," that is, to an equitable sharing of the costs (or benefits) of demographic transition between citizens. Still, every parent who has tried to explain to younger children why it is "fair" that they are put to bed before their older siblings knows that determinations of what is equitable are often highly contested. It is not surprising, then, that the contemporary notion of "intergenerational equity" and its range of application should also be contested (Laslett and Fishkin 1992). In some contexts, the concept is used to discuss point-in-time differences between generations or cohorts currently alive (the old, the young), while in other contexts it pertains more to the legacy that one generation (all those now living) will leave to future generations (those not yet born). Here I make use of both senses of the term (see text below). The range of outcomes considered also varies. Should policies aimed at effecting equity between generations be applied only to the activities of government or to the entire social, economic, and natural infrastructure left to future generations?

8. It is important to recall that we are describing a fixed contribution model in a *pay-as-you-go* design, not to be confused with a fixed contribution model in a funded scheme where benefits reflect contributions plus (or minus) realized gains (or losses) on invested contributions. Few readers outside of France will be familiar with the pay-as-you-go FCR model.

9. The FRP principle, however, would not satisfy a concept of fairness defined by the notion that each generation ought to pay the same proportion of salary to get the same level of pension rights during retirement. On a three-generational "family farm," for example, the *share* or proportion of output required to support aging parents in retirement under FRP will be larger when there are two producers in the working-age generation than when there are four.

10. This is not the place to engage in an in-depth discussion of the normative merits of reciprocity and equiproportional burden sharing. In line with Musgrave's original approach, stated in terms of the political viability of social security arrangements, I rather note that proportionality indeed often acts as a focal point in negotiation problems (thus lending support to FRP as a benchmark). Political viability, or a policy's sustainability, is not an intrinsic feature of an ideal normative conception of justice. But it is a desideratum, and an important one, when pragmatically implementing a theory of justice. See Vandenbroucke (2001) for a further elaboration of this last point.

11. It should be clear that implementation of FRP does not preclude

passing judgment on the current distribution (e.g., that it is too high or too low), making adjustments accordingly, and applying FRP thereafter.

12. Hence, the FRP design can be distinguished from solutions that index benefits but not contributions to the higher retirement costs that result from increased longevity, the latter being essentially an FCR strategy.

13. As Musgrave (1986, pp. 107–8) observes, at any given point in a cohort's life course, those motivated by their immediate (i.e., myopic) self-interest are likely to make choices that depart from the FRP design. For young workers entering the labor force with foreknowledge that the population is aging, a "self-interested" response from a cohort concerned mainly with its immediate living standards (i.e., myopic choice) would lead to a preference for a model based on a fixed contribution rate because their contributions to support the retired would not rise during their working years. These preferences, however, would undoubtedly change as they approach retirement because now they would face an impoverished old age relative to earlier retiree cohorts.

14. The choice of principles might well vary according to the *source* of change in retirement costs. Thus, the FRP principle might be applied to distribute the costs that result from "demographic change" (i.e., past changes in fertility), while the FCR principle might be adopted to accommodate any decline in retirement ages, and some mix of the two to changes that result from greater longevity.

15. For purposes of this discussion, we adopt the standard assumption that payroll taxes, even when borne by the employer, are additions to labor costs, which are ultimately borne by labor, typically in the form of lower wages.

16. Every NIT model is defined by three parameters: the *guarantee level* (the level of benefit provided to people with no other income; the *tax-back rate* (the rate at which benefits are reduced as the recipient gains income); and the *break-even point* (the income level at which benefits disappear). A high guarantee level is desirable to provide people with adequate incomes, and a low tax-back rate is desirable to encourage people to work. But such a combination means that the break-even point is very high and so are the costs. In practice, virtually all NIT proposals are broken into two tiers in order to contain costs and to maintain work incentives. One tier is intended for people who are not expected to work (such as elderly persons) with a high guarantee level, a high tax-back rate, and a low break-even level. The second tier, for those expected to work, typically has a lower tax-back rate and a higher relative break-even point but a lower guarantee level.

17. For working-age families, the level at which social benefits affect work incentives is a function of the wage distribution. When wage inequality in the lower tail of the distribution (e.g., when low-paid workers

earn about 40 percent of the median wage), a high guarantee level will have more disincentive effects than when wage inequality is more modest (e.g., where low-paid workers earn about 70 percent of the median).

18. I do not preclude the possibility that there may be significant advantages to a system of "earmarked" Social Security contributions so long as such contributions are based on total income and provide for some degree of progressivity, especially in the lower tail of the distribution, and provide adjustments for family size.

19. I hasten to add, however, that there is no intrinsic reason why second-tier employer pensions cannot incorporate interpersonal transfers to achieve desirable social objectives.

References

Barr, N. 2001. *The Welfare State as Piggy Bank: Information, Risk, Uncertainty and the Role of the State.* Oxford: Oxford University Press.

Bonoli, G. 1996. Politics against convergence?: Current trends in European social policy. Paper presented at the conference on the Distributive Dimension of Political Economy, Center for European Studies, Harvard University, March 1–3.

Bonoli, G. 1997. Switzerland: institutions, reforms and the politics of consensual retrenchment. In J. Clasen, ed., *Social Insurance in Europe.* Bristol: Policy Press.

Diamond, P., and J. Hausman. 1984. Individual retirement and savings behavior. *Journal of Public Economics* 23:81–114.

Haber, C., and B. Gratton. 1994. *Old Age and the Search for Security: An American Social History.* Bloomington: Indiana University Press.

Hauser, R. 1997. *Adequacy and Poverty Among the Retired.* Paris: Organization for Economic Cooperation and Development.

Hernes, G. 1976. Structural change in social processes. *American Journal of Sociology* 32:513–47.

Laslett, P., and J. Fishkin (Eds.). 1992. *Justice between Age Groups and Generations.* New Haven: Yale University Press.

Meyer, M. H. 1996. Making claims as workers or wives: the distribution of Social Security benefits. *American Sociological Review* 61:449–65.

Musgrave, R. 1986. *Public Finance in a Democratic Society.* Volume 2: *Fiscal Doctrine, Growth and Institutions.* New York: New York University Press.

Myles, J. 2002. A new social contract for the elderly. In G. Esping-Andersen, D. Gallie, A. Hemerijck, and J. Myles, eds. *Why We Need a New Welfare State.* Oxford: Oxford University Press.

Myles, J., and P. Pierson. 1997. Friedman's revenge: the reform of liberal welfare states in Canada and the United States. *Politics and Society* 25:443–72.

Myles, J., and P. Pierson. 2001. The comparative political economy of pension reform. Pp. 305–33 in *The New Politics of the Welfare State,* edited by P. Pierson. Oxford: Oxford University Press.

Organization for Economic Cooperation and Development 2001. *Aging and Income: Financial Resources and Retirement in Nine OECD Countries.* Paris: OECD.

Orszag, P., and J. Stiglitz. 1999. Rethinking pension reform: ten myths about social security systems. World Bank, Washington, D.C., September.

Schokkaert, E., and P. Van Parijs. 2003. Social justice and the reform of Europe's pension systems. *Journal of European Social Policy* 13:245–63.

Sinn, H. W. 2000. Why a funded pension system is useful and why it is not useful. *International Tax and Public Finance* 7(4/5):383–410.

Smeeding, T., and D. Sullivan. 1998. Generations and the distribution of economic well-being: a cross-national view. Luxembourg Income Study, Working Paper Series, No. 173.

Thompson, L. 1998. *Older and Wiser: The Economics of Public Pensions.* Washington, D.C.: Urban Institute.

Tuchszirer, C., and C. Vincent. 1997. Un consensus presque parfait autour de la reforme du systeme du retraite. *Chronique Internationale de l'IRES* 48:26–30.

Vandenbroucke, F. 2001. Forward: Sustainable social justice and "open coordination" in Europe. In G. Esping Andersen, D. Gallie, A. Hemerijck, and J. Myles, eds., *Why We Need a New Welfare State.* Oxford: Oxford University Press.

Wolfson, M., G. Rowe, X. Lin, and S. Gribble. 1998. Historical generational accounting with heterogeneous populations. Pp. 107–26 in *Government Finances and Generational Equity,* edited by M. Corak. Ottawa: Statistics Canada.

4. Decreasing Welfare, Increasing Old Age Inequality
Whose Responsibility Is it?
Madonna Harrington Meyer

Who is responsible for taking care of the elderly? For the better part of a century, the U.S. answer has emphasized the model of a three-legged stool. One-third of old age security should come from the welfare state, through universal and poverty-based benefit programs. One-third should come from the corporate sector, through employment-based benefits. The remaining one-third should come from the savings and investments of older individuals themselves. But since the early 1980s, policymakers have restricted supports provided through the welfare state, employers have cut benefits provided through jobs, and many older people and their families have watched their stocks and investments diminish in value. Long considered a sacred cow, old age security is once again contested terrain.

Since the early 1980s, conservative policymakers in the United States have been in the midst of an effort to dismantle the welfare state. Recent efforts to push responsibility for old age security onto the shoulders of individuals and their families are not without precedent. Historically, most societies have placed the burden of any sort of dependency squarely on the family. But between the mid-1800s and mid-1900s, modern welfare states became increasingly involved in taking responsibility for the provision of at least some basic needs, particularly for elderly citizens. Welfare states offered health insurance, income security, and various family benefits partly because officials recognized that filial responsibility had real limits (Katz 1986; Harrington Meyer 1996). The elderly came to be defined as the deserving poor, and policymakers recognized that filial responsibility concentrated risk, privatized cost, and maximized inequality between families.

In comparison to most other developed Western nations, the United States was slow to form programs and exceptionally restrictive with the benefits that were offered (Quadagno 1999b). Nonetheless, between the 1930s and the 1970s the United States implemented and expanded poverty-based welfare programs such as Medicaid and Supplemental Security Income, and two universal programs, Social Security and Medicare. A major point of U.S. exceptionalism, however, was the tendency to rely heavily on corporate and market-based, rather than welfare state–based, benefits. Particularly when universally distributed, benefits offered by welfare states potentially spread risk; share costs; and reduce gender, race, and class inequality (Korpi and Palme 1998). By contrast, benefits offered through employers or markets tend to help only those with sufficiently strong links to the labor force to receive the benefits (Harrington Meyer and Pavalko 1996). To the extent that they have weaker links to the labor force or are less rewarded for their efforts in the labor force, women, persons of color, and part-time or low-wage workers are significantly less likely to reap the rewards of employment-based benefits (Estes 2001; Korpi and Palme 1998).

Though the U.S. welfare state has never even come close to catching up to our peer nations, we have begun dismantling in earnest. As costs for welfare state benefits and employment-based benefits alike have spiraled, cost containment, privatization, and retrenchment have become a central preoccupation (Estes 2001). Over the past two decades many welfare state policies have been left unattended even though they are seriously outdated, while others have been reconfigured to restrict eligibility and reduce benefits. Alarmingly, during that same time period employment-based benefits such as health insurance and pensions have also been cut dramatically. The call to return to individual and filial, rather than corporate or welfare state supports, is deafening.

No matter what the rhetoric, at the root of dismantling efforts is the goal of shifting responsibility from welfare states to corporate sites, from employers to employees, from collectives to individuals (Estes 2001). Rather than provide benefits through the welfare state or through employment-based programs, the goal of twenty-first-century individualist policies is to minimize corporate taxes and expenditures, minimize individual income taxes, and rely on a "free" market for the provision of services to frail elderly persons (Moon and Herd 2002). (This trend is captured nicely in the comic strip in Fig. 4.1.) The conservative agenda is to encourage each of us invest for our own old age and then let each of us face the consequences. That some earn too little to make such investments, others will be displaced or downsized out

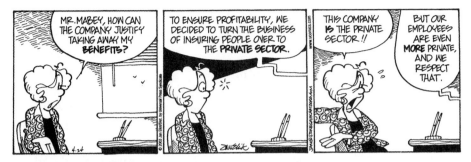

Fig. 4.1. One view of privatization. Source: Stone Soup © 2003 Jan Eliot. Reprinted with permission of Universal Press Syndicate. All rights reserved.

of the market, many will have needs that far outpace their resources, and nearly all of us will watch our stock values plummet, is of little concern to proponents of individualistic market solutions (Baker and Weisbrot 1999). Those with sufficient economic resources can weather the impact of financial, physical, and other sorts of downturns, but those with more modest resources can not. We already have the highest levels of old age inequality among advanced Western nations; the surest outcome of our shrinking welfare- and employment-based safety nets is increased inequality (Street and Wilmoth 2001).

Health Care

A key source of old age inequality is inadequate health care coverage. The United States is the only Western nation that fails to provide health insurance to all of its citizens, and nearly 17 percent, or 44 million Americans, are uninsured (Quadagno 1999a; EBRI 1994; Seccombe and Amey 1995). Instead of national health insurance, U.S. employers receive tax incentives aimed at encouraging the provision of health insurance through jobs. These tax breaks amounted to $57 billion in lost revenues in 1997 alone (Quadagno 1999a). Thus, as taxpayers we are already paying for health insurance as a social benefit, but because we are distributing it through employment-based rather than welfare state mechanisms, we have little control over how the benefits are distributed (Estes 2001). As a social experiment in providing a basic necessity through employment rather than through the welfare state, the U.S. health care system is revealing. The same sorts of gender, race, and class inequalities that emerge from the market are replicated and amplified by the market-based distribution of benefits.

Employee-Based Health Insurance

For the most part, we rely on corporate or employment-based health insurance coverage in the United States (Harrington Meyer and Pavalko 1996). Already spotty, health insurance coverage by employers has been declining steadily for two decades. Between 1979 and 1992, the proportion of working men of all ages with insurance through their own jobs declined from 65 to 52 percent, while the proportion of women with insurance through their own jobs declined from 47 to 37 percent (EBRI 1994, Harrington Meyer and Pavalko 1996). Coverage varies by gender, race, and marital status. Whites, men, and full-time and high-paid workers are most likely to have health insurance, while persons of color, women, and part-time and low-waged workers are more likely to be uninsured or rely on poverty-based programs (Harrington Meyer and Pavalko 1996).

Employment-Based Retirement Health Insurance

Similarly, employment-based health insurance for retirees has dropped significantly in recent years. A U.S. GAO report shows that even among large employers, who are most likely to offer retiree health insurance, the proportion who offer retiree health benefits has dropped from over 50 percent in 1993 to 37 percent in 2000. In 1999 only 37 percent of retirees aged 55 to 64, and about 26 percent of those age 65 and older, had employer-sponsored health coverage (U.S. GAO 2001). White, male, full-time, and highly paid workers are more likely to accrue these retiree health benefits, but even for those groups, coverage is on the decline, and the GAO expects these declines to continue. Moreover, employers who still offer retiree coverage are pushing more of the costs onto retirees and tightening restrictions on benefits.

Medicare

Since 1965 Medicare has provided universal health care benefits to aged, blind, and disabled persons. Before the program began, just 56 percent of the aged had hospital insurance. In 2001, more than 95 percent of all older persons in the United States had hospital coverage (Harrington Meyer and Bellas 1995; SSA 2002). The entire system operates at prohibitively high costs, yet many kinds of health care remain out of reach for many. Recent policy initiatives have shifted costs back to elderly persons and to their families.

Medicare costs rose dramatically from the moment the program was implemented (Marmor 1970; Moon and Herd 2002). Between 1980 and 2001, Medicare Part A costs rose 470 percent. Even more dramatically, Part B costs rose by 800 percent (SSA 2002). To curb runaway costs, in 1984 the Health Care Financing Administration implemented a prospective payment system aimed at reducing unnecessary medical treatment and cutting costs. By certain measures the effort succeeded: hospital stays were shortened dramatically, and the rate at which total costs were rising slowed measurably (Estes 1989; 2001). But studies also revealed that hospitals and clinics increased the extent to which they exported unprofitable care, discharged clinically unstable patients, and made multiple readmissions (Glazer 1990; Estes 2001).

In the wake of the prospective payment system, the demand for post-acute care rose dramatically. Nursing homes and convalescent facilities met some of the demand, but much of it was shouldered by family members. Between 1988 and 1997, home health care payments rose from $1.9 billion to $16.7 billion. However, after the Balanced Budget Act of 1997, which reduced payments to hospitals ands shifted home health care from Part A to Part B, the commitment to home health care plummeted (Moon and Herd 2002). Under Medicare, the number of licensed, participating home health agencies dropped 37 percent between 1997 and 2001 (SSA 2002). Total Medicare expenditures on home health care for elderly persons dropped 32 percent between 1997 and 1998 (SSA 2002, p. 301). In that same year, the number of persons receiving home health care benefits under both Part A and Part B actually increased; thus, the per person benefit dropped 41 percent for Part A and 32 percent for Part B (SSA 2002, p. 301).

Care work changed as hospitals discharged patients quicker and sicker, and Medicare and Medicaid coverage of home care dried up (Glazer 1990; Hooyman and Gonyea 1995). With little training, families are often expected to take on highly technical work such as chemotherapy, apnea monitoring, phototherapy, oxygen tents, tubal feedings, and dressing changes (Glazer 1990). Estes (1989) calculated that in the first five years of Diagnostic Related Groups (DRGs), more than 21 million days of care work had been transferred to families from hospitals. Glazer (1990) estimated that that the medical industry saves at least $10 billion in wages annually because of the unpaid care work provided by family members. The reduction in health care coverage under Medicare has shifted responsibility to families, increasing the dependence of elderly persons on informal caregivers and causing many older persons to do without needed care (Estes 2001, Harrington Meyer and Kesterke-Storbakken 2000; Moon and Herd 2002).

Although Medicare is nearly universal in terms of eligibility, it is hardly universal in its benefit coverage. Gaps in Medicare coverage include long-term care, preventive care, dental care, vision and eyeglasses, Part B premiums, deductibles, co-payments, and any amount that surpasses the allowable charges (Harrington Meyer and Bellas 1995; SSA 2002). Recent estimates suggest that Medicare covers just over 40 percent of old age health care costs (Quadagno 1999a). Medicare's benefits are so spotty, and exclude so many of the very benefits that elderly persons are likely to need, that Margolis (1990) quips that Medicare must have been created for some group other than the elderly. Certainly, the coverage is less than most Americans count on from their employer-based plans; one study found that fully 82 percent of employer-based plans had more generous coverage than Medicare (Moon and Herd 2002).

Cost sharing by elderly persons is enormous and rising. With respect to nursing home care, Medicare covers portions of the first 100 days of nursing home care, but the benefits are quite limited. After day 20, the co-pay was $105 a day in 2003, making the monthly co-pay over $3,000. With respect to Medicare Part B, the premium increased 244 percent between 1980 and 1990 (Waxman 1992). In 1993 the Part B premium was set at 25 percent of the cost of Part B services, and the 1997 Balanced Budget Act (BBA) made this a permanent condition. Thus the Part B premium is expected to continue rising at rates much higher than the cost of living. Because the Part B premium is deducted from Social Security benefits before the checks are mailed, the net effect may be smaller Social Security benefits across the board. In addition to premiums, Medicare deductibles and co-payments have risen sharply. For example, between 1980 and 2003, the Part A deductible for a hospital stay increased by 470 percent (Waxman 1992; SSA 2002). Additionally, Medicare reimbursement rates have been curtailed since the 1997 BBA, and providers are transferring costs above the assigned rate to patients (Moon and Herd 2002). Aware that out-of-pocket expenses are particularly burdensome for lower-income old people, Medicare implemented Medicare savings programs, but as a result of the complexity and burdens of the program, less than half who are eligible are enrolled (Moon and Herd 2002; Quadagno 1999a).

In an attempt to determine whether the private market could provide more comprehensive medical care at controlled costs, Medicare turned to capitated HMO and managed care plans. The Balanced Budget Act of 1997 created Medicare plus Choice (M+C), which permits Medicare recipients to enroll in PPOs, HMOs, and other managed private plans (Moon and Herd 2002). Enrollment in Medicare PPOs and HMOs rose between 1992 and 2000 from 1.6 million to 6.3 million beneficiaries. Still, at its zenith, M+C accounted for only 16 percent of the total Medicare population (Kaiser Foundation 2003b). By 2000, M+C plans had pulled out of many service areas, cut benefits, and raised premiums. Enrollment in the privatized system dropped. By 2004, just 4.6 percent of Medicare enrollees remained in the program. Initially M+C did not charge enrollees a premium over the part B premium, but by 2002, 62 percent charged premiums averaging $60.50 a month (Kaiser Foundation 2003b). Critics of M+C options warned that private firms skim the healthiest elderly persons for these programs to keep costs down and that the care may be inferior to that under traditional fee-for-service plans. Evidence on the quality of care is mixed and suggests that those with many health problems do not tend to fare well in M+C plans (Kaiser Foundation 2003b; Moon and Herd 2002; Quadagno 1999a). Hopes that privatizing Medicare through M+C might reduce Medicare expenditures have not been met. A 2001 U.S. GAO report shows that Medicare paid an average of 13 percent more per person in M+C plans than it would have if those persons had received care under the traditional Medicare program. Part of the problem is that while HMOs typically report administrative costs between 20 and 25 percent, Medicare keeps administrative costs at just 2 percent (SSA 2002). Despite all this evidence that privatizing Medicare does not appear to be working, many legislative proposals currently under consideration attempt to privatize Medicare costs through similar sorts of capitated plans.

Indeed, the failure of M+C did not deter Congress from trying to privatize another aspect of Medicare. Until very recently, Medicare did not cover prescription drugs. This was particularly problematic because, on average, older people take 3.8 medications per day and prescription drug costs have risen sharply (Palmer and Dobson 1994). In December 2003, Congress created an optional Medicare Part D through which beneficiaries select from a slate of private market drug insurance policies. Once implemented in 2006, program beneficiaries will pay approximately $35 in monthly premiums, a $250 annual deductible, and then a 25 percent co-pay for all drug costs from $251 to $2,250. Most seniors would then pay all of the next $2,850 in drug costs before an emergency benefit kicks in that pays annual drug costs in excess of $5,100 (Kaiser Foundation 2004).

State Medicaid expenditures should diminish as primary responsibility for drug coverage for poor elderly persons shifts from Medicaid to Medicare; however, the legislation has many shortcomings. First, out-of-pocket expenses may be as high as $3,600 a year. Second, only prescriptions on an approved list would be covered and counted in the benefit coverage. Third, because lawmakers wanted to be sure that beneficiaries would bear some of the costs, seniors will be prohibited from purchasing any Medigap policies that would cover uncovered drug costs. Finally, it appears that the most immediate beneficiaries of the new legislation will be the HMOs who take Medicare patients; serving only 4.6 million seniors, they will receive an additional $1.3 billion in 2004 and 2005. Urban Institute analyst Robert Berenson suggests that the Bush administration is so keen to maintain or even increase HMO coverage of Medicare recipients that by 2006 Medicare will pay HMOs 25 percent more than the traditional Medicare costs for the same beneficiaries (*Post Standard* 2003). Given the sharp rise and fall of M+C, it seems likely that Part D beneficiaries will quickly see their premiums rise, benefits dissipate, and out-of-pocket expenses increase.

Thus, we are four decades into the program, and the costs of health care for elderly persons are a greater burden than before the program began. In 1965, older people spent 15 percent of their annual incomes on health care. In 1998, the average older person spent 22 percent of income on health care expenses not covered by Medicare. By 2025, out-of-pocket health care expenses are expected to reach 30 percent (Moon and Herd 2002). Each year, one-third of the near poor are reduced below the poverty line by out-of-pocket health care expenses. Because they have poorer health and lower incomes, older women, blacks, and Hispanics are particularly likely to be made poor by their out-of-pocket health care expenses (Moon and Herd 2002; Angel and Angel 1997). Medicare provides universal health care to nearly all older Americans, but the program is not well tailored to the health needs of elderly persons. Congress is preoccupied with trying to privatize this social benefit. Meanwhile, the costs of old age health care are increasingly shifted back to elderly persons and their families. The poor and those with chronic illnesses have great difficulty making do, even with Medigap or supplemental insurance policies in place.

Supplemental Insurance

Because Medicare leaves so many costs uncovered, 66 percent of Medicare beneficiaries pay premiums on supplemental policies that cover Medicare premiums, co-pays, deductibles, and exclusions such as long-term care, eye exams, and hearing aids (U.S. HCFA 1998). Whites are more likely to have supplemental coverage, even when poor. While 48 percent of poor whites had Medigap coverage, only 17 percent of poor blacks and Hispanics had coverage (HCFA 1998; Harrington Meyer and Herd 2001). Recent studies show that access will become increasingly difficult because supplemental insurance premiums have risen significantly and are expected to continue to do so (Alecxih et al. 1997). Between 1992 and 1996, rates rose between 20 to 40 percent in certain states, leaving even more women and older minorities without supplemental insurance (Moon and Herd 2002). Selecting a plan can be overwhelming because prices and benefits vary enormously, premiums tend to rise over time, and coverage of pre-existing conditions is difficult to locate after the six-month period of open enrollment (U.S. GAO 2001). The result is that many older people are often stuck in plans with exorbitant premiums or inadequate coverage, denied coverage for certain conditions, or forced to go without supplemental coverage at all (Moon and Herd 2002; U.S. GAO 2001).

Reductions in employment-based health insurance and retiree insurance as well as persistent gaps in Medicare coverage leave older Americans little choice but to try to fill the gaps with private supplemental policies. The problem is that as consumers they face a dizzying selection with little leverage. Despite some government oversight, they are often unprotected from rising premiums, dropped coverage, increased deductibles, decreased coverage, caps, exclusions, fraud, and mismanagement (U.S. GAO 2001). The reliance on private supplemental policies shifts responsibility for elderly persons out of the welfare state, and out of the corporate sector, and squarely onto the shoulders of older individuals. Those with the fewest resources, who often have the poorest health, are least likely to be able to obtain and retain private insurance and are increasingly likely to do without insurance and, at times, without needed care.

Medicaid

Since 1965, Medicaid has provided comprehensive coverage of health care for poor aged, blind, and disabled persons. Most elderly Medicaid recipients are dually enrolled with Medicare as the principal insurer; thus, Medicaid covers only expenses Medicare does not: the Medicare Part B premium, nursing home care, prescription drugs, copays, and deductibles (Kaiser Foundation 2003a; SSA 2002; Harrington Meyer 2000; Quadagno 1999a). Because full coverage is so comprehensive, and because health care providers are prohibited from charging costs above the allowable rates to Medicaid recipients, full Medicaid coverage reduces out-of-pocket expenses from 20 percent to just 5 percent of annual income for dual enrollees (Kaiser Foundation 2003a). However, it is important to note that the effort to transfer long-term care back to the jurisdiction of family caregivers is just as pronounced under Medicaid as it is under Medicare. In the year following the 1997 Balanced Budget Act, the number of Medicaid recipients receiving home health care dropped 34 percent, the total Medicaid dollars devoted to home health care dropped 78 percent, and the average annual Medicaid dollars per home care recipient dropped 66 percent (SSA 2002).

The proportion of older people on Medicaid has dropped from 16 percent in 1970 to less than 13 percent in 2000 (Quadagno 1999a; SSA 2002). This is partly due to Medicaid's restrictive income and asset tests. Federal guidelines for full Medicaid benefits set the income test well below the federal poverty line, at just 73 percent (Kaiser Foundation 2003a). Many states have established more generous provisions, but few have established limits that approach the federal poverty line (SSA 2002). Moreover, the asset tests for full benefits, set at $2000 for an individual and $3000 for a couple and never indexed to inflation, have been in effect since 1989.

A smaller subset of dual Medicare and Medicaid enrollees receive limited Medicaid coverage under new rules that relax eligibility guidelines. Since 1998, Medicare recipients with incomes below 100 percent of the federal poverty line and assets up to $4,000 for an individual and $6,000 for a couple may be eligible for the Qualified Medicare Beneficiary Program (QMB). QMB covers the Medicare Part B premium and most deductibles and co-pays for those with incomes below 100 percent of the federal old age poverty line. Those with incomes between 100 and 120 percent of the poverty line and assets up to $4000 for an individual and $6000 for a couple may be eligible for the Specified Low Income Medicare Beneficiary (SLMB) program, which covers the Part B premiums (Kaiser Foundation 2003a). For those who are enrolled, QMB and SLMB benefits help by reducing out-of-pocket costs to 13 percent of total annual incomes.

The process of applying is so arduous and stigmatizing, and the rules of eligibility are so restrictive, that less than one-third of poor elderly persons actually receive Medicaid. In fact, only half of those who are eligible for Medicaid receive the benefit (U.S. House Committee on Ways and Means 2000; Moon and Herd 2002; Kaiser Foundation 2003b; February 2003a). QMB and SLMB are reported to be even more complex and burdensome to apply for and use. Only 55 percent of those who qualify for QMB actually participate, and only 16 percent of those who qualify for SLMB actually participate (Moon and Herd 2002; Quadagno 1999a).

Because Medicaid is a poverty-based program, health care providers are generally not permitted to charge patients amounts over Medicaid assignment. As a result, many doctors, clinics, labs, hospitals, and nursing homes refuse to treat Medicaid patients or use a variety of mechanisms to cap the proportion of Medicaid patients they see. Between 1980 and 1997, nursing homes and other health care providers could sue the state on the grounds that Medicaid reimbursement rates were too low, using provisions in the Boren Amendment to the federal Medicaid statute in the Social Security Act. But that amendment was repealed with the 1997 Balanced Budget Act. As Medicaid rates stalled out, private pay rates continued to rise. One result is that hospitals, clinics, nursing homes, and other providers became even more likely to eliminate or limit Medicaid admissions. Another result is that private payers in all types of health care facilities are subsidizing the costs of care to Medicaid patients in their same facility. Because older women, blacks and Hispanics, and unmarried persons are more likely to be on Medicaid, they are more likely to face denial of, or delays in, treatment or admission (Wallace et al. 1998; Harrington Meyer and Kesterke-Storbakken 2000).

Those who wish to bypass paying for nursing home care out-of-pocket or through Medicaid can purchase private long-term care insurance policies that cover home care, community-based care, or institutional care. Selecting a plan is burdensome because cost and benefits vary dramatically by the type of coverage, age and health of the insured, and state or region of the country. Despite some government regulation, the plans have proven fairly unstable. Put off by spiraling premiums, fraud, overcharges, and general mismanagement, many people simply will not purchase the coverage (Angel and Angel 1997; Estes 2001).Moreover, those with serious health care problems often find that no plan will accept them (Quadagno 1999a; Angel and Angel 1997). Estimates are that as many as 40 percent of elderly persons could probably afford private long-term care insurance premiums if the market were more reliable and better managed; that means some 60 percent probably could not. Women, blacks and Hispanics, and unmarried older persons are particularly likely to have old age incomes so low that such premiums would be formidable (Angel and Angel 1997; Hooyman and Gonyea 1995). In yet another example of how the provision of health care coverage through the market has not worked to date, most estimates are that only 5 to 7 percent of elderly persons have private long-term care insurance (Moon and Herd 2002).

The strength of Medicaid is that it provides comprehensive health care services to poor older persons. The weakness is that the eligibility guidelines are strict and outdated, and that reimbursement rates are low and becoming proportionately lower. Medicaid retrenchment has primarily taken the form of gatekeeping. Income and asset requirements as well as provider reimbursement rates have not kept pace with cost of living increases, and the overall effect is to minimize the proportion of elderly Americans who are eligible and minimize access to benefits among beneficiaries. With long-term care needs left unmet by both the welfare state and by market insurance options, the pressure is even greater on families to provide care to frail elderly persons.

Shifting Care Work

Retrenchment and cost-shifting in the health care arena transfers the responsibility for, and costs of, old age health care to families, notably women. Women have higher rates of chronic illness, longer life expectancies, and fewer resources than older men, thus they are more likely to need long-term care. Moreover, due to the gendered division of labor and lower earnings, they are more likely to perform long-term care (Herd and Harrington Meyer 2002; Estes 2001; Quadagno 1999a). Indeed, women perform as much as 75 percent of all long-term care in the United States.

While care work can be emotionally rewarding, it often takes a toll on care workers in terms of the economic, physical, emotional, and social health of those doing the care work. Many spouses and adult sons and daughters reduce their work hours to accommodate care work. One study showed that 21 percent reduced work hours and 19 percent took time off without pay (Scharlach 1994). Ward (1990) estimates that families lose $8 billion a year in lost wages due to care work. In addition to lost wages, care workers who reduce hours miss out on pensions and Social Security, making them particularly vulnerable in their own old age.

The effects of prolonged caregiving can include physical and psychological distress, sleeplessness, exhaustion, inadequate exercise, increases in chronic conditions, and drug misuse (Baumgarten et al. 1992; Pavalko and Woodbury 2000). Care workers often have lower physical and mental health than their peers (National Alliance for Caregiving 1997; Commonwealth Fund 1999). Mothers providing unpaid care work full-time, along with women who have disproportionate burdens of household labor, have high levels of stress and depression (Bird 1999). In addition, numerous studies document that caregivers for developmentally disabled persons as well as elderly persons have poorer self-reported health, including higher levels of depression, sleeplessness, and exhaustion; lack of exercise; higher rates of chronic illnesses; and drug misuse (Hoyert and Seltzer 1992). Emotionally and socially, the costs can be high as well. Caregivers report loneliness, anxiety, depression, and tension with spouses and children (Stephens and Franks 1995; Pavalko and Woodbury 2000). Finally, caregivers often face problems accessing health care services for themselves. Compared to noncaregivers, caregivers were twice as likely to forego needed medical care and to miss filling a prescription due to cost. When costs are shifted from public and corporate coffers, they do not disappear (Herd and Harrington Meyer 2002). They weigh heavily on older persons and their families.

Economic Security

The path to economic security in old age is clear. Those with good educations, good family connections, good jobs and fringe benefits, and good health are particularly likely to be able to stash away savings and investments. By contrast, those with less education, few family connections, low-wage jobs, and meager fringe benefits are significantly less likely to have the savings and investments needed for a comfortable old age. Their chances are even smaller if they are women who have juggled paid and unpaid work with only the twelve weeks of unpaid family leave; blacks and Hispanics who are subject to racial discrimination in the labor market; or sick or disabled persons who are without good health insurance or meaningful disability benefits (Harrington Meyer 1996; Moon and Herd 2002; Hooyman and Gonyea 1995). Older people who reach old age with only spare economic resources generally do so because, across the life course, they have not been well tended by the welfare state nor well rewarded by the market. They have often faced cumulative disadvantages with little social or corporate support. Robust universal old age welfare state policies can offset some of the inequalities due to different life course trajectories—unless, of course, they are dismantled (Korpi and Palme 1998; Harrington Meyer 2000).

Social Security

Until recently, the history of Social Security was primarily one of liberal expansion. When the program was enacted in 1935 to provide monthly income to aged Americans, elderly persons were more likely than other age groups to be poor. But by the mid-1980s, primarily because of Social Security, poverty rates for aged persons actually dropped below poverty rates for other ages. The initial legislation, which excluded agricultural and domestic workers; the self-employed; and employees of religious, charitable, and educational organizations, covered just half of all workers and relatively few women and blacks.

With time, coverage was expanded, and now 95 percent of older persons are covered by Social Security (Quadagno 1984; Abramovitz 1988, Harrington Meyer and Bellas 1995; Century Foundation 1998). Social Security comprises about 40 percent of the income for all those aged 65 and older; one-fourth of elderly persons rely on it for 90 percent or more of their income (SSA 2002). Because of reduced access to private pensions and private savings, African Americans and Hispanics rely on Social Security for 48 and 44 percent of their annual incomes respectively (Grad 1994; Angel and Angel 1997).

Initially, only those who contributed to Social Security were eligible to receive benefits. The retirement test was strict; retirees who earned more than $15 a month forfeited the entire benefit. But expansion of the program began before the first benefits were even distributed (Harrington Meyer 1996). By 1939 spouses and widows were granted benefits equal respectively to 50 percent and 100 percent of their husband's benefit. In 1950 Congress made the rule gender neutral, and men gained the right to spouse and widower benefits as well. As divorce became more common, the rule that spouses had to be currently married was changed to one requiring twenty years of marriage before a divorce. By 1977 the marriage requirement had been lessened to ten years (SSA 2002). The earnings test was also lessened over time to the point that now there are no limits on earnings for those age 65 and older. Earnings limits remain only for early retirees. In 2000, those aged 62–65 may earn up to $10,080 a year without penalty, though they lose $1 in benefits for each $2 earned over that amount (SSA 2002).

Social Security is funded through the FICA tax at the rate of 6.2 percent per employer and employee. This tax is regressive because of a ceiling set on taxable earnings. In other words, lower-wage workers, predominately women, blacks, and Hispanics, were paying a higher proportion of their wages in taxes than higher-wage workers with earnings above the ceiling. In 1965, for example, 36 percent more women than men paid taxes on all of their earnings (Harrington Meyer 1996). Over time, that ceiling was raised significantly, so that now nearly all workers pay the tax all year. Raising the ceiling on taxable earnings reduced the regressiveness of the tax and reduced gender, race, and class inequality in the system.

Social Security is well known for its progressive benefit structures. Benefits redistribute resources from high to low lifetime earners

(Walzer 1988; Ozawa 1976). A high-wage earner receives benefits that replace 28 percent of pre-retirement income, while a low-wage earner receives benefits that replace 78 percent (Koitz 1996; Century Foundation 1998). But only the retired worker component of Social Security is redistributive. Most women actually receive benefits as spouses or widows of retired workers, and those benefits are not progressive. My earlier work shows that middle- and upper-class married white women are the most likely to receive noncontributory Social Security benefits (Harrington Meyer 1996). With more women working and fewer women married for a qualifying ten-year marriage, what was once an important safety net for lower-income retirees has turned into a marriage bonus with the greatest value for traditional families in higher income brackets. Dozens of possible fixes have been proposed through the years, but the only one that is adequately progressive and takes into account declining marital rates is a minimum benefit set near the federal poverty line (Harrington Meyer 1996).

The provision of noncontributory spouse and widow benefits on the basis of marital status provides an important example of how Social Security policy has not been responsive to major demographic changes. But other changes in Social Security policy have been introduced specifically to reduce benefits and constrain program costs. One rather subtle example is that benefit formulas and bend points have been recalculated in ways that cause each successive cohort to receive a smaller return on their contributions. Early retirees contributed for fewer years and at lower tax rates; more recent retirees have contributed for more years at higher FICA tax rates. Benefits are indexed to cost of living increases, but the overall benefit-to-contribution ratio has declined steadily and will continue to do so (Century Fund 1998).

A bolder move to cut costs by reducing benefits involved the elimination of the minimum benefit. Before 1982, Social Security had a minimum monthly retired worker benefit equal to $20 a month in 1940 and $110 a month before it was eliminated. Social Security still has a special minimum benefit, but relatively few older people qualify for it, and many receive amounts below this threshold. The elimination of the minimum benefit introduced an important source of gender and race inequality into Social Security. Restoration of a minimum, set near the federal poverty line, would significantly reduce poverty and inequality in old age (Harrington Meyer 1996; SSA 2002).

One of the most dramatic moves to sustain solvency of the Social

Security trust funds was to raise the age for full retirement. Beginning in 2003, the age of eligibility for full benefits gradually increases from 65 until the year 2027, when it will be 67. The age for early retirement remains age 62, but the penalty for taking early benefits, which most men and nearly all women take, has increased. Currently, those who take benefits before age 65 receive 20 percent less than their full benefit for the remainder of their lives; by 2022, they will receive 30 percent less (SSA 2002). Hardest hit are those who are unable to continue working due to poor health or unemployment. Women, blacks, and Hispanics are more likely to be affected by both (Moon and Herd 2002; Harrington Meyer 1996; Angel and Angel 1997).

Without a doubt, the biggest threat to Social Security looms just before us in the form of privatization. Conservative policymakers are determined to divert some funds into individual accounts that rise or fall based on individual investment decisions. The debate has taken many forms and has gone on for more than twenty years, but those opposed to universal benefits for elderly persons are trying to dismantle Social Security (Baker and Weisbrot 1999; Quadagno 1999b; Street and Wilmoth 2001). I argue that the reasons to uphold universal Social Security far outweigh any arguments for privatization. Social Security has a progressive benefit formula unmatched in the world of private pensions and impossible in the world of private investments. Social Security is highly efficient. The administrative costs of Social Security are less than 1 percent of the total budget, whereas the administrative costs for employer-based private pensions hover between 12 and 14 percent (Century Fund 1998). The estimated administrative costs of privatizing even small portions of Social Security range from 15 to 20 percent, perhaps higher, assuming consumers want sufficient oversight to prevent fraud, theft, and mismanagement (Baker and Weisbrot 1999). The current system spreads risk, whereas a privatized system will isolate risks related to economic and investment downturns.

Social Security has reduced poverty rates among elderly American dramatically, and supporters argue that without it, poverty rates will approach 50 percent (Harrington Meyer 1996; Quadagno 1999a). Solvency of the Social Security trust fund is a serious issue, but several analysts suggest a solution as simple as a 1.1 percent rise in the FICA tax as sufficient to help us ride the wave of baby boomers passing through old age. Some fear that a 1.1 percent rise in the tax might be burdensome, but more than twenty nations already have higher Social

Security taxes than the United States (Quinn 1997; Quadagno 1999b; Harrington Meyer and Herd 2001; Baker and Weisbrot 1999).

Supplemental Security Income

Supplemental Security Income (SSI) has provided monthly cash benefits to aged, blind, and disabled poor persons since it was created in 1972. Under federal guidelines, those who qualify for SSI receive enough benefits to raise their monthly incomes to roughly 77 percent of the federal poverty level. Many states provide supplemental benefits, but only a few provide enough of a supplement to meet the poverty line (Neuschler 1987; Harrington Meyer and Bellas 1995). Generally, SSI use is on the decline among elderly Americans. The proportion of elderly persons receiving SSI dropped from about 10 percent in 1975 to about 4 percent in 2001 (SSA 2002). Because women live longer and are more likely to be poor, nearly two-thirds of elderly SSI recipients are women (SSA 2002). Because of lifelong lower earnings and higher rates of chronic illness and disability, blacks are also more likely than whites to rely on SSI. Though they comprised only 8 percent of the elderly population in 2000, blacks accounted for 24 percent of SSI recipients ages 55 to 64, and 20 percent of SSI recipients age 65 and older (Himes 2001; SSA 2002).

SSI benefits have been indexed to cost of living increases since the implementation of the program and have risen steadily each year. In 2001, federal maximum benefits were $545 a month for a single person and $817 for an aged couple (SSA 2002). Maximum benefits are about 77 percent of the federal poverty line for single beneficiaries and 87 percent of the federal poverty line for older couples (Quadagno 1999a). States are permitted to supplement these benefits and many do, though few approach the federal poverty line. The size of the maximum benefit is somewhat moot, however, because most people do not receive the maximum. In 2001 the average monthly payments to single poor older people were just $307 and to couples $695 (SSA 2002). For 40 percent of SSI recipients, SSI is their only source of old age income. Among the 58 percent of older SSI recipients who also receive Social Security, the average SS benefits are fairly low, just $408 (SSA 2002).

As with most poverty-based programs, SSI is underused. Between 30 and 50 percent of those who are eligible do not apply because they are either unaware of the benefits, overwhelmed by the cumbersome eligibility forms, or too stigmatized to "endure the humiliating scrutiny of a means-test" (Quadagno 1999a, p. 83; Harrington Meyer and Bellas 1995). Because SSI is a poverty-based program, applicants must prove that they meet the income and asset tests, and their benefits can be garnished depending on living arrangements and other sources of income. Less than 2 percent of SSI recipients report earnings, in part because the earnings test is strict (SSA 2002). Unlike Social Security, SSI considers all earned and unearned income in calculating benefits. Under federal guidelines, the first $65 in earned income, along with an additional $20, is disregarded each month. Any additional earnings decrease benefits by $1 for every $2 earned. Assets, excluding a house, car, and burial funds under certain conditions, must be below $2000 for individuals and $3000 for couples. Additionally, SSI reduces payments by one-third if the recipient lives with someone, sharing food and shelter. The Social Security Administration (2002) reports that it does this rather than calculate the in-kind support and maintenance. Benefit reductions due to co-residence become increasingly problematic as people age and face declining income and health. SSI's modest income disregards have been in place since 1981; the asset maximums have been in place since 1989 (SSA 2002). Neither has been linked to cost of living, and neither can be raised except by congressional legislation. By failing to adjust the income disregard and the asset maximums for over twenty years of inflation, SSI has been retrenched more by default than by explicit policy changes. But the overall effect of many SSI policies in the last few decades is to disqualify many and to lower benefits for others.

Private Pensions

Receipt of a private pension greatly reduces the chances of being poor in old age, but employer-based pensions are on the wane (Harrington Meyer and Herd 2001). Among those aged 65 and older in 1992, private pensions accounted for only 10 percent of total income (Grad 1994). In 1994, 48 percent of older men, compared to only 30 percent of older women, had private pensions (National Economic Council 1998). Historically, the main determinants of pension coverage have included income, tenure, full-time status, and union membership (Evan and MacPherson 1998). But even in professions with high rates of pension coverage, women were less likely to be covered than men (DeVinney 1995). Recently, however, the gender gap in pension coverage has diminished—not because women's coverage is increasing, but because men's coverage is decreasing. Among men ages 21–36, 62 percent were covered in 1979, compared to only 49 percent in 1993. Among women of comparable ages, 46 percent were covered in 1979 and 48 percent in 1993 (Quadagno 1999a). Though younger women are now nearly as likely as men to be covered by private pension, their pension size is smaller. Women's private pensions average just 70 percent of men's (Hooyman and Gonyea 1995). Racial differences in pension coverage are persistent. In 1997, blacks earned on average 70 percent of what whites earned, and black men were two to three times more likely to be unemployed (U.S. Bureau of Census 1998). As a result, pension coverage and pension size are significantly less for blacks than for whites.

Even among those who do have pension coverage through their jobs, the very meaning of a private pension has changed. The shift from defined benefit to defined contribution plans has placed a great deal of the responsibility for employer-based private pensions onto individuals. Defined benefit plans paid a certain benefit when the worker reached a certain age. The cost of the benefits, including investment risks, fell with the employer. Defined contribution plans involve both employer and employee contributions to the old age pension, but the full weight of the investment risk falls on the individual. There is no guarantee that there will be a benefit there at all by the time the person reaches old age. The percentage of the workforce with defined benefit plans declined from 39 in 1975 to 26 in 1992. The percent with defined contribution rose from 14 to 37 percent (Quadagno 1999a). Increased reliance on IRAs and 401Ks means that employer contributions and responsibilities diminish, and individual contributions and responsibilities expand. With increased responsibility comes increased vulnerability. Those with a lifetime of sufficiently high wages and adequate investments can compensate for meager private pensions and unfortunate investments; those with a lifetime of relatively low wages generally have few savings and even fewer investments to draw on to compensate for inadequate private pensions.

Discussion

The cornerstone of exceptionalism in the U.S. welfare state is our stubborn insistence on the corporate or privatized provision of what might otherwise be social benefits. Our social experiment of relying on the market to provide social benefits has been in place for decades, and the evidence that it is failing has been accruing rapidly. Employee-based health insurance, employee-based retirement health insurance, supplemental health insurance, long-term care insurance, and most recently M+C are all on the decline. They provide the greatest benefits to those who need them least, and they do little to relieve gender, race, class, and other forms of socioeconomic inequality. Nonetheless, conservative policymakers plough ahead, creating a privatized drug coverage plan through Medicare Part D and lobbying for privatization of Social Security.

In many respects, retrenchment of the U.S. welfare state has been accomplished through benign neglect. Outdated rules and policies have simply not been revised to match changing demographic patterns. In other respects, retrenchment has been accomplished with a knife. Formulas, rules, and regulations have all been cut to restrict eligibility and curtail benefits. Resources have been shifted from elderly persons to private venues such as HMOs. There is no mystery about what the effects will be if we return to the individualistic and filial-based notions of the previous centuries. Those with ample resources will be fine; those without will not. Gone will be the welfare state safety nets and corporate benefits that millions of voters and workers demanded. Gone will be the mechanisms to spread the costs and risks of dependency across the entire population.

It is ironic that policymakers are retrenching and devolving even our universal programs at a time when the vast majority of Americans think we are doing too little for elderly persons. Between 70 and 90 percent of poll respondents report that they would be willing to pay higher taxes to keep universal old age benefits and that they favor universal health insurance for all (Century Fund 1998). It is not middle-class, working-class, or poor people in the United States who favor privatization or devolution or retrenchment. The proponents are generally conservatives, neoliberal policymakers, and think tank members who prioritize individual gain over the collective good.

While it is easy to point the finger at the conservative agenda that has prevailed through much of the past two decades, I find it more constructive to demand a liberal agenda that will (1) implement family-based policies that match family demographics in the twenty-first rather than the nineteenth century; (2) redistribute resources through universal programs in ways that constrain rather than escalate gender, race, and class inequality; and (3) spread the costs and risks of old age dependency across families rather than concentrating them within families. The welfare state represents a great opportunity to ameliorate inequalities—unless, of course, we dismantle it.

Acknowledgments

I appreciate the assistance and editorial advice of Pam Herd, Sara Smits, Janet Wilmoth, Emily Napier, and Christine Caffrey.

References

Abramovitz, M. 1988. *Regulating the Lives of Women: Social Welfare Policy from Colonial Times to the Present*. Boston: South End Press.

Alecxih, L. M. B., S. Lutzky, P. Sevak, and G. Claxton. 1997. *Key Issues Affecting Access to Medigap Insurance*. Washington, D.C.: Commonwealth Fund.

Angel, R. J., and J. L. Angel. 1997. *Who Will Care for Us? Aging and Long Term Care in Multicultural America*. New York: New York University Press.

Baker, D., and M. Weisbrot. 1999. *Social Security: The Phony Crisis*. Chicago: University of Chicago Press.

Baumgarten, M., R. N. Battista, C. Infante-Rivard, J. A. Hanley, R. Becker, and S. Gauthier. 1992. The psychological and physical health of family members caring for an elderly person with dementia. *Journal of Clinical Epidemiology* 45:61–70.

Bird, C. E. 1999. Gender, household labor, and psychological distress: The impact of the amount and division of housework. *Journal of Health and Social Behavior* 40:32–45.

Century Foundation. 1998. *Social Security Reform*. New York: Century Foundation.

Commonwealth Fund. 1999. *Informal Caregiving*. Washington, D.C.: The Commonwealth Fund.

DeVinney, S. 1995. Life course, private pension, and financial well-being. *American Behavioral Scientist* 39:172–85.

Employee Benefit Research Institute. 1994. *EBRI Issue Briefs*. Washington, D.C.: Employee Benefit Research Institute.

Estes, C. 1989. Aging, health and social policy: Crisis and crossroads. *Journal of Aging and Social Policy* 1:17–32.

Estes, C., and Associates. 2001. *Social Policy and Aging: A Critical Perspective*. Thousand Oaks, Calif.: Sage.

Evan, W. E., and D. A. MacPherson. 1998. Racial and ethnic differences in pension coverage and benefit levels. Working Paper Series Number 53. Tallahassee, Fla.: Pepper Institute on Aging and Public Policy.

Glazer, N. 1990. The home as workshop: Women as amateur nurses and medical care providers. *Gender and Society* 4:479–99.

Grad, S. 1994. Income of the Population 55 or Older, 1992. Publication No. 13-11871. Washington, D.C.: Social Security Administration, Office of Research and Statistics.

Harrington Meyer, M. 1996. Making claims as workers or wives: The distribution of Social Security benefits. *American Sociological Review* 61(3):449–65.

Harrington Meyer, M., ed. 2000. *Care Work: Gender, Labor, and the Welfare State.* New York: Routledge Press.

Harrington Meyer, M., and M. Bellas. 1995. U.S. old age policy and the family. Pp. 263–83 in *Handbook on Aging and the Family,* ed. V. Bedford and R. Blieszner. New York: Academic Press.

Harrington Meyer, M., and M. Kesterke-Storbakken. 2000. Shifting the burden back to families? How Medicaid cost-containment reshapes access to long-term care in the U.S. Pp. 217–28 in *Care Work: Gender, Labor and the Welfare State,* ed. M. Harrington Meyer. New York: Routledge Press.

Harrington Meyer, M., and P. Herd. 2001. Aging and aging policy in the U.S. Pp. 375–88 in J. Blau, ed., *Blackwell Companion to Sociology.* Oxford, UK: Blackwell Publishers.

Harrington Meyer, M., and E. Pavalko. 1996. Family, work, and access to health insurance among mature women. *Journal of Health and Social Behavior* 37 (December):311–25.

Herd, P., and M. Harrington Meyer. 2002. Carework: Invisible civic engagement. *Gender and Society* 16(5):665–88.

Himes, Christine L. 2001. "Elderly Americans." Population Bulletin 56, no 4. Washington, D.C.: Population Reference Bureau.

Hooyman, N., and J. Gonyea. 1995. *Feminist Perspectives on Family Care: Politics for Gender Justice.* Volume 6, Family Caregivers Application Series. Thousand Oaks, Calif.: Sage.

Hoyert, D. L., and M. M. Seltzer. 1992. Factors relating to well-being and life activities of family caregivers. *Family Relations* 41(1):74–81.

Kaiser Foundation. 2003a. "Dual Enrollees: Medicaid's Rose for Low-Income Medicare Beneficiaries." Washington, D.C.: Henry J. Kaiser Family Foundation

Kaiser Foundation. 2003b. Medicare Fact Sheet: Medicare+Choice. Washington, D.C.: Henry J. Kaiser Family Foundation.

Kaiser Foundation. 2004. "Prescription Drug Coverage for Medicare Beneficiaries." Washington, D.C.: Henry J. Kaiser Family Foundation.

Katz, M. 1986. *In the Shadow of the Poor House: A Social History of Welfare in America*. New York: Basic Books.

Koitz, D. 1996. *The Entitlement Debate*. Washington, D.C.: Congressional Research Service.

Korpi, W., and J. Palme. 1998. The paradox of redistribution and strategies of equality: Welfare state institutions, inequality, and poverty in the Western countries. *American Sociological Review* 63:661–87.

Margolis, R. 1990. *Risking Old Age in America*. Boulder, Colo.: Westview.

Marmor, T. 1970. *The Politics of Medicare*. New York: Aldine.

Moon, M., and P. Herd. 2002. *A Place at the Table: Women's Needs and Medicare Reform*. New York: The Century Foundation.

National Alliance for Caregiving. 1997. *Family Caregiving in the U.S.: Findings from a National Survey, Final Report*. Washington, D.C.: National Alliance for Caregiving and AARP.

National Economic Council. 1998. *Women and Retirement Security*. Washington, D.C.: NEC.

Neuschler, E. 1987. "Medicaid Eligibility for the Elderly in Need of Long Term Care." Contract No. 86-26. Washington, D.C.: National Governor's Association Congressional Research Service.

Ozawa, M. 1976. Income redistribution and Social Security. *Social Service Review* 50:209–23.

Palmer, H., and K. Dobson. 1994. Self-medication and memory in an elderly Canadian sample. *Gerontologist* 34:658–64.

Pavalko, E., and S. Woodbury. 2000. Social roles and process: Caregiving careers and women's health. *Journal of Health and Social Behavior* 41(2):91–105.

Post Standard. 2003. Medicare law helps HMOs before seniors. December 10, A8.

Quadagno, J. 1984. Welfare capitalism and the Social Security Act of 1935. *American Sociological Review* 49:632–47.

Quadagno, J. 1999a. *Aging and the Life Course*. New York: McGraw Hill College.

Quadagno, J. 1999b. Creating a capital investment welfare state: The new American exceptionalism. *American Sociological Review* 64:1–11.

Quinn, J. B. 1997. Social Security in better shape than many say. *Washington Post*, May 3, 1C.

Scharlach, A. 1994. Caregiving and employment: Competing or complementary roles. *Gerontologist* 34:378–85.

Seccombe, K., and C. Amey. 1995. Playing by the rules and losing: Health insurance and the working poor. *Journal of Health and Social Behavior* 36:168–81.

Social Security Administration. 2002. *Annual Statistical Supplement to the Social Security Bulletin.* Washington, D.C.: Social Security Administration.

Stephens, M. A. P., and M. M. Franks. 1995. Spillover between daughter's roles as caregiver and wife: Interference or enhancement? *Journal of Gerontology Series B: Psychological Sciences and Social Sciences* 50: B9–17.

Street, D., and J. Wilmoth. 2001. Social insecurity? Women and pensions in the U.S. Pp. 120–41 in *Women, Work and Pensions,* ed. J. Ginn, D. Street, and S. Arber. Philadelphia: Open University Press.

U.S. Bureau of the Census. 1998. Poverty in the United States, 1997. *Current Population Reports.* Series P60-201. Washington, D.C.: Government Printing Office.

U.S. General Accounting Office. 2001. "Retiree Health Benefits: Employer-Sponsored Benefits May be Vulnerable to Further Erosion." Publication GAO-01-374. Washington, D.C.: U.S. GAO.

U.S. Health Care Financing Administration. 1998. *A Profile of Medicare: Chart Book, 1998.* Washington, D.C.: Government Printing Office.

U.S. House Committee on Ways and Means. 2000. *The Green Book.* Washington, D.C.

Wallace, S., L. Levy-Storms, R. Kington and R. Andersen. 1998. The persistence of race and ethnicity in the use of long-term care. *Journal of Gerontology: Social Sciences* 53B:S104–12.

Walzer, M. 1988. Socializing the welfare state. Pp. 13–26 in *Democracy and the Welfare State,* ed. Amy Gutmann. Princeton, N.J.: Princeton University Press.

Ward, D. 1990. Gender, time and money in caregiving. *Scholarly Inquiry for Nursing Practice.* 4:223–39.

Waxman, J. 1992. Testimony before the Joint Hearing of the Select Committee on Aging and the Congressional Black Caucus. U.S. House of Representatives. 102nd Congress, First session, September 13, 1991. Aging Commission, Publication No. 102-846. Washington, D.C.: Government Printing Office.

5. Social Security and the Paradoxes of Welfare State Conservatism

Steven M. Teles

At times an unbridgeable gap seems to separate the policy sciences from the practical world of politics. Politicians complain that policy analysis is not "useful" to them, and policy analysts lament what they see as politicians' ignorance of even the most rudimentary analytical principles. This gap is not simply a matter of willful obscurity on the one side or policy illiteracy on the other. Rather, it reflects a conscious choice of policy experts to eschew political and institutional analysis in favor of a more pure science of policy.

The costs of this choice can be seen most clearly when analyzing the largest U.S. social-welfare program—Social Security. Critics of social insurance make arguments that are by now commonplace; their techniques of analysis are almost always dependent on an accepted, but morally and politically suspect, set of assumptions. Moreover, these assumptions are radically utopian and thus are a dangerous foundation for reasoning about social institutions like the modern welfare state, which are deeply embedded in social life. I will lay out, in the context of a discussion of pensions, a way of approaching welfare-state questions that differs from modern libertarian arguments and also from the "progressive" arguments that have dominated welfare-statist approaches up to the present.

My argument is that one of the outcomes of public policy is the politics it creates. Policies are more than mechanisms for the solving of problems. They are also contexts in which future policy battles will be fought. Put another way, policies do not simply operate *within* a context—after they are implemented, they *are* the context. If this is true, it is impossible to design policies rationally without taking politics into account. If the outcomes of public policies are both their effects on clients *and* on the character of public debate and institutional development, then the artificial academic division of labor between "policy analysis" and "policy process" must be collapsed.

Politics and Policy Analysis

What is the relationship between politics and policy analysis? Policy analysts are not "philosopher kings," handing down perfect policies to a waiting world; in fact, politicians regularly ignore our recommendations. One approach is for analysts simply to ignore the world of politics, to hide behind the mask of science. Isn't it our job to discover the truth, and if the world ignores it, so much the worse for the world? This solution is far less rare than my (admittedly cartoonish) description might suggest. But policy analysts are *not* basic scientists: our job is to make recommendations, and the very act of recommending requires that those being advised be taken into account.

A second approach would view the political world as a series of obstacles to best practice. That is, policy analysts should start out by determining "the truth," but then account for the need to have their proposal passed by real legislators and administered by real bureaucrats. The job of the policy analyst, in this model, is to discover how to shape policies that are attractive to legislators, while ensuring that they are not warped by the bureaucrats in charge of implementation.

This approach is an enormous improvement over the first, but there is still something unsettling about it. It makes the critical assumption that the relationship between policy analysis and politics is one in which all reason flows in a single direction, from those with "knowledge" to those with "power," from what "ought to be" to what "is." In a nontrivial set of cases, however, those with power have information that those who claim to have knowledge should pay heed to, and what "is" is at least as trusty a guide to what "ought to be" as arguments based on abstractions. In these cases, policy analysis that reasons backwards from what is to what should be is superior to its opposite.

The Problem with Abstract Reason

Typically, policy analysts compare existing policies with an abstract ideal and then make recommendations to implement the ideal. The problems with this should be obvious but usually aren't. We know a great deal about existing policies. Their very existence allows us to discover how they work in a complex world and influence those in charge of their continued existence. Experience can tell us relatively accurately how a policy exists *in time*. About ideal policies, however, we can have much less certain knowledge. In the ideal, policies are carried out as the analyst suggests, are supported politically as he wishes, and are not deformed or diminished over time. In the real world, of course, this is not the case.

Clearly, there are times when reasoning from first principles to policy recommendations is unavoidable, as when there is no tradition or "existing practice" on which to draw, or when existing practice is manifestly unacceptable. To argue otherwise would be to counsel inaction in the face of pressing need. But the more common situation is one of tolerably sufficient existing policies. In these cases, the first instinct of the policy analyst should be to reason backward from existing practice to policy recommendations.

The first question of the policy analyst in this mode is, "Is this program adequately supported?" That is, is it capable of sustaining its legitimacy, garnering enough resources, and generating sufficient consent from society to perpetuate itself? Second, does the program generate any clearly pathological consequences? Before asking whether it does much good, therefore, the policy analyst should ask whether it does any harm. Third, does the program adequately serve at least some of the multiple tasks expected of it? In many cases, the answer to these questions would be yes or, "sure, for the most part." In these cases, the existing policy should be the starting point. One should ask how to improve it at the margins, operating within its own assumptions, rather than judging it from the outside. Piecemeal reform would make sense, since radical surgery on its faults would very likely disable what it does well, and so do more harm than good.

The obvious criticism of this approach is that it is conservative. Quite so. But this is not to say that policy analysts should just pack their bags and go home—that all is for the best in the best of all possible worlds. Far from it. The critical question is where policy analysis starts from. And true, the problems inherent in starting from abstract reason were once well understood, especially by conservatives. Earlier, it was the Left that lost itself in utopian policymaking, but today it is conservatives who are most likely to push for grand, abstract schemes. The disjuncture between the real and the ideal now weighs more heavily on those who would "privatize" or radically reform the welfare state than on those who would defend it.

Ideal Policy and Pensions

Too often analysts comfortable with a "political" approach to policy analysis demonstrate the dangers of abstract reason by criticizing policy positions they oppose; the position critiqued typically becomes little more than an easily dismissed straw man. Instead of a straw man, I will use my own ideal policy preference to illustrate the political approach to policy analysis, showing how my own "abstract" preference for pensions policy should generally be disregarded, or at the very most applied differently, depending on national context.

Were I in an abstract, apolitical mode of analysis, my preference would be for a pensions policy with a flat "first tier" set at a reasonably generous percentage of average wages (say 30 percent) and funded from general revenue. In my view, a flat first tier is preferable to a means-tested system in that it minimally distorts savings behavior. It is also preferable to an earnings-related system for two principled reasons, one egalitarian and the other libertarian. The egalitarian reason is that given the same revenue, a flat-rate system is by definition more redistributive. The libertarian reason is that I view the provision of pensions beyond the poverty line as impinging on a function that is properly private: there is no reason for governments to hold a large portion of retirement savings when other forms of collective provision are possible. My reasons for preferring general revenue as to wage-based contributions are simple: wage-based revenue sources discourage hiring, promote off-the-books employment, and are highly regressive.[1] That is, they necessarily harm the welfare of those most in need.

Most advanced industrialized countries have at least two tiers of pensions. In the United States, the first tier (Social Security) is income-related and modestly redistributive, while in Britain, the first tier is made up of the Basic Pension (flat) and means-tested assistance. Both countries have a second tier as well. In the United States, this second tier takes the form of voluntary but highly regulated and subsidized company pensions, IRAs, 401(k)s, and other devices. In Great Britain, the second tier is mandatory and consists either of the state earnings-related pension (SERPS) or the "opted-out" company or personal pensions.

Advocates of Social Security privatization essentially wish to collapse the first tier into the second by turning Social Security into a form of mandatory private savings. On the other hand, many pension analysts, concerned with low levels of national savings and the unwillingness of workers to put aside enough for retirement, counsel expanding the second tier through mandates and increased incentives while not materially changing the first.

My ideal pensions policy would go in neither of these directions. Any form of compulsory private savings necessarily pulls the government into a very close—and illiberal—relation with private finance. By requiring private savings, the government pursues essentially public goals through the use of private instruments. This "public use of private markets" has been voguish for at least two decades now, and yet the concept is deeply problematic. First, partnership and regulation go hand in hand: the more private markets are depended on to pursue public functions, the more they must be actively reshaped in the image of their regulators. On the other side, such "partnerships" mean that the state enters into a dependent relationship with private actors, with the significant risk that it will be forced into a "boosterism" rather than a "referee" role vis-à-vis private actors. More classically republican analysts would call this corruption. Of even greater danger, the more the line between what is "state" and what is "private" erodes, the greater the political incentives for blame-shifting and evasion of responsibility, undermining effective democratic governance.

Finally, there seems to me no reason for any publicly recognized second tier. In a liberal society, whether people do or do not save for their retirement should be up to the individual. Flat-pension systems make a retirement without poverty available to all but make any greater comfort the result of individual or voluntary collective action. It seems hard to square any more expansive state role with even my own very activist form of liberalism.

The Beveridge Plan

So much for my account of the "ideal" pension scheme. The rest of this essay will be devoted to demonstrating why my ideal is fraught with political flaws and would tend, over the long term, to serve its own ends less well than alternative schemes that start from a much different point.

My ideal is, in fact, quite close to the original Beveridgian model that undergirded the postwar reconstruction of the British welfare state. Beveridge wanted to base the welfare state on a model of flat, "subsistence" pensions because, on the whole, he was a liberal (Harris 1994, pp. 30–31). He wanted simultaneously to relieve need and to encourage self-reliance and voluntary, unplanned cooperative action among citizens. Looking back, however, it becomes clear that his model for old age pensions was inherently unstable. The basic flat-rate pension he developed was incapable of generating sufficient political support to keep it high enough to alleviate poverty, and eventually it was overtaken by means-tested benefits. In Britain today, because the threshold for means-tested benefits is above the flat-rate pension, for those with very low income the basic pension is purely notional: they live in a world of means-tested benefits. What is more, the basic pension was unable to maintain itself at a high enough level to forestall the creation of a state-run earnings-related pension on top of it, albeit one that (because of the development of private pensions) has been reserved mainly for the poorest workers. The consequence is that a system designed primarily to avoid means-testing is, in fact, dominated by it.

Beveridge hoped that his flat-rate benefits would provide a sturdy foundation for British citizens to develop their own self-managed and self-owned systems of private insurance. This was a critical assumption, for the chief virtue of his liberalism was self-reliance. Individuals learned to be citizens by making the major decisions of their lives. It was this sort of private sector, not one dominated by insurance companies, that Beveridge wanted to encourage. However, in practice, what Britain ended up with was quite different: friendly societies managed by workers themselves withered; insurance companies and large pension firms grew; and the room Beveridge left for private effort was filled by interests that delayed implementation of an income-related second pension, which would have at least preserved contributory principles, until the 1970s. What is more, the susceptibility of the basic pension to low-visibility cuts has created substantial pressures to regulate private pensions, a decision that has led, paradoxically, to a massive expansion of government control (Fawcett 1996). In short, my "ideal" has decomposed, in the not idiosyncratic laboratory of Great Britain, into its opposite.

What of the United States? From the perspective of my "ideal" pension policy, there is much to dislike about the U.S. pension system. It imposes a very high payroll tax, the revenue from which is used both for redistribution and income replacement. The United States subsidizes and regulates private pensions fairly substantially, thus potentially creating serious problems from the interweaving (and thereby blurring) of public and private.

The great difference between the British and U.S. systems, over time, turns out to be not their initial differences but their contrary political trajectories. The British system evolved away from its original conception into a much less desirable one. Moreover, it has become increasingly unpopular and unstable, leading to recurrent waves of "reform," few of which have stuck. The U.S. system, on the other hand, has evolved toward a greater concern with "adequacy" (redistribution) and a diminished concern for "equity" (the relationship between contributions and benefits), in part because the presence of some equity functions provided political cover for an increasing focus on adequacy. What is more, the relatively strong income-related nature of Social Security has meant that no party has seen the need to create a mandatory second tier, keeping all government interference in private markets limited to voluntary encouragement and oversight.

In short, the U.S. system serves more of the functions that the British system intended, in part because it pursued those goals indirectly. In retrospect, Beveridge's approach was too pure, too principled, one might say, and this purity of principle has led to an inferior outcome.

United States versus Britain

The core (and probably by now rather tired) claim of the politics of policy analysis field is that "policy makes politics"—that policies contain within themselves "rules of the game," incentives or disincentives for political organization, self-defensive mechanisms, and so on. To discover why the "ideal" pension policy devolved into something altogether unsatisfying, while a pension policy less than ideal evolved into something quite satisfactory, we need to examine the political pitfalls of the Beveridgian structure.

The primary reason for the sustainability of the U.S. system and the collapse of the British system is, to use political scientist Paul Pierson's useful terminology, the comparative policy "lock-in" of the two systems (1994). Income-related pension systems accompanied by "trustfunds" that must maintain actuarial balance tend to generate popular feelings of entitlement. In addition, they create substantial "transition costs" in order to move to another, "funded" alternative. This means that once they have been in operation for a substantial period, it is almost impossible to renegotiate the fundamentals of the policy. Moreover, policies like Social Security are inherently expansive, since funding problems can most easily be solved by extending the policy to new groups rather than cutting back benefits or fundamentally restructuring. Flat pensions without trust funds do not have these benefits and are therefore more susceptible to benefit reduction or fundamental renegotiation.

Even more basically, there are reasons to think that any pensions policy that leans too heavily on either the equity or the adequacy side is likely to be renegotiated in the future. Heavily insurance-based systems tend over time gradually to incorporate greater redistributive components, while more redistributive systems seem gradually to incorporate more insurance-like elements. So classically Bismarckian systems like Germany and the United States have slowly changed in a more redistributive direction, while more egalitarian systems like Sweden, Australia, and Britain have added an earnings-related tier.

This inherent tendency toward a blending of functions drives economists and public-choice analysts crazy. By definition, no single system can optimize on both equity and adequacy. As a result, it is easy to demonstrate that hybrid systems are insufficiently redistributive or fail to generate as high a "rate of return" as private market instruments. But such analysis fails to grapple with the political imperative of hybridity. Failing to accept this imperative, the analysts risks his recommendations morphing into something he cannot control and would never approve of. Simply as a matter of professional ethics, the policy analyst needs to hold himself responsible for the actual consequences of his recommendations, not merely what he intended. If this is the case, the "political" approach to policy analysis becomes unavoidable.

Reforming Social Security

Given that public pensions already exist, policy analysis must begin with the question: "Is there something here worth conserving?" This is followed by: "What are the dangers associated with policy alternatives?" As the political approach to policy analysis would predict, asking these two questions first leads to very different policy recommendations for the United States and Britain.

The reform of state pensions is at the top of the policy agenda in both countries, but for very different reasons. In the United States, the issue has been driven, not by any structural flaw in the program, but by the likelihood that its current tax rate will be insufficient to cover its future liabilities. A few aspects of this problem deserve mention. First, the problem is forward-looking, in the sense that it is driven by problems that analysts believe will occur in the future, rather than by tangible problems in the present. Second, it is speculative, driven by calculations about the future that may or may not be correct. These two facts violate most of what political scientists believe about the U.S. political system, namely, that it is shortsighted and incapable of planning. As Eric Patashnik (2000) observes, due to the peculiarities of trust-fund financing, the politics of pensions in the United States is perhaps more forward-looking than in any other advanced industrial country.

The "crisis" that Social Security advocates decry threatens to overshadow the program's many successes. Whatever its flaws—and some of these were suggested earlier—Social Security provides reasonable retirement security to nearly all Americans. Old age retirement is now a small-scale problem in the United States, and few older Americans are forced to rely on means-tested assistance. Furthermore, Social Security is politically stable. Despite recent attacks and the prediction that it will "go bust," Social Security has never missed a payment and has maintained its benefit level and the political coalition that sustains them. The arguments against it, therefore, are premised on claims that some other system would be even better or that the system cannot maintain itself in the future. What opponents cannot claim is that Social Security has not pursued a defensible goal with tolerable success, the standard I defended earlier.

This is not to say that no changes in Social Security are advisable. Clearly, it is worth reining in somewhat the level of benefits, especially for higher earners. In addition, it may be worth adding a new tier of retirement savings on top of, but not completely independent from, Social Security, in the form of individual accounts.[2] But these changes are incremental, and the critical reason for making only incremental changes has to do with the "transition costs" of moving to a different system.

In the Social Security debate, the concept of "transition costs" typically refers to only the program's unfunded liabilities, which must be paid off in order to move to a funded system of pensions. One generation will pay taxes twice: once to pay off the old system and then again to build up their own pensions.[3] Thinking of transition costs in this way is excessively rationalistic. It suggests that all of the costs of moving from the current system to another one can be accounted for. But when we use the concept in a more political sense, the costs of transition appear significantly higher.

First and most important, Social Security is deeply embedded in the structure of American society. Company pensions assume the presence of Social Security, as do individual investors. Individuals are able to be riskier in their private savings because Social Security provides them a safety-net that they could not purchase in the open market. Furthermore, the presence of Social Security has removed the need for large numbers of Americans to invest for their own retirement at all, thereby reducing the transaction costs and the worry associated with private investment.[4] More broadly, the relations between old and young, and between men and women, have been dramatically altered by Social Security. It is impossible to predict how they would be changed by the various privatization proposals.

Even more critically, the advocates of structural reform in Social Security, whether liberal or conservative, tend to underestimate the political uncertainties that accompany their proposals. On the left, many "defenders" of Social Security have proposed investing part of the surplus in equities so as to increase the "return" on payroll taxes. There is a perfectly good economic argument against this: Social Security is a government program, and any of its funds that do not purchase government debt must be replaced by other taxes that will. If other taxes are not raised, the government is simply borrowing to purchase equities—in other words, buying on leverage. This is nothing more than a dangerous shell game, since it would put the government in the position of raising revenue, not through taxation, but through owning—literally—the means of production. The argument that "states own stocks for their employees' retirement systems, so why shouldn't Social Security" is difficult to take seriously. There is an enormous difference between the government purchasing stocks in its position as an employer for its employees' retirement and doing so as part of a universal social program.

The main argument against such an approach, however, is that it makes an enormous political gamble for less than compelling reasons. No one knows how turning the federal government into a major shareholder of every company in the United States would change American politics. Since every cost the government imposed on business would show up on its books not just in foregone tax revenue but also in lower stock prices, it could have a powerfully conservative influence. Literally no decision—from regulating tobacco companies and HMOs to changing corporate taxation and capital gains—could be made without regard to the government's ownership role in the affected companies. Those who doubt this should take note of how the states, once sworn enemies of "big tobacco," now seek to shield it from further litigation, since their settlement money is contingent on the companies' continuing viability. Introducing such a relationship in Social Security would be a strange outcome for a policy pushed by liberals.

Having the government own a large share of equities would also make stock market fluctuations even more of a political issue than they are now. Fluctuations in stock prices would impinge directly on government budgets (as opposed to indirectly through capital gains and other taxes), creating even greater pressure for measures such as the "collars" inadvisably put on stock markets after the 1987 crash.

Privatization, favored by conservatives, would face similar political problems. The pressure to reduce stock market fluctuations would be even more severe under privatization than if the government invested the surplus in equities, since fluctuations would directly affect the resources individuals would have in their private accounts on retirement. The decision to retire just a few weeks sooner or later could mean a substantial difference in retirement income for two individuals with similar earnings. The obvious equity problem this raises would create pressure to "do something" about the necessary ups and downs of the market. What is more, privatization would mean that stock market investing would no longer be a voluntary decision. In attempting to develop a more "libertarian" system of social insurance, conservatives would actually be empowering government, granting it a wholly novel authority to coerce private investment. This would, in all likelihood, substantially alter the nature of financial regulation in the United States, forcing regulators to assume much lower levels of investor sophistication, leading to the possibility of more prescriptive (as opposed to disclosure-based) regulation.

Finally, splitting up the insurance and redistributive aspects of Social Security, as all privatization programs must, may lead to programmatic instability. Advocates of privatization can promise that their system will lead to even more redistribution than Social Security; but it is impossible to know whether, once the functions have been divided and exposed, the political coalition in support of redistribution will hold. The experience from the United Kingdom is mixed, but it suggests that levels of support for the poorest elderly persons will fall and that the system will become predominantly means-tested over time. So even if some form of privatization is the best policy, political considerations may render it worse than the current program.

The foregoing surely reads like an unrealistic premonition of doom. And it well may be. The government will find ways of adapting to the problems that I have predicted, as will individuals themselves. But at what cost? Who is to say that my list is exhaustive? It is literally impossible for any analyst to specify the consequences of major change to such a deeply embedded social institution.

Reforming the British System

The British case presents a different set of problems. The value of both the basic pension (which is flat-rate) and SERPS (which is income-related) has fallen and will continue to do so in the future, even by the current government's estimation. Taken together, the Basic Pension and SERPS will decline from 35 percent of national average income in 2003 to 28 percent in 2025 (Pensions Policy Institute 2003, p. 27). As a consequence, increasing numbers of older Britons are being pushed onto means-tested assistance, while a majority of Britons have "opted out" of SERPS and now expect to receive the great majority of their retirement income from a private (either individual or company) pension. Most middle-class individuals barely consider themselves part of the state pension system, and there seems to be little support for returning to more generous state benefits.

Moreover, the current system of private pensions, because it is still linked (through opting out) to the state system, is incredibly complex. Individuals have to make decisions between SERPS, company pensions, personal pensions, and the recently introduced "stakeholder pension." The results of this complexity are very high transaction and marketing costs, and a recent scandal that severely damaged the reputation of the pensions industry.[5] Pensions have been reformed over and over again since the early 1980s. None of the reforms seems to have cut into the system's simultaneous failure to provide for the poorest pensioners while still baffling those opting for the private sector.

Even by the fairly high hurdle laid out earlier in this chapter, the British system is sufficiently troubled to justify the turmoil that would accompany root-and-branch reform. Constructing an income-related system of social insurance along the lines of the United States is not in the cards. It is simply too far from the existing consensus. Any reform that is to get a serious hearing will build on some form of individual account. The critical questions are: How do you structure a privatized system that generates sufficient redistribution while not collapsing into widespread means-testing? And next, how do you introduce pension instruments that generate policy lock-in, so that individuals and institutions can establish reasonable expectations about the future?

Privatized systems hold two great dangers: first, redistribution becomes more difficult to maintain over time; and second, the financial system becomes socialized as much as the welfare state becomes privatized. That is, the main concerns have to do with the unintended political consequences of reform. As I suggested earlier, the problems are sufficiently severe to risk these consequences as well as others that an analyst cannot predict. But there are ways in which these dangers might be minimized.

The redistribution problem might be tackled by obfuscating the link between taxes and contributions in privatized accounts. By paying for the entire pension system through general taxation, the government could contribute to private accounts in a more egalitarian manner than if the revenue were raised by payroll taxes. Unfortunately, this would mean that all contributions had to flow through the government accounts, and one of the main motivations for privatization (among New Labour supporters, at least) is to get pensions off the government's accounts. This means that there are few alternatives to a system of mandatory private (and off the government's books) savings with a government "top up" or subsidy for those with low earnings. In such a case, it makes more sense to have the government top-up low-wage earners' pensions year by year rather than at the end of their working lives, even if this would involve the same level of redistribution. The former system would make redistribution more difficult to retract than under the latter system, when the amount of the "top up" could be changed any time and all at once.

The other problem is that coerced private investment inevitably leads to a shift in the structure of government financial regulation. Suffice it to say that privatization of the welfare state usually translates into the partial socialization of private markets, since the latter are now being used for public purposes. How is it possible to avoid excessive entanglement? The British government should set up the equivalent of the American Federal Employee Retirement System (FERS) of private, indexed accounts centrally administered by the government (off the books), which could be used by workers for their retirement account. Those who wished could pick alternatives to the centralized system, although few who understood the system would. Since anyone would have the option of using the government-organized system, pressure to regulate private providers would be limited.[6]

Ultimately, what will determine the success or failure of changes in the British pension system will be their degree of irreversibility, which is a political, not a technical, problem. How one can do so within a privatized system is a question of the first order for policy analysts, but also one difficult to raise within the current policy paradigm.

Democracy versus Welfare-state Conservatism

I have argued up to now that if it is true that "policy creates politics," then politics must be part of policy analysis. Politics is not merely a matter of how to "sell" one's preferred policies. Rather, it must be a major criterion in the shaping of policy itself. Policy analysts would not hesitate to shape their policies to reflect the likely behavior of clients; not to do so would be tantamount to professional misconduct or at least incompetence. But policies also create feedback from political institutions and policymakers. They either create the conditions necessary for policy resilience and expansion or render policies politically weak and in danger of contraction. Such feedback would affect whether the design of policies was, in fact, in the interests of the clients they serve.

If the maintenance of political support and the maximization of policy goals always pointed in the same direction, analysts would not have to consider political variables. But public policy typically involves tragic choices. The best policy in programmatic terms may be unsustainable in political terms. In other words, the real outcome of the best policy may be worse, after it has been processed through political institutions, than would be the second best if the second best were more likely to generate politically protective mechanisms. Where this is the case, the policy analyst must, as a matter of professional duty, recommend the second best.

But there is a further complication. So far I have argued that although political considerations must be taken into account, the ultimate goal is the clients' welfare. We move to the second-best, not because we care about politics per se, but because we care about the clients themselves. Such an approach, however, is incomplete.

As I argued regarding Social Security, concern for the welfare of older citizens requires that we adopt the second-best policy of social insurance, as opposed to the first-best policy of flat-rate pensions paid out of general revenue. But such a policy has costs, not so much to the consumers of the policy but to the political system itself. The second-best works because it generates mechanisms that make it very hard to change the policy substantially after it has been put in place. It protects the interests of older Americans by, in effect, closing off the possibility for politicians to rethink the policy. This is what we mean when we call Social Security the "third rail" in American politics. Social Security works primarily by deflecting discussion away from the policy's core and toward peripheral or system-maintenance concerns.

Such a policy is not good for politics conceived as an end unto itself. Recently, "deliberation" has become a voguish concern among American liberals, an antidote to what is taken to be the ossified, bureaucratized, and technocratic character of the politics of social policy. But what must be given up to make such deliberation possible? Deliberation is typically taken to be the outcome of particular institutional forms, but rarely is it suggested that policies themselves may either facilitate or close off deliberation. If deliberation is taken to be an end unto itself, the possibility that social policies themselves may be antideliberative should be of the gravest concern. But the liberal advocates of a more deliberative politics barely mention this possibility.

The reason is that what makes the social policies favored by liberals viable is precisely their antideliberative aspect. In particular, it is Social Security's great success at closing off or at least limiting debate that has made it the most stable element of the American welfare state. To enhance deliberation would mean shaping policies such that they could be reconsidered. But reconsideration is the last thing liberal defenders of Social Security (or any other major element of the welfare state) would want.

I close, therefore, on a dour note, or at least a point of paradox. To incorporate political variables into the consideration of social policies is necessary if we wish to ensure those policies' success, but to do so may be at the expense of politics taken as an end unto itself. The "welfare state conservatism" I have defended and democratic accountability are, necessarily, in tension. The choice between these two is itself inherently political, not subject to any technical calculus. To choose requires a consideration of the fundamental ends of the polity and thus a turn to the basic questions of political philosophy. This requires a political education that, sadly, most policy analysts lack. More fundamentally, it requires that policy analysts recognize that their work is not an alternative to, but an extension of, the political enterprise.

Notes

An earlier version of this chapter appeared in *The Public Interest*. Previously published material is reprinted with permission. Copyright, *The Public Interest*, No. 141, Fall 2000, Washington, D.C.

1. There are technical economic reasons why these patterns may not apply further up the wage scale, but these are beyond the scope of this chapter.

2. I must admit my strong disagreement with such a policy, however. It seems unlikely that such a policy would increase retirement savings. Its more likely effect would be simply to divert funds that would be saved in some other way into the new accounts. Its only effect would be on those who are not currently saving, and for these individuals (who tend to be poorer) it would be tantamount to a new tax on labor.

3. It may be possible to spread these liabilities more widely through longer-term debt mechanisms or through consumption taxes (which would hit current elderly persons, who have a high propensity to consume relative to young workers).

4. Conservatives typically argue that government should take into account individual and corporate compliance costs when judging the value of regulations or the tax system. The off-the-books cost of educating oneself in the financial market—which cannot be seen as a collateral benefit, since there is no intrinsic value to knowing the merits of different mutual funds— clearly have to be counted as losses.

5. For details, see Steven Teles, "Pensions, Social Citizenship and the Ubiquity of the State: The Relevance of the British Privatization Experience in the United States and Beyond," unpublished manuscript.

6. A more detailed description of such a plan and its justification can be found in S. Teles and P. Agulnik, "How to Fund a Happier Retirement," *New Statesman,* 12 February 1999.

References

Fawcett, H. 1996. The Beveridge strait-jacket: Policy formation and the problem of poverty in old age. Pp. 20–42 in M. Kandiah and A. Seldon, eds., *Ideas and Think Tanks in Contemporary Britain*. London: Frank Cass.

Harris, J. 1994. Beveridge's social and political thought. In J. Hills, J. Ditch, and H. Glennerster, eds., *Beveridge and Social Security: An International Retrospective*. Oxford: Clarendon Press.

Patashnik, E. 2000. *Putting Trust in the US Budget: Federal Trust Funds and the Politics of Commitment*. Cambridge: Cambridge University Press.

Pensions Policy Institute. 2003, February. The pensions landscape, p. 27. www.pensionspolicyinstitute.org.uk/uploadeddocuments/PPI-_14_Feb_03-_The_Pensions_Landscape.pdf

Pierson, P. 1994. *Dismantling the Welfare State?* Cambridge: Cambridge University Press.

II. Age-Based Policy
and Population Dynamics

6. When Old Age Begins
Implications for Health, Work, and Retirement
Angela M. O'Rand

Life expectancy at birth in the United States increased more than 60 percent over the twentieth century, from 47 years in 1900 to approximately 77 years in 2000 (Himes 2001). Even more dramatic has been the more recent growth of the population aged 85 and older (referred to as the "oldest old" since 1984). The ascendance of the oldest age category is attributed to reduced morbidity and mortality at younger ages, although the oldest subgroup is characterized by the highest prevalence of morbidity, disability, and institutionalization. Thus, besides increased life expectancy, the extension of "active life expectancy"—defined as the expanding portion of the disability-free life span—appears to be rescheduling the *average* onset of disabled old age to later ages. As such, the traditional categorization of the aged population as 65 and older is arbitrary and, at best, now obsolete.

Arguably, the 65 and older category has always been arbitrary and defined more by historically anchored institutional (Social Security and Medicare) schedules than by demographic factors related to health, productivity, and wealth. The age 65 threshold is blind to health and economic disparities in the population that can begin earlier in the life course and lead to highly variable active life expectancies within older cohorts. As such, the institutional designation of *any* age as a new threshold to old age would also ignore variability in the onset of disability, frailty, and health decline at younger ages across subgroups of the population and the relationship of this variability to economic inequality. Moreover, attaching the designation of old age to the onset of disability at *any* age may ignore the capacities of individuals to "manage disability" with the assistance of medical resources and insurance support systems.

Hence, the answer to the question of when old age begins tends to move away from exclusive and universal chronological designations and toward demographic and socioeconomic criteria, which are gauged, respectively, by two defining sets of interdependent parameters in aging cohorts: (1) relative functional capacities and vulnerabilities to health risks, and (2) relative economic status and vulnerabilities to economic risks, across a wide range of ages. The linkage of these two sets of factors underlies the variability in when old age begins in the population, making universal chronological criteria arbitrary. This chapter addresses the question of when old age begins by focusing on life course variability in the process of aging and the lifelong impact of interdependent health and economic disparities on the aging process. State and market policies bear on these outcomes throughout the life course. Recent policy proposals, which call for increased privatization and individualization of employment and health insurance risks, provide both promise and threat to the well-being of diverse aging cohorts in the U.S. population who follow highly variable life course trajectories.

Time to Disability or Death

Chronological age has provided a convenient standard for state policymaking for more than a century. Actuarial estimates of average life expectancy (mean age of mortality) have driven assumptions underlying age-related policies. Meanwhile, compulsory years of schooling until an assigned age and the ages of early or normal retirement (Social Security) or social health insurance (Medicare) eligibility are the two most obvious and pervasive sets of age-dependent policies in the United States. And indeed, these policies institutionalized the life course over the last half of the twentieth century, regulating the average timing of transitions from youth to adulthood and from adulthood to old age in light of average life expectancies.

A significant share of the increase in life expectancy over the past century has occurred for those reaching the age of 65, who at this time can expect to live an average of 18 more years in the white population and a little more than 16 more years in the black population. Those from both groups who reach age 85 can expect to live an average of more than 6 additional years (Federal Interagency Forum on Aging-Related Statistics 2003), and in the 2000 U.S. Census, approximately 50,000 were reported as centenarians.

These trends have sparked debates in the demographic and actuarial literatures regarding longevity, or the upper limits of the duration of life. Some argue that real longevity is rising and that recent reductions in mortality reflect a "stream of continuing progress" over the century, stemming from advances in nutrition, sanitation, education, income, health, and related factors (e.g., Oeppen and Vaupel 2002, p. 1029). Cases of extreme longevity evident in the surge of centenarians across societies fuel this argument (e.g., Vallin and Mesle 2001).

Alternatively, critics of this position raise two distinct sets of counterarguments. One is principally methodological and challenges conventional measures of life expectancy that overestimate how long we live. For example, Bongaarts and Feeney (2002) argue that when the average age at death is rising, conventional calculations of life expectancy at birth tend to overestimate life expectancy as a result of a "tempo effect" (when calculations of minor fluctuations in mean age at death lead to larger fluctuations in life expectancy). The second set of arguments advocates instead a fixed limit to the life span and a "compression of morbidity"—a postponement and shorter duration of disability before death (e.g., Fries 2002). The National Long Term Care Survey (NLTCS) estimated annual declines in disability in elderly persons of 1.7 percent between 1982 and 1999, with an increased tempo of annual decline between 1994 and 1999 of 2.6 percent (Manton and Gu 2001). Another stunning finding of this report is that blacks age 65 and older experienced an even more rapid annual decline in disability of 4 percent per year in the last five years of the survey. When the NLTCS sample is stratified according to disability criteria introduced by the Health Insurance Portability and Accountability Act of 1996 (HIPAA) that distinguish the mild/moderate from three levels of the severe disability, the overwhelming majority of long-term care costs (92%) are incurred during episodes of severe disability with a ratio of 2.8 to 1 in female to male expected per capita lifetime costs (Stallard 2001).

In short, the latter findings (e.g., Crimmins, Hayward, and Saito 1996) are refocusing the debate from mean mortality rates to factors associated with the extension of "active life expectancy" (also referred to as the disability-free, or "quality-adjusted" life expectancy), which estimates the average onset of functional limitations across subgroups of the population and the trajectory of moderate to severe disabilities.

However, the chief limitation of many of the excellent studies in this area (see Freedman, Martin, and Schoeni 2002 for a summary of these studies) is that they continue to focus nearly exclusively on the 65 and older population and thereby ignore earlier phases of the life course (especially midlife) when chronic disease and functional limitations emerge unevenly across educational, occupational, ethnic, and gender subgroups (Martin and Soldo 1997). Indeed, other studies have identified some recent increases in morbidity and disability prevalence among younger adults (Clancy and Andresen 2002) and higher risks for the onset of morbidity and disability among the "uninsured" population under age 65 in the United States (Institute of Medicine 2003). These observations call for an emphasis on health expectancy (including mental health expectancy) and its contingencies as opposed to an age-dependent focus on mortality risks alone (see also Pearlin 1999; Wagener et al. 2001). Health disparities begin early and can cumulate over the life span of a cohort (House et al. 1994). Functional disability begins earlier and increases with age among ethnic minorities; African Americans and Hispanics exhibit the highest levels at the oldest ages and encounter their onset earlier (Bradsher 1996). In short, the onset, duration, and trajectories of disability in the U.S. population are correlated with age but with considerable variation across population subgroups displaying age-variant disability and related employment patterns.

The Variable Life Course and Emergent Old Age

The life course in the United States is not a universal sequence of social roles and transitions highly correlated with age. The period since World War II has included a growing heterogeneity in life course trajectories that do not readily conform to the triphasic model of the life course historically associated with industrial societies. The age-differentiated model of the life course was aptly captured in Riley and Riley (1994). Figure 6.1 is an expanded version of their model, which originally identified three age-graded role domains that defined the life course and the social policies that regulated them: education for the young, work for adulthood, and leisure for old age. This model assigned education strictly to the young phase of the life course, followed sequentially by work in midlife and then leisure (retirement) in old age. While this "normal life course" may never have been entirely universal within U.S. cohorts living throughout the twentieth century, it nevertheless reflected public and private policy assumptions influencing the three role domains of interest. Figure 6.1 adds two other role do-

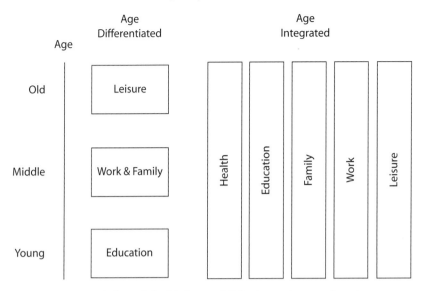

Fig. 6.1. Expanded model of Riley and Riley's age integration theory

mains to the Riley model—family and health—that also fit with policy assumptions about the patterns of lives. Arguably, family has been allocated to midlife in a gendered pattern based on a breadwinner model in which traditional family arrangements in adulthood divide market and household responsibilities. So too, health policies have been predicated on age-graded expectations to direct health policies to the young in preventative efforts to protect against infectious diseases and to the old in the management of morbidity and mortality.

Riley and Riley (1994) argued that the prevalence of deviations from the age-graded model has steadily increased in the population and that social policies and structural arrangements in both the public and private spheres are "lagging behind" significant demographic trends, especially increased average active life expectancy. They implied that these shifts were introducing pressures in the direction of another policy logic that they termed "age integration" (i.e., policies supporting social and market institutions sensitive to age-variant patterns of role incumbency and status transitions across the life course). Accordingly, as the right panel in Figure 6.1 illustrates, social roles and status transitions can occur across the life course in all domains and can impinge on each other at any time across the life span, given different life circumstances. Health status can influence the course of life from the beginning and emerge as a consequential factor over the entire life span; health status can change throughout the life course in response to short-term and long-term experiences in other role domains, such as family or work. Education can recur in midlife in response to job loss, divorce, economic downturns, or even employer sponsorship. Family roles and responsibilities can recur throughout life from youth to old age. Similarly, work may begin earlier in the life course in adolescence; may be interrupted over time by health, family, or market events; and may be renewed after initial retirement. And so on.

This view of the life course leads to a highly contingent and variable definition of the onset of "old age." *Old age is a variably emergent, not a fixed status* that reflects the cumulative impact of several inter-related factors over time. Net of genetic predispositions, earlier and chronic exposures to life course risks, and stressors can accelerate the aging process (Pearlin 1999), but significant variability has been observed (Manor, Matthews, and Power 2003). Social and economic supports can ameliorate stressors and "manage" or reverse disabilities to facilitate productive activities such as employment and extended life expectancies. Alternatively, access to structures of support (forms of insurance) can have protective effects by reducing risks and delaying the onset of old age.

Life Course Capital and Life Course Risks

The emergence or timing of old age is a product of the interaction of resources and risks over the life course, which I defined above as the interdependent and variable sequences of social statuses across life domains (health, education, family, work, and leisure among others) over the life span. Individuals face opportunities (positive risks) and hazards (negative risks) across the life span and respond to them behaviorally and attitudinally following patterns in which later responses are conditioned by earlier responses. Higher resources (e.g., advantaged social origins) and positive risks (e.g., access to higher education) earlier in the life course predict higher economic gains (wages and health insurance coverage) and longer life and health expectancies (e.g., House et al. 1994; Wagener et al. 2001; Elman and O'Rand 2003). Lower resources (e.g., poverty) and negative risks (e.g., high school dropout) predict lower economic attainment and shorter life and health expectancies.

Resources can be conceptualized as forms of *life course capital*: stocks of resources inherited, attributed, and/or accumulated and also divested and deployed over the life span to satisfy basic human needs and wants, including economic, social, and psychophysical (health) well-being (O'Rand 2001, 2003a). Several forms of life course capital have been defined for individuals, including levels of:

- human capital—education, skill, and experience that define labor market (wage) value
- social capital—social integration and support that can be mobilized from personal networks
- psychophysical capital—physical and mental health
- personal capital—social competence, self-esteem, and positive identity.

These forms of life course capital are interdependent and influence each other over the life span. Socioeconomic status, education, income, and health are mutually dependent over time and lead to patterns of cumulative advantage and disadvantage over the life course.

Even collective or shared levels of capital can be identified (see O'Rand 2001):

- status capital—race/ethnic, social class, or gender status
- community capital—community-level resources in the market (employment and wage levels), state (access to services), and neighborhood (poverty)
- institutional capital—sharing or spreading of resources by those who will benefit by them (otherwise known as social insurance).

The report on unequal health insurance coverage by the Institute of Medicine (2003) endorses this conceptualization with its own definition of "health capital" as the value of individual health over future years of life, including the subjective value of being alive and healthy, earning potential, and physical and mental development from birth.

The levels of life course capital are conditioned by *life course risks*, defined above as the differential likelihoods of exposure to hazards and opportunities over time that lead to the accumulation, protection, or depletion of forms of life course capital. Positive and negative risks (exposures to opportunities and hazards, respectively) are unevenly distributed in cohorts systematically over time. This unequal distribution is regulated by institutional structures that "spread," "share," "protect against," or "assign" risks at critical life transitions.

Social insurance policies were traditionally formulated as "institutionalized solutions to individual risks" (O'Rand 2003b). That is, public education, social and private retirement pensions and health insurance, worker's compensation, disability, Medicare/Medicaid, and other forms of insurance were developed to spread risks, following a principle of "equity" (i.e., collective allocation of resources to those who need and will benefit by them). However, even these institutions failed to reach large segments of the working and nonworking population. For example, private pensions have never covered more than three-fifths of the workforce (Costa 1998), and health insurance does not cover 15 percent of the total population at any given time (suggesting actual higher risks for noncoverage for everyone over time) (Institute of Medicine 2003). Moreover, public education's wider access has been eclipsed by the highly unequal quality of schools and school systems. The inequalities in exposures to risks generated by these systems have contributed to the life course variability, health and wealth disparities, and differential onset of old age.

Today, welfare reforms and proposals in response to some of these failures follow a different policy logic than traditional reforms. Instead, current policies and proposals are seeking "individualized solutions for institutional risks" (O'Rand 2003a). Vouchers in education, managed care "options" in health insurance, and individual retirement and health accounts for income maintenance—all indicate a shift to the individualization of risk. In this context, risks are considered to be endogenous to the individual and framed in the language of "choice." Consequently, normal and exceptional life course risks associated with education, health, and employment devolve to individual capacities and prerogatives. And the implications of this individualization for the onset of old age become more complex.

In the changing insurance landscape, individuals and organizations (such as states and corporations) tend to take risks to avoid costs rather than to make gains (Heimer 2002). Employers and insurers are making workers bear a greater portion of their life course risks in health and employment. Some workers are assigned higher burdens of risk-bearing than others because they present putatively higher long-term costs to insurers. Patterns of risk aversion also lead workers to avoid costs, but their costs are often assessed on shorter time horizons conditioned by current levels of life course capital.

Work and Retirement in the New Economy: New Worker Risks

Patterns of work and retirement at the turn of the twenty-first century provide a window on the complex implications of diverse life course patterns. The dominant pattern of retirement over the post–World War II period until the 1990s was a two-pronged trend toward *early retirement*. Two streams of early retirees emerged over the period: one set retired voluntarily in response to employer pension incentives (primarily defined benefit plan schedules) available to professional, managerial, and skilled (manufacturing, communications, and transportation sector) workers constituting what some economists have called "pension elites" during the 1970s and 1980s. A second, more heterogeneous stream "retired" early as a result of either plant closings and dislocations (some with early retirement packages) or high risks for unemployment, underemployment, and disability leading to increased rates of dependence on disability benefits and early retired-workers' benefits at ages 62 to 64 under Social Security (Burkhauser, Couch, and Phillips 1996).

Early retirees in the second stream came overwhelmingly from disadvantaged labor markets until well into the 1990s. Two recent studies provide evidence for these patterns. First, a recent publication using longitudinal data from the New Beneficiary Survey (NBS) of the Social Security Administration provides a profile of these retirees and their first ten years following early retirement (Haveman et al. 2003). Individuals aged 62 and older who first received Social Security retired worker benefits between 1980 and 1981 were interviewed in 1982 and re-interviewed in 1991. First, age at receipt of first benefits and gender (female) were negatively associated with worker and spouse earnings, asset income, family income, and income-to-needs ratios and positively associated with poverty (or near poverty) across initial (1982) and surviving (1991) subgroups. Second, the patterns of relative decline in economic resources over the decade paralleled those originally observed in 1982. Those retiring early had lower economic status; ten years later, their age-related disadvantage increased, particularly among female early retirees.

The second study used two waves of the Health and Retirement Study to track the labor market transitions of workers age 51 to 61 in 1991 between 1992 and 1994 (Flippen and Tienda 2000). The purpose of the study was to examine interwave labor market transitions by race, Hispanic origin, and sex among four states: employment, unemployment, retirement, and out of the labor force. All else being equal (controlling for education, health, and occupational characteristics), black, Hispanic, and female adults under age 62 were both less likely to be working at the first wave and more likely to have experienced involuntary separation from work between the two waves. Importantly, this involuntary job loss eventuated in retirement.

The major implications of these findings are that pathways to retirement may include other portals besides pension eligibility. Instead, subgroups of the older worker population may exhibit transitions to Social Security benefit receipt via unemployment, disability, and other portals. Other studies suggest that disability is perhaps the most expanding alternative portal to retirement among disadvantaged groups (e.g., Santiago and Muschkin 1996; Tapay and Smolka 1999). These findings and the well-established negative association between retirement income, prior disability status, and lower life expectancy reveal the life course risks at retirement faced by disadvantaged workers (Martin and Soldo 1997).

A Reversal of Early Retirement

Evidence emerged in the mid-1990s that the trend toward early retirement may have halted or perhaps reversed (Quinn 1997; Costa 1999). Explanations for these putative changes are different for subgroups of workers. Some economists project that employees are beginning to remain at work longer than in recent decades because of pecuniary and nonpecuniary incentives to remain at work, especially flexible benefits (health insurance, child and elder care assistance, educational enhancements), commitments to careers, and better health (see, e.g., Mitchell, Blitzstein, and Gordon 2003) and the growing predominance of defined contribution pension plans that require workers to manage their own pension savings portfolios, leading them to be responsive in their labor supply to market fluctuations (Mitchell and Schieber 1998). For workers without flexible benefits, defined benefit plans, or expectations of adequate Social Security benefits, these trends suggest that for those who need to work as long as possible, early or normal retirement are not clear options in the current economy (Mutchler et al. 1997). While these are all preliminary estimates and tentative explanations relevant to future trends, they are notable in light of the question at hand about the onset of old age.

Parnes and Somers (1994), who have examined general trends in the labor supply of older male workers using the National Longitudinal Study (NLS) of older men, have examined the factors that predict why older workers continue to work. Multivariate analyses suggest that education, health, and positive attitudes toward work increase the likelihood of working past early and normal retirement ages. Their results lead them to argue that, on average, nonpecuniary concerns drive elderly labor supply more than economic needs.

My examination of labor force data provided by the U.S. Bureau of Labor Statistics (2002) illuminates a very complex picture of changes in labor force participation rates by subgroups of workers since 1980 that suggests that minority subgroups with less advantage are also increasing their labor supply (although their shares of older labor are relatively smaller). Figures 6.2 and 6.3 are based on estimates of the change in labor force participation among age groups of workers between 60 and 80 and older years of age. Figure 6.2 compares the rates of change in labor for participation of age groups of men and women between 1980 and 1990, 1980 and 2000, and 1990 and 2000, respectively. The annual prevalence rates among these groups are not high, but some have experienced increases in labor force participation ranging between 10 and 80 percent. About 15 percent of persons over the age of 65 were employed in 1999; approximately 16 percent of men and 10 percent of women. However, these participation levels reflect general declines among men and increases among women over two decades. Overall, men's participation generally appears to have declined across the three period comparison provided here, with the highest overall rates of change for men in the 62 to 64 age range between 1980 and 2000; while over the most recent decade (1990–2000, when data for age groups 75 and older are available at the BLS Web site) the greatest rates of decline have been among the two oldest groups. Alternatively, women's rates of change increased generally across age groups, with the lowest rate increases in the 62 to 64 age

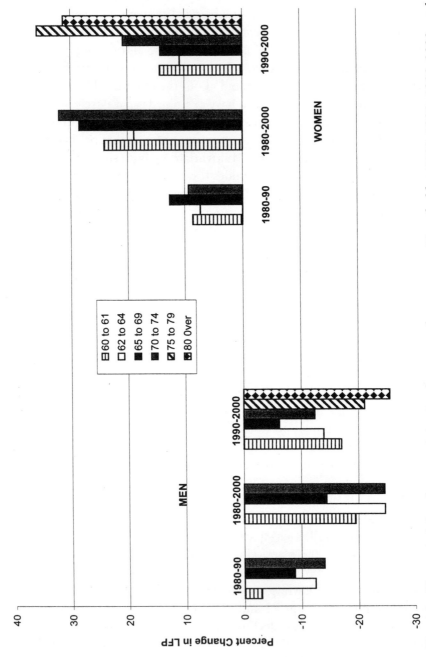

Fig. 6.2. Change in labor force participation by men and women age 60 and older, 1980–1990, 1980–2000, and 1990–2000. Source: Data from U.S. Bureau of Labor Statistics 2003

range. Over the 1990s, the oldest age groups displayed the most significant changes in their labor participation (more than a 33% increase among women 75 to 79 and a 31% increase among women over 80).

Figure 6.3 provides the same period and age group comparisons for black men, black women, and Hispanic men. The stunning results are that the oldest age groups experienced the highest rates of change in participation in the 1990s, with Hispanic men over the age of 62 especially more likely to have increased their labor supply. These figures suggest that despite the average lower relative base rates of participation at older ages among these groups when compared to white men, women and minority ethnic subgroups of workers are also contributing to the trend away from early retirement.

Declining Medical Benefits

The role of health insurance coverage in the timing of retirement over the 1990s appears to be increasing. Declines in retiree health insurance before Medicare eligibility may also account for the reversal in early retirement. Figure 6.4, drawn from Fronstin and Salisbury (2003) at the Employee Benefits Research Institute, is based on a national survey of employer-sponsored health plans in 2002 among employers of 500 or more workers conducted by William M. Mercer, Inc., of New York. It documents the trend away from employer health insurance coverage of both early retirees and Medicare-eligible retirees over the 1990s.

Fronstin and Salisbury further report that in 2000 only 11 percent of all U.S. private establishments offered retiree health benefits to Medicare eligible retirees and only 12 percent offered them to retirees under age 65. Even fewer retirees in the future can expect these benefits to be offered by employers. Rising health costs and changing accounting rules establishing long-term liabilities for employers have motivated these shifts. A consequence of the changes may well be the reversal of early retirement for advantaged and disadvantaged workers.

These institutional changes in the workplace imply that old age officially begins at age 65 when the public health insurance system begins to accept some responsibility for the health of workers who, if previously covered by employer plans, cared for themselves and their families, or who, if previously not covered by employer plans, either paid out of pocket for health care, qualified for means-tested assistance

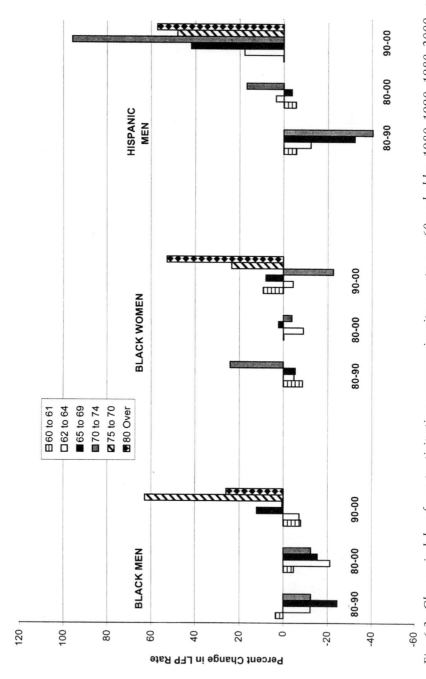

Fig. 6.3. *Change in labor force participation among minority groups age 60 and older, 1980–1990, 1980–2000, and 1990–2000.* Source: Data from U.S. Bureau of Labor Statistics 2003

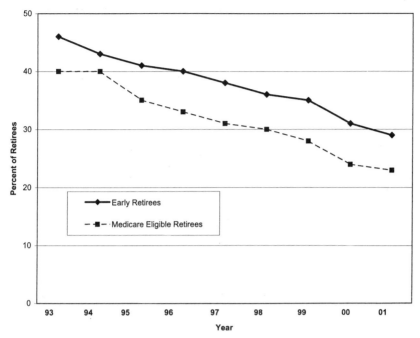

Fig. 6.4. Provision of retiree health benefits for current and future retirees by employers with 500 or more employees, 1993–2001. Source: Mercer Human Resources Consulting, Inc., as cited by Fronstin and Salisbury, EBRI 2003

(through Medicaid), or were constrained to delay or to forego health care altogether. The costs of noninsurance for subgroups of workers over the life course are diminished health and longevity for individuals and spillover losses to society as a whole in the form of human capital, productivity, and foregone health (Institute of Medicine 2003).

Discussion and Conclusions

The answer to the question of when old age begins is a challenge for researchers and policymakers alike. It may be the fundamental question that all researchers concerned with aging in society ultimately confront. Social welfare systems have historically defined old age using chronological age markers as readily convenient and purportedly efficient ways of managing the well-being of aging populations. However, while the convenience of age-based policies for large systems has some logical and empirical gravity, the ultimate efficiency of these systems is less supportable when the disparate outputs of the system are evaluated. In spite of increased life expectancy in the population, health disparities that bear on the aging process emerge early in the lives of cohorts, long before universal age-based support structures are accessible. By late adulthood, life and health expectancies have diverged significantly in the population, making subgroups arriving at the same chronological age—say, 62—quite unequal in levels of health functioning and economic independence. Trajectories of health and wealth diverge even more dramatically after these ages.

I have used a framework that links life course capital and life course risks to consider the mechanisms by which the experience of aging varies in the population. It is particularly useful in accounting for how inequalities emerge over the life course. Forms of life course capital stemming from education, social integration, health, and self-esteem interact over time to produce inequalities. Also, these individual forms of life course capital are embedded in wider contexts of collective capital, such as unequally distributed institutional sources of health insurance and retirement pension coverage. Over time, cumulative processes of advantage and disadvantage across different institutional contexts of capital stratify the fortunes of cohorts.

The dependence on employer-sponsored insurance systems that increasingly place more responsibility on workers and their families to choose whether and how much to be covered by insurance may exacerbate this system of divergent fortunes. These institutional changes are framed in the language of choice and option and thus depend on the capacities and prerogatives of individuals and families to make appropriate and feasible decisions vis-à-vis their own welfare. Risk-taking and risk-aversion pervade these decisions and promise to yield growing inequalities and diversities in the aging process.

References

Bongaarts, J., and G. Feeney. 2002. How long do we live? *Population and Development Review* 28:13–29.

Bradsher, J. 1996. Disability among racial and ethnic groups. *Disability Statistics Abstract* 10:1–4.

Burkhauser, R. V., K. A. Couch, and J. Phillips. 1996. Who takes early social security benefits? The economic and health characteristics of early retirees. *Gerontologist* 36:789–99.

Burtless, G., and J. F. Quinn. 2000. *Retirement Trends and Policies to Encourage Work Among Older Americans.* WP 2000–03. Center for Retirement Research. Chestnut Hill, Mass.: Boston College.

Clancy, C., and E. Andresen. 2002. Meeting the healthcare needs of persons with disabilities. *Milbank Memorial Fund Quarterly* 80:381–91.

Costa, D. 1998. *The Evolution of Retirement: An American Economic History, 1880–1990.* Chicago: University of Chicago.

Costa, D. 1999. "Has the early retirement trend reversed?" Conference paper for the Centers for Retirement Research of Boston College and University of Michigan. Available at: www.bc.edu.centers/crr/papers/cp_quinn.pdf.

Crimmins, E., M. Hayward, and Y. Saito. 1996. Differentials in active life expectancy in the older population of the United States. *Journal of Gerontology—Social Sciences* 51B:S111–20.

Elman, C., and A. M. O'Rand. 2003. The race is to the swift: Childhood adversity, adult education, and wage attainment. *American Journal of Sociology* (forthcoming).

Employee Benefit Research Institute. 1997. *EBRI Handbook on Employee Benefits,* fourth edition. Washington, D.C.

Federal Interagency Forum on Aging-Related Statistics. 2003. *Older Americans 2000: Key Indicators of Well-Being.* Hyattsville, Md.: Federal Interagency Forum on Aging-Related Statistics.

Flippen, C., and M. Tienda. 2000. Pathways to retirement: Patterns of labor force participation and labor market exit among the pre-retirement population by race, Hispanic origin, and sex. *Journal of Gerontology-Social Sciences* 55B :S14–27.

Freedman, V. A., L. G. Martin, and R. F. Schoeni. 2002. Recent trends in disability and functioning among older adults in the United States: A systematic review. *Journal of the American Medical Association* 288(24): 3137–46.

Fries, J. F. 2002. Reducing disability in older age. *Journal of American Medical Association* 288(24):3164–66.

Fronstin, P., and D. Salisbury. 2003. *Retiree Health Benefits: Savings Needed to Fund Health Care in Retirement.* EBRI Issue Brief No. 254. Washington, D.C.: Employee Retirement Research Institute.

Haveman, R., K. Holden, K. Wilson, and B. Wolfe. 1999. The changing economic status of U.S. disabled men: Trends and their determinants, 1982–1991. *Empirical Economics* 24:571–98.

Haveman, R., K. Holden, K. Wilson, and B. Wolfe. 2000. The changing economic status of disabled women, 1982–1991.

Haveman, R., K. Holden, K. Wilson, and B. Wolfe. 2003. Social security, age of retirement and economic well-being: Intertemporal and demographic patterns among retired worker beneficiaries. *Demography* 40:369–94.

Heimer, C. A. 2002. Insuring more, insuring less: The costs and benefits of private regulation through insurance. Pp. 116–45 in T. Baker and J. Simon, eds., *Embracing Risk: The Changing Culture of Insurance and Responsibility*. Chicago: University of Chicago Press.

Himes, C. L. 2001. *Elderly Americans*. Population Bulletin Vol. 56/4. Washington, D.C.: Population Reference Bureau.

House, J. S., J. M. Lepkowski, and A. M. Kinney. 1994. The social stratification of aging and health. *Journal of Health and Social Behavior* 35(3):213–34.

Institute of Medicine. 2003. *Hidden Costs, Value Lost: Uninsurance in America*. Washington, D.C.: National Academy Press.

Manor, O., S. Matthews, and C. Power. 2003. Health selection: The role of inter- and intra-generational mobility on social inequalities in health. *Social Science and Medicine* 57:2217–27.

Manton, K. G., and X. Gu. 2001. Changes in the prevalence of chronic disability in the United States black and nonblack population above age 65 from 1982 to 1999. *Proceedings of the National Academy of Sciences* 98:6354–59.

Martin, L. G., and B. J. Soldo, eds. 1997. *Racial and Ethnic Differences in the Health of Older Americans*. Washington, D.C.: National Academy Press.

Mitchell, O. S., and S. J. Schieber. 1998. *Living with Defined Contribution Pensions: Remaking Responsibility for Retirement*. Philadelphia: Pensions Research Council, University of Pennsylvania Press.

Mitchell, O. S., D. S. Blitzstein, M. Gordon, and J. F. Mazo, eds. 2003. *Benefits for the Workplace of the Future*. Philadelphia: Pension Research Council, University of Pennsylvania Press.

Mutchler, J. E., J. A. Burr, A. M. Pienta, and M. P. Massagli. 1997. Pathways to labor force exit: Work transitions and work instability. *Journal of Gerontology-Social Science* 52B:S4–12.

Oeppen, J., and J. W. Vaupel. 2002. Broken limits to life expectancy. *Science* 296:1029–31.

O'Rand, A. M. 2001. Stratification and the life course: The forms of life-course capital and their interrelationships. Pp. 192–216 in R. H. Binstock and L. K. George, eds., *Handbook of Aging and the Social Sciences,* 5th ed. New York: Academic Press.

O'Rand, A. M. 2003a. "Life course capital and life course risks." Paper presented at the 98th Annual Meeting of the American Sociological Association, Atlanta, Ga.

O'Rand, A. M. 2003b. "The future of the life course: Late modernity and life course risks." Pp. 693–701 in J. T. Mortimer and M. J. Shanahan, eds., *Handbook of the Life Course*. New York: Plenum.

O'Rand, A. M. 2002. "Retirement patterns." Pp. 1201–7 in D. J. Eckerdt, ed., *Macmillan Encyclopedia of Aging*. New York: Macmillan.

Parnes, H., and D. Somers. 1994. Shunning retirement: Experience of men in their seventies and eighties. *Journal of Gerontology-Social Sciences* 49B:S117–24.

Pearlin, L. I. 1999. The stress process revisited: Reflections on concepts and their interrelationships." Pp. 395–415 in C. S. Aneshensel and J. C. Phelan, eds., *Handbook of the Sociology of Mental Health*. New York: Plenum.

President's Commission to Strengthen Social Security. 2001. *Strengthening Social Security and Creating Personal Wealth for All Americans*. Washington, D.C.: Government Printing Office.

Quinn, J. 1997. Retirement trends and patterns in the 1990s: The end of an era? Pp. 10–14 in *Public Policy and Aging Report*. Washington, D.C.: National Academy on Aging.

Riley, M. W., and J. W. Riley. 1994. Structural lag: Past and future. Pp. 115–36 in M. W. Riley, R. L. Kahn, and A. Foner, eds., *Age and Structural Lag*. New York: Wiley.

Santiago, A. M., and C. G. Muschkin. 1996. Disentangling the effects of disability status and gender on the supply of Anglo, black and Latino older workers. *Gerontologist* 36:299–310.

Stallard, E. 2001. Estimates of the incidence, prevalence, duration, intensity and cost of chronic disability among the U.S. elderly. Paper presented at the Annual Meeting of the Population Association of America, Washington, D.C.

Tapay, N., and G. Smolka. 1999. *Disabled Medicare Beneficiaries under Age 65: A Review of State Efforts to Provide Access to Medicare Supplemental Insurance*. Working Paper No. 9915. Washington, D.C.: American Association of Retired Persons, Public Policy Institute.

U.S. Bureau of Labor Statistics. 2002. *Employment Cost Index: Historical Listing. National Compensation Survey*. Office of Compensation Levels and Trends. Washington, D.C. Available at: www.bls.gov/ncs.

U.S. Bureau of Labor Statistics. 2003. Labor Force (Demographic) Data, 1980–2000. Washington, D.C. Available at: www.bls.gov/emp/emplab1.htm.

Vallin, J., and F. Mesle. 2001. Living beyond the age of 100. *Population et Societes*. Paris: Institut National d'Etudes Demographique.

Vaupel, J. W. 2002. Life expectancy at current rates vs. current conditions: A reflexion stimulated by Bongaarts and Feeney's "How do we live?" *Demographic Research* 7, no. 8. Rostock, Germany: Max Planck Institute for Demographic Research.

Vigdor, E. R. 2003. *Coverage Does Matter: The Value of Health Forgone by the Uninsured*. Durham, N.C.: Duke University, Sanford Institute of Public Policy.

Wagener, D. K., M. T. Molla, E. M. Crimmins, E. Pamuk, and J. H. Madans. 2001. Summary measures of population health: Addressing the first goal of healthy people 2010, improving health expectancy. *Healthy People 2010 Statistical Notes, No. 22*. Hyattsville, Md.: National Center for Health Statistics.

Walker, A. 1999. The future of pensions and retirement in Europe: Towards productive ageing. *Hallym International Journal of Aging* 1:3–15.

7. Minority Workers and Pathways to Retirement

Chenoa A. Flippen

Age has long been a defining criterion for both public and private retirement benefit systems. The aging of the baby boom cohort and the acute strain on Social Security that it portends have motivated numerous public policies to encourage later employment. However, these policies, most notably raising the minimum age for full Social Security eligibility from age 65 to 67, are overwhelmingly supply oriented and are likely to have a disparate impact by race and Hispanic origin, owing to stark differences across groups in work histories, health, and employment opportunities. Specifically, minority workers' more discontinuous work histories and poorer health put them at increased risk for involuntary job loss in the years proximate to retirement. From a public policy perspective, it is extremely important to evaluate how constraints on late-aged employment will shape minority workers' response to changing retirement incentives. These responses are critical to financial security in retirement and have the potential to exacerbate already large racial and ethnic disparities in economic well-being among aged Americans.

While the vulnerability of black male workers to involuntary job loss at older ages is relatively well established (Gibson 1987; Burr et al. 1996; Hayward, Friedman, and Chen 1996), far less research has examined the process of Hispanic labor market withdrawal. Though one of the fastest growing segments of the U.S. elderly population (Wykle and Kaskel 1991), we know surprisingly little about Hispanic aging and retirement behavior, largely due to a lack of adequate Hispanic representation in previous nationally representative surveys of aged Americans. Elderly Hispanic persons experience high rates of poverty and are often more disadvantaged than their black peers with respect to employment history characteristics (Quinn and Kozy 1996;

Santiago and Muschkin 1996). This economic marginality, coupled with the accelerating growth of the Hispanic elderly population, make it essential to anticipate whether and how Hispanic retirement behavior differs from that of blacks and whites in both its precursors and its consequences.

Previous research, furthermore, hints at an important interaction between race and gender in structuring labor market outcomes in the preretirement years (Gohmann 1990; Ruhm 1996). Among men, whites have the highest and blacks the lowest labor force participation rates through the life span. And both black and Hispanic men are disadvantaged relative to white men in terms of their employment characteristics such as pension coverage and employment stability. Among women, blacks have the highest and Hispanics the lowest rates of labor force participation. Also, because black women are considerably more likely than white women to have worked steadily most of their adult lives, they actually compare favorably to white women on several employment outcomes (Belgrave 1988; Ruhm 1996). However, studies that consider both race and gender differences in pathways out of the labor market *and* that distinguish between retirement and other forms of labor market exit remain rare.

Accordingly, the study reported here compares patterns of labor force participation among white, black, and Hispanic men and women approaching retirement age. Using the first four waves of the Health and Retirement Study (HRS), I analyze labor force transitions in a multistate framework and estimate the demographic, human capital, employment history, and health sources of differential employment patterns across groups. The analysis recognizes the considerable heterogeneity of workers' pathways to retirement, distinguishing between full-time work, part-time work, unemployment, retirement, partial retirement, and nonparticipation. The first part of the analysis describes aggregate differences in labor force status across groups and uses the HRS baseline survey to examine factors associated with employment decisions by race, Hispanic origin, and sex. The second part of the analysis examines changes in employment status across waves of the HRS and documents how pathways out of the labor market differ across groups. Results suggest considerable constraints on labor force participation among older low-skill and minority workers that render age-based welfare systems problematic.

Multiple Pathways to Retirement

The traditional conception of retirement as a single transition from a full-time career job to full-time retirement in response to pension and Social Security incentives is increasingly being recognized as inadequate, particularly for minority workers. Based largely on the experiences of white, middle-class males, the research overemphasizes the "pull" factors that entice advantaged workers into retirement to the relative neglect of "push" factors such as diminished job opportunities and poor health that are often more influential in the labor market exit decisions of minority workers.

Over the past decade, researchers have identified multiple pathways out of the labor force, each associated with diverse long-term work and health career patterns (Hayward and Grady 1990; Quinn and Kozy 1996; Mutchler et al. 1999; Quinn 1999). The more complex view of retirement recognizes the influences of individual work, health, and family histories that move individuals toward retirement or final labor exit at variable rates and via different routes, which may include pension or Social Security–based retirement, disability, part-time work or partial retirement, unemployment, and nonparticipation.

These issues are particularly salient for minority workers, many of whom leave the labor market before they are eligible for Social Security or pension benefits and in spite of very low levels of retirement savings (Boaz 1988; Mitchell, Levine, and Phillips 1999). Minority workers are more likely to have had less stable work histories, comprised of multiple voluntary and involuntary shifts among jobs of shorter duration and frequent or prolonged work interruptions over the career (O'Rand and Henretta 1999). Minorities also average lower levels of education and are differentially distributed across industrial sectors and occupational groups that encounter uneven risks for involuntary job loss, job displacement, and unemployment (Gibson 1987, 1993; Hayward, Friedman, and Chen 1996).

In fact, research on older black workers suggests that the term "retirement" may have little meaning for working-class blacks who display continuous instability in employment throughout their lives until death or full disability (Gibson 1987; Burr et al. 1996). Comparable research on Hispanic workers is relatively scarce, but existing studies show that like blacks, many Hispanic workers exhibit lifetime patterns of employment instability that lead to the gradual lengthening of non-work episodes with age (Zsembik and Singer 1990; Santiago and Muschkin 1996). Older nonwhites are not only more vulnerable to job displacement but also more adversely affected by it. Specifically, they experience lower rates of re-employment, lower personal and household incomes, and lower rates of health insurance coverage following displacement than white workers with similar levels of education and job tenure (Couch 1998).

Minority retirement is further complicated by their poorer average health (Wray 1996; Martin and Soldo 1997; Smith and Kington 1997). Despite recent declines in chronic disability among the elderly population (Manton and Gu 2001), minority workers' lower socioeconomic status, concentration in manual labor with greater exposure to hazardous work conditions, and higher lifelong health vulnerabilities result in elevated levels of disability and mortality relative to whites (Manton and Stallard 1997; Hayward and Heron 1999). Older black workers therefore spend a greater portion of their lives disabled than whites (Hayward et al. 1989), and race differences in health and functional ability account for a large part of the race gap in employment (Hayward and Grady 1990; Bound, Schoenbaum, and Waidman 1995).

The greater vulnerability to involuntary job loss through displacement and disability calls into question older minority workers' ability to meet age-based eligibility criterion for retirement benefits, particularly as they are expected to adjust their labor supply upward in response to changing Social Security requirements. This chapter contributes to the understanding of ethnoracial and gender differences in labor force withdrawal in several ways. In addition to including Hispanics, a group generally neglected in studies of minority aging, in our analysis, ethnoracial and gender differences in labor market exit are simultaneously considered. The analysis takes into account the considerable complexity in late-aged employment patterns, distinguishing between full-time work, part-time work, unemployment, retirement, partial retirement, and nonparticipation. By combining longitudinal and cross-sectional data, we trace the actual pathways of black, white, and Hispanic men and women out of the labor market, distinguishing between voluntary and involuntary forms of labor market exit, which are especially important for low-skill and minority older workers.

The Present Study

The data for the empirical analyses are drawn from the first four waves of the Health and Retirement Study (HRS), a nationally representative, longitudinal survey of the preretirement population and their spouses or partners, with oversampling of Hispanics and African Americans. The survey was constructed to follow a cohort of adults born between 1930 and 1941, and therefore aged 51 to 61 at the time of initial interview, through the retirement process and into old age. The baseline survey was conducted in 1992, and additional waves of data were collected every two years. This chapter is based on data from 1992, 1994, 1996, and 1998.

In addition to copious demographic and background characteristics, the HRS collected extensive information about labor force participation, including occupation, industry, firm size, job tenure, career employment stability, and numerous other characteristics of current or most recent job for all respondents. Other core topics covered by the HRS include health status, family structure, individual and household income by source, and a broad range of wealth indicators, including pension, housing, and other assets.

The HRS is ideally suited for a study of ethnoracial and gender variation in preretirement employment patterns for several reasons. First, the HRS is one of the only nationally representative surveys of older populations to oversample Hispanics in addition to blacks. While a rapidly growing segment of the U.S. population in general and of the older U.S. population in particular, very few nationally representative surveys of older Americans contain enough Hispanic respondents to allow for their separate analysis. This is a critical advantage of the HRS over other data sources. Wave I contained 12,654 respondents, 16.6 percent (2,096) of whom were black and 9.3 percent (1,174) of whom were Hispanic. By Wave IV, 11,302 of the original respondents remained in the sample, 15.1 percent (1,634) of whom were black and 8.8 percent (949) of whom were Hispanic.

A second important feature of the HRS is its longitudinal design. The panel data obtained from the HRS allows us to formulate a more dynamic model of labor market exits. Rather than a single event, the transition into retirement is often the result of a complex process of labor market changes. Tracking the labor market position of individuals at each wave, the HRS allows us to better capture the often fluid nature of employment behavior and identify different pathways that eventually culminate in permanent labor market withdrawal.

The Model

The focus of this study is the process of labor market exit among the pre-retirement population. The *dependent variables* in the analyses are discrete, categorical outcomes that represent diverse transitions out of employment via part-time employment, unemployment, partial retirement, retirement, and other nonparticipation (which includes both disabled and discouraged workers and, among women, significant numbers of homemakers). Models across waves also include survey exit as an employment outcome resulting from both death and sample attrition.[1]

Independent variables in the analyses follow the literature described above and include characteristics that measure both the push and pull factors affecting retirement pathways. The first set of variables includes ascribed characteristics such as race and ethnicity to determine the extent to which these factors continue to influence retirement patterns after socioeconomic conditions are taken into account. In addition, the model controls for age to reflect the age dependence of retirement behavior.

The analysis also includes human capital characteristics such as years of education and marital status. Given the increasing labor market payoff to education and skill that characterized the 1980s and 1990s (Murphy and Welch 1993), we expect more highly educated workers to remain in the labor market longer and to follow a more traditional pathway from full-time employment to retirement. The same applies to married workers, although this effect is expected to vary considerably by gender. Health status is another critical aspect of human capital that structures employment opportunities at all ages, but particularly as workers approach retirement. We include two measures of health status: whether workers experience limitations in Activities of Daily Living (ADLs), and whether they experience mobility and large muscle limitations.[2]

The next set of characteristics included in the models reflects aspects of employment history that determine a worker's vulnerability to involuntary job separation. A dummy variable for white-collar occupations tests whether this type of employment offers greater opportunities for remaining employed, either through greater job security or because the less physically demanding work conditions allow workers to moderate their environment to adjust for physical limitations. Conversely, employment in industrial sectors most adversely affected by deindustrialization and in smaller firms may expose older workers to involuntary labor market exit. We therefore distinguish between employees in professional industries (professional services, finance, and public administration) from those in agriculture/mining, manufacturing/transportation, services (business, repair, and personal services), and sales industries and include a dummy variable for employment in large (more than 500 employees) firms. Likewise, a history of unstable employment during prime-aged years could increase the risk of instability in later years. To measure employment instability, we use the number of times a person was laid off over a career.

Finally, to represent retirement savings available for postemployment consumption, we index whether workers are covered by a pension and include a measure of household net financial assets. Both pension coverage and financial assets are expected to facilitate transitions into retirement and protect workers from involuntary labor market outcomes such as unemployment or part-time work.

The empirical analysis is separated into two steps. First, we model employment status in Wave I to better understand the selection process that sorts groups into different employment categories at survey baseline. This model is estimated using multinomial logistic regression techniques. Second, pooling the four waves of data together, we model labor force transitions in a multistate framework to investigate the demographic, human capital, and employment history sources of differential labor market experiences across groups over time. Because independent variables are measured in the previous wave, the time lag built in these models makes them particularly suitable for capturing the causal mechanisms behind employment outcomes.

Results

Labor Force Status in the First Wave of the HRS

Table 7.1 presents the employment status of white, black, and Hispanic HRS respondents across the first four waves of the HRS separately by sex. Focusing for the time being on differences across groups in Wave I employment, minority labor market disadvantage relative to whites is apparent in their lower rates of full-time employment and

Table 7.1 Aggregate trends in employment status across Waves I–IV, by race, Hispanic origin, and sex

| | Employed | | | | | Disabled/ Out of | | |
	Full Time	Part Time	Un- employed	Partly Retired	Retired	Labor Force	Exit Survey	N
Men								
White								
Wave I	72.2	4.7	2.3	4.8	12.5	3.5	—	3,386
Wave II	59.0	3.5	1.7	5.7	17.7	2.9	9.5	
Wave III	47.4	2.7	1.1	8.7	22.3	2.9	14.9	
Wave IV	37.6	2.6	0.7	9.4	27.5	3.2	19.1	
Black								
Wave I	57.6	6.7	4.4	3.0	17.5	10.9	—	707
Wave II	40.9	6.2	3.4	4.4	21.2	8.1	15.8	
Wave III	36.1	3.8	1.3	4.5	23.2	8.4	22.8	
Wave IV	28.0	2.6	0.6	5.5	24.5	9.7	29.3	
Hispanic								
Wave I	63.5	7.3	4.6	1.2	11.4	12.0	—	411
Wave II	48.9	5.6	3.7	2.9	13.1	7.8	18.0	
Wave III	39.2	5.1	2.2	4.4	16.8	9.3	23.1	
Wave IV	36.0	4.4	2.0	4.1	22.1	7.1	24.3	
Women								
White								
Wave I	43.6	15.2	2.0	3.0	13.4	22.9	—	3,635
Wave II	35.6	12.9	1.6	4.4	20.0	17.3	8.2	
Wave III	29.5	8.5	1.3	6.2	24.7	18.0	11.8	
Wave IV	22.9	8.3	0.9	6.5	28.4	17.8	15.2	
Black								
Wave I	44.6	13.3	1.9	2.9	17.6	19.7	—	979
Wave II	33.6	11.6	2.9	3.5	24.1	14.3	10.1	
Wave III	26.9	9.6	1.4	3.8	25.2	16.6	16.5	
Wave IV	22.4	7.0	0.9	5.4	25.8	17.7	20.8	
Hispanic								
Wave I	32.2	12.2	4.0	0.6	8.4	42.5	—	501
Wave II	23.6	9.2	5.0	1.6	12.4	32.0	16.4	
Wave III	20.4	9.2	2.6	1.0	13.8	34.4	18.8	
Wave IV	16.8	8.4	0.8	3.4	16.6	30.4	23.8	

higher levels of unemployment, part-time work, and nonparticipation. However, racial and ethnic differences in employment are far more pronounced among men than among women. White and black women exhibit very similar patterns of employment owing to the historically high rates of labor force participation among black women. Hispanic women, on the other hand, are less likely to be employed full time and are more likely to be unemployed or out of the labor force than white women. In general, women are less likely than men to be employed full time or retired and more likely to be out of the labor force (primarily homemakers).

A key question is whether these employment disparities reflect racial and ethnic differences in human capital, employment, and health characteristics, or whether race exerts a direct effect on retirement pathways net of these factors. To address this question, Tables 7.2 and 7.3 present results from multinomial logit models predicting labor force status in the first wave of the HRS for men and women, respectively. Results confirm that significant racial and ethnic differences in labor force status remain even net of human capital, health, and employment characteristics. As predicted, these effects differ by sex. Black men are more likely than their white counterparts to be working part-time, unemployed, retired, and out of the labor force relative to working full-time. Hispanic men are less likely than whites to be partially retired and, like black men, are more likely to be out of the labor force. Although more likely to be retired than white women, black women do not exhibit the same pattern of labor market disadvantage evinced by their male counterparts. They are neither more likely to be unemployed nor out of the labor force than white women.[3] Hispanic women, on the other hand, are significantly more likely to be unemployed and less likely to be retired than white women with similar socioeconomic and labor market characteristics.

Tables 7.2 and 7.3 also demonstrate the importance of human capital, health, employment history, and savings characteristics on late-aged labor force activity. Older age is associated with a lower likelihood of employment, reflecting the positive effects of pension and Social Security on retirement. Education insulates workers from nonparticipation and encourages partial retirement. Marital status also influences late-aged employment, though differently for men and women. Married men are significantly more likely to be employed full-time than their unmarried counterparts, and they experience lower

Table 7.2 Multivariate models predicting Wave I Employment Status: Men

	Employed Part Time		Unemployed		Partly Retired		Retired		Out of Labor Force	
Ascribed characteristics										
Black	0.368**	(0.189)	0.798***	(0.240)	-0.187	(0.254)	0.476***	(0.139)	0.947***	(0.196)
Hispanic	0.058	(0.239)	0.351	(0.302)	-1.255***	(0.473)	-0.160	(0.200)	0.542**	(0.244)
Age	-0.010	(0.022)	0.047	(0.030)	0.142***	(0.026)	0.188***	(0.017)	-0.002	(0.026)
Achieved (human capital) characteristics										
Education	-0.013	(0.025)	-0.029	(0.031)	0.090***	(0.031)	-0.012	(0.018)	-0.079***	(0.025)
Married	-0.565***	(0.171)	-0.675***	(0.225)	-0.192	(0.213)	-0.621***	(0.133)	-0.837***	(0.182)
Health										
ADL lim	0.793*	(0.438)	0.864	(0.537)	1.046**	(0.431)	1.803***	(0.234)	2.003***	(0.262)
Mobility lim	0.014	(0.195)	0.196	(0.249)	0.406**	(0.205)	1.477***	(0.116)	2.001***	(0.182)

	Model 1		Model 2		Model 3		Model 4		Model 5	
Employment characteristics										
White collar occupation	−0.311	(0.196)	0.393	(0.251)	−0.407**	(0.196)	−0.300**	(0.136)	−0.222	(0.256)
Industry (ref = professional)										
Agriculture/Mining	0.179	(0.227)	0.152	(0.338)	−0.639**	(0.263)	−0.614***	(0.195)	−0.024	(0.314)
Manufacturing	−0.623***	(0.233)	0.534*	(0.304)	−0.776***	(0.254)	0.385***	(0.140)	0.554**	(0.281)
Sales	−0.121	(0.246)	0.407	(0.350)	−0.501**	(0.255)	−0.612***	(0.203)	0.228	(0.323)
Service	0.075	(0.258)	−0.249	(0.465)	0.021	(0.249)	−1.194***	(0.304)	−0.063	(0.393)
Missing	−0.600	(1.048)	−2.933***	(0.504)	−0.289	(0.667)	−2.858***	(0.335)	4.080***	(0.411)
Large Firm	−0.184	(0.188)	−1.663***	(0.298)	−0.082	(0.217)	−1.195***	(0.125)	−1.794***	(0.254)
No. of times laid off	0.142***	(0.029)	0.228***	(0.033)	−0.041	(0.060)	−0.023	(0.035)	0.064	(0.041)
Savings characteristics										
Pension coverage	−1.044***	(0.180)	−0.107	(0.213)	−2.333***	(0.251)	0.575***	(0.123)	0.074	(0.190)
NFA ($10,000s)	−0.005	(0.006)	−0.026**	(0.013)	0.003	(0.003)	0.005***	(0.002)	−0.005	(0.010)
Constant	−0.841	(1.334)	−5.259***	(1.776)	−10.411***	(1.570)	−12.076***	(1.043)	−2.210	(1.532)

Chi-squared = 1350.79   N = 4497

*** p < .01
**p < .05
*p < .10

Table 7.3 Multivariate models predicting Wave I Employment Status: Women

	Employed Part Time		Unemployed		Partly Retired		Retired		Out of Labor Force	
Ascribed characteristics										
Black	0.088	(0.128)	0.288	(0.296)	0.386	(0.252)	0.586***	(0.136)	0.154	(0.147)
Hispanic	0.017	(0.179)	0.628**	(0.316)	-1.083*	(0.603)	-0.432**	(0.217)	0.239	(0.181)
Age	0.033**	(0.014)	0.027	(0.032)	0.143***	(0.029)	0.175***	(0.016)	0.012	(0.016)
Achieved (human capital) characteristics										
Education	0.009	(0.021)	-0.024	(0.042)	0.159***	(0.045)	-0.029	(0.022)	-0.070***	(0.021)
Married	0.827***	(0.107)	0.045	(0.218)	0.842***	(0.222)	0.551***	(0.114)	0.968***	(0.120)
Health										
ADL lim	-0.008	(0.351)	0.559	(0.533)	0.766	(0.571)	1.916***	(0.224)	1.473***	(0.238)
Mobility lim	0.078	(0.106)	0.226	(0.231)	0.122	(0.215)	1.009***	(0.109)	0.789***	(0.110)

Employment characteristics

	Coef.	SE	Coef.	SE	Coef.	SE	Coef.	SE	Coef.	SE
White collar occupation	-0.523***	(0.114)	-0.049	(0.258)	-0.343	(0.228)	0.070	(0.129)	-0.392***	(0.126)
Industry (ref = professional)										
Agriculture/mining	-0.353	(0.297)	-0.755	(0.790)	0.550	(0.445)	-0.441	(0.360)	0.075	(0.283)
Manufacturing	-1.167***	(0.171)	0.583**	(0.288)	-0.407	(0.333)	0.499***	(0.144)	0.176	(0.158)
Sales	0.308***	(0.126)	0.307	(0.310)	0.365	(0.254)	0.491***	(0.147)	0.655***	(0.145)
Service	0.091	(0.137)	0.101	(0.318)	0.154	(0.265)	-0.334*	(0.178)	-0.189	(0.164)
Missing	-0.911	(0.664)	-1.951***	(0.601)	-0.285	(1.071)	3.062***	(0.353)	4.589***	(0.337)
Large Firm	-0.199*	(0.104)	-1.843***	(0.339)	-0.158	(0.222)	-1.807***	(0.139)	-1.601***	(0.159)
No. of times laid off	0.093***	(0.034)	0.237***	(0.043)	0.017	(0.082)	-0.072	(0.048)	-0.067	(0.046)
Savings characteristics										
Pension coverage	-1.032***	(0.108)	-0.786***	(0.248)	-2.202***	(0.268)	-0.250**	(0.117)	-1.553***	(0.139)
NFA ($10,000s)	0.018***	(0.004)	-0.019***	(0.006)	0.012*	(0.007)	0.021***	(0.004)	0.020***	(0.004)
Constant	-2.782***	(0.854)	-4.048**	(1.894)	-12.469***	(1.774)	-11.270***	(0.977)	-1.242	(0.950)

Chi-squared = 1728.87   N = 5068

*** p < .01
**p < .05
*p < .10

rates of part-time work, unemployment, retirement, and nonparticipation. For women, on the other hand, the opposite pattern is found. Married women are more likely to work part-time, to be fully or partly retired, and to be out of the labor force rather than employed. These findings are consistent with prior research that suggests a positive effect of marriage on men's well-being (Waite 1995). For women, on the other hand, marriage confers financial security that discourages labor force participation. The fact that women tend to marry men that are on average older than themselves and that couples tend to make retirement decisions at least somewhat jointly (O'Rand, Henretta, and Krecker 1992) also discourages labor force participation among older married women.

Functional ability is a crucial determinant of labor force participation among the preretirement population. For both men and women, ADL or mobility limitations are associated with lower full-time employment. Not surprisingly, physical impairment raises the odds of being out of the labor force (which includes disabled workers) in Wave I. But those with impaired physical function are also more likely to be partially or fully retired than their unimpaired peers.

Job characteristics also influence preretirement employment opportunities. Older men employed in white-collar occupations are less likely to be retired, and older white-collar women are less likely to work part-time or to be out of the labor force than their peers in other occupations. Thus, for both men and women, white-collar work is associated with extended employment opportunities. Industry is also importantly related to employment prospects in the preretirement years. As expected, men and women with a history of employment in manufacturing and transportation industries are significantly more likely to be unemployed, retired, and, among men, out of the labor force, than workers in professional industries. This finding reflects recent trends toward deindustrialization and the concomitant decline in manufacturing employment that have pushed many older workers, especially men, out of the labor market (DeViney and O'Rand 1988). Several other industries, such as agriculture, sales, and services, offer diminished opportunities for retirement and part-time work, particularly among men. For women, the sales field also stands out as being less hospitable to continued employment, as women employed in sales are more likely to work part-time, to retire, or to be out of the labor force than women in professional fields.

Firm size also structures labor force participation in the years proximate to retirement. Employees of large firms experience lower odds of unemployment, nonparticipation, and retirement than employees of smaller firms. This is likely due to the relationship between productivity, income, and age. While average income rises steadily with age, productivity generally levels off or even declines slightly, making older workers more expensive to retain than younger workers. Smaller companies are less able or less willing to bear these extra costs, and workers with a history of employment in such firms leave the labor market at younger ages, on average, than their peers at larger firms.

Men and women with prior lay-off experience have higher odds of unemployment than other workers. Previous research suggests that these workers are most vulnerable to premature withdrawal from the market (Diamond and Hausman 1984; Hayward et al. 1998). But a history of employment instability is also associated with higher odds of part-time employment. Thus, workers with unstable work histories are simultaneously more vulnerable to continued labor market disruptions as they age and less able to depart through traditional retirement pathways. Instead, they may be forced into part-time employment and "bridge" jobs, which generally have lower salaries, benefits, and stability than career jobs (Doeringer 1990).

Finally, pension coverage and private savings represent important "pull" factors that affect late-aged labor force participation among both men and women. Pensioned older men are more likely to be retired and less likely to work part-time than their unpensioned counterparts, while women who work in jobs that offer retirement benefits are more likely to be working full-time than women who lack such benefits. Private savings render men and women less likely to be unemployed and more likely to be retired, and encourage nonparticipation and part-time work among women.

Thus, even in the cross-section, numerous challenges stand out to age-based retirement benefit systems. All respondents included in the analysis were 61 or younger in the first wave of the HRS and thus were not eligible even for early Social Security benefits. Nevertheless, significant numbers had already left the labor market. Moreover, racial and ethnic minorities were more likely to have left full-time employment by Wave I, and increased vulnerability to involuntary forms of joblessness was also evident among the less-educated and those with less favorable employment history characteristics.

Labor Market Pathways across Waves of the HRS

We next extend this cross-sectional view by examining employment pathways across the first four waves of the HRS. Referring back to Table 7.1, we see important differences between minorities and whites in movement out of the labor force across waves of the HRS. Among men, whites exhibit the traditional patterns of labor force participation, with a low incidence of part-time work, disability, and unemployment and with a steady decline in full-time employment and concomitant rise in retirement across waves. Minority men present a very different picture. They begin the period with significantly lower full-time employment, particularly for blacks. Rates of disability are higher than for whites and grow more dramatically over time. Unemployment is also more prominent among minority men. While full-time work falls steeply over time, retirement does not rise as rapidly as it does for whites. Relative to blacks, Hispanics exhibit higher rates of labor force participation and significantly lower rates of retirement, most likely due to their limited rates of pension eligibility.

Overall, women exhibit lower rates of full-time and higher rates of part-time work and nonparticipation (primarily homemaking) than men. Once again, racial and ethnic differences among women are much more modest than among men. White and black women exhibit similar levels of full-time and part-time work across waves. However, black women are significantly more likely than their white counterparts to be disabled and less likely to be out of the labor force/homemakers (not shown). Hispanic women have much lower labor force participation than either black or white women and experience a steeper drop in participation across waves. In sharp contrast to white and black women, Hispanic women are more likely to be out of the labor force (homemakers) than employed full time across all waves of the survey.

To understand the factors undergirding group differences in pathways out of the labor market, we estimate multinomial logit models predicting change in employment status across waves. The key question from these analyses is whether minorities are at greater risk than whites of exiting the labor market via unemployment and nonparticipation. The results, reported in Tables 7.4 and 7.5 for men and women, respectively, exclude those who were fully retired or out of the labor force in Wave I, since these individuals were very unlikely to reenter the labor market across waves.

Empirical estimates show significant race and ethnic effects on pathways out of the labor market across waves, again with important differences by gender. Among men, older African Americans are more likely than their white counterparts to move into part-time work and unemployment, and are less likely to partially retire. Hispanic men are also more likely to become unemployed across waves, but are significantly less likely than whites to move into either full or partial retirement. Among women, racial and ethnic disparities in employment pathways are much more modest. Older black women are more likely to move into part-time work over time, but are otherwise similar to white women. Hispanic women, on the other hand, are significantly more likely to become unemployed over time and are less likely to retire than white women. It is important to note that minority men and women are also significantly more likely than their white peers to exit the survey over time.

Taken together, the preceding analyses demonstrate that minorities are both more likely to be unemployed and out of the labor force in the cross-section and more likely to become unemployed over time. Previous research using the first two waves of the HRS shows that once unemployed, black workers are also more likely than similarly situated whites to exit unemployment by withdrawing from the labor force. Hispanic workers are more likely to remain unemployed relative to becoming reemployed (Flippen and Tienda 2000). Once again, these results underscore the salience of race and ethnicity in structuring pathways out of the labor market. They confirm that blacks and Hispanics, but particularly blacks, are disadvantaged relative to whites in their ability to maintain labor force attachment leading up to retirement age. The income consequences of premature labor market withdrawal, especially in the absence of adequate pension supports, point to larger race and ethnic economic inequality in the future as greater numbers of minorities reach retirement age.

The effects of education, marital status, and health status on change in labor force participation across waves closely parallel those reported for the cross-sectional analysis. For both men and women, the likelihood of retirement rises with age. Education encourages later labor force participation, reducing the odds of part-time work, retirement, and nonparticipation. Once again, marital status influences the employment decisions of men and women in markedly different ways. Older married men are less likely to become unemployed, to retire, and

Table 7.4 Multivariate models predicting change in employment statues, Waves I–IV: Men

	Employed Part Time		Unemployed		Partly Retired		Retired		Out of Labor Force		Survey Exit	
Ascribed characteristics												
Black	0.439***	(0.150)	0.416*	(0.234)	-0.255*	(0.149)	-0.059	(0.115)	0.311	(0.216)	0.502***	(0.105)
Hispanic	0.144	(0.192)	0.584**	(0.271)	-0.330*	(0.200)	-0.396***	(0.161)	-0.077	(0.280)	0.432***	(0.130)
Age	0.022	(0.017)	-0.014	(0.027)	0.188***	(0.013)	0.252***	(0.012)	-0.036	(0.026)	0.034***	(0.012)
Achieved (human capital) characteristics												
Education	-0.043**	(0.020)	-0.008	(0.031)	0.025	(0.018)	-0.049***	(0.015)	-0.095***	(0.028)	-0.046***	(0.014)
Married	-0.086	(0.151)	-0.454**	(0.212)	-0.023	(0.131)	-0.275***	(0.106)	-0.884***	(0.186)	-0.471***	(0.099)
Health												
ADL lim	0.195	(0.316)	0.158	(0.468)	-0.076	(0.267)	0.289	(0.193)	1.145***	(0.306)	-0.156	(0.249)
Mobility lim	-0.096	(0.150)	0.152	(0.219)	-0.024	(0.120)	0.536***	(0.090)	0.396**	(0.198)	0.185*	(0.099)
Employment characteristics												
White collar occupation	0.226	(0.136)	0.287	(0.207)	0.064	(0.107)	0.027	(0.090)	-0.234	(0.214)	0.086	(0.093)
Industry (Ref = professional)												
Agriculture/mining	0.340**	(0.176)	0.598**	(0.302)	0.059	(0.154)	0.087	(0.133)	0.822***	(0.302)	0.114	(0.128)
Manufacturing	-0.374**	(0.178)	0.239	(0.271)	-0.040	(0.126)	0.128	(0.102)	0.631**	(0.288)	-0.037	(0.107)
Sales	0.194	(0.179)	0.557*	(0.295)	0.169	(0.142)	-0.109	(0.134)	0.637**	(0.325)	-0.049	(0.130)
Service	0.364*	(0.190)	0.690**	(0.317)	0.241	(0.153)	-0.039	(0.149)	0.616*	(0.351)	0.011	(0.147)

	(1)		(2)		(3)		(4)		(5)		(6)	
Large firm	-0.111	(0.144)	0.199	(0.211)	0.206**	(0.106)	0.534***	(0.089)	-0.297	(0.213)	-0.061	(0.092)
No. of times laid off	0.099***	(0.025)	0.103***	(0.037)	0.042	(0.027)	0.026	(0.023)	0.022	(0.039)	0.007	(0.023)
Savings characteristics												
Pension coverage	-0.606***	(0.133)	-0.264	(0.204)	-0.154	(0.104)	0.267***	(0.092)	-0.202	(0.195)	-0.105	(0.090)
NFA ($10,000s)	0.003*	(0.002)	-0.030***	(0.012)	0.004***	(0.001)	0.001	(0.002)	-0.015	(0.012)	0.000	(0.002)
Previous wave employment status												
Part time	2.451***	(0.137)	1.412***	(0.279)	1.431***	(0.173)	1.064***	(0.162)	1.397***	(0.251)	0.879***	(0.150)
Unemployed	1.496***	(0.261)	2.793***	(0.248)	1.468***	(0.256)	1.911***	(0.185)	2.268***	(0.261)	0.944***	(0.214)
Partially retired	1.598***	(0.223)	1.667***	(0.354)	3.615***	(0.127)	2.354***	(0.137)	1.472***	(0.343)	1.430***	(0.167)
Constant	-3.793***	(1.016)	-3.353**	(1.620)	-13.917***	(0.847)	-16.339***	(0.754)	-0.455	(1.550)	-3.144***	(0.712)

Chi-squared = 2951.21   N = 9226

*** p < .01
**p < .05
*p < .10

Table 7.5 Multivariate models predicting change in employment statues, Waves I–IV: Women

	Employed Part Time		Unemployed		Partly Retired		Retired		Out of Labor Force		Survey Exit	
Ascribed characteristics												
Black	0.231**	(0.104)	0.197	(0.231)	0.000	(0.146)	0.062	(0.109)	0.112	(0.159)	0.249**	(0.123)
Hispanic	-0.056	(0.154)	0.739***	(0.262)	-0.237	(0.245)	-0.306*	(0.179)	0.310	(0.201)	0.557***	(0.157)
Age	0.018	(0.012)	0.030	(0.026)	0.242***	(0.016)	0.250***	(0.013)	-0.011	(0.018)	0.041***	(0.014)
Achieved (human capital) characteristics												
Education	-0.018	(0.017)	-0.014	(0.036)	0.043*	(0.024)	-0.014	(0.018)	-0.043*	(0.025)	-0.041**	(0.020)
Married	0.400***	(0.085)	-0.044	(0.174)	0.352***	(0.113)	0.421***	(0.086)	0.320***	(0.127)	0.171*	(0.097)
Health												
ADL lim	-0.073	(0.251)	0.556	(0.395)	0.366	(0.279)	0.495***	(0.199)	0.819***	(0.252)	0.204	(0.263)
Mobility lim	-0.159*	(0.085)	-0.011	(0.185)	0.156	(0.110)	0.391***	(0.083)	0.245**	(0.125)	0.025	(0.100)
Employment characteristics												
Professional occupation	-0.281***	(0.094)	0.054	(0.208)	-0.233*	(0.128)	-0.107	(0.100)	-0.493***	(0.142)	-0.083	(0.115)
Industry (Ref = professional)												
Agriculture/mining	-0.059	(0.238)	-0.522	(0.747)	0.091	(0.317)	0.098	(0.261)	0.650**	(0.301)	0.212	(0.299)
Manufacturing	-0.606***	(0.135)	0.113	(0.253)	-0.182	(0.171)	0.086	(0.113)	0.027	(0.185)	0.176	(0.129)
Sales	0.136	(0.108)	0.591***	(0.227)	0.238	(0.145)	-0.008	(0.121)	0.368**	(0.172)	0.370***	(0.133)
Service	0.098	(0.115)	0.363	(0.248)	0.155	(0.154)	0.013	(0.130)	0.557***	(0.163)	0.205	(0.145)

Large firm	−0.112	(0.088)	−0.027	(0.194)	0.031	(0.117)	0.159*	(0.087)	−0.116	(0.142)	−0.022	(0.102)
No. of times laid off	0.027	(0.029)	0.127***	(0.044)	−0.015	(0.043)	−0.008	(0.032)	0.042	(0.038)	−0.021	(0.037)
Savings characteristics												
Pension coverage	−0.423***	(0.091)	−0.617***	(0.201)	−0.288**	(0.121)	0.138	(0.093)	−0.805***	(0.151)	−0.075	(0.108)
NFA ($10,000s)	0.007***	(0.002)	−0.001	(0.008)	0.006**	(0.003)	0.007***	(0.003)	0.000	(0.006)	0.002	(0.004)
Previous wave employment status												
Part time	2.967***	(0.088)	1.211***	(0.218)	2.141***	(0.130)	1.383***	(0.107)	1.626***	(0.140)	1.021***	(0.123)
Unemployed	1.680***	(0.213)	2.756***	(0.246)	1.761***	(0.281)	1.855***	(0.199)	2.435***	(0.212)	1.115***	(0.243)
Partially retired	2.657***	(0.199)	1.524***	(0.454)	4.174***	(0.190)	3.061***	(0.182)	2.249***	(0.264)	1.889***	(0.234)
Constant	−2.874***	(0.725)	−5.259***	(1.570)	−17.457***	(1.024)	−16.581***	(0.790)	−1.749	(1.103)	−4.187***	(0.861)
Chi-squared = 3399.21		N = 8063										

*** p < .01
**p < .05
*p < .10

to move out of the labor force over time than unmarried men. Older married women, on the other hand, are less likely to remain employed full-time, experiencing higher odds of moving into part-time work, partial or full retirement, or nonparticipation across waves. These results buttress the conclusions drawn earlier from Tables 7.2 and 7.3, and highlight continued gender differences in the determinants of retirement.

Physical limitations encourage retirement and nonparticipation for both men and women. Hence, for older workers in better financial circumstances, failing health could induce early retirement; while among those with less fortuitous economic prospects, functional limitations could precipitate labor market withdrawal, either with or without disability benefits.

Several employment characteristics also significantly influence labor force pathways for older workers. For women, white-collar occupations offer a protected environment, insulating them from movement into part-time work, partial retirement, and nonparticipation. Men and women in professional industries are also significantly less likely than their peers in agriculture, manufacturing, sales, and service fields to move out of the labor force over time. Among men, agricultural and service workers, and among women, sales workers, are more likely to become unemployed across waves. Employees of large firms, while less likely to be retired in the first wave, are more likely to move into retirement across waves than employees of smaller firms. Those with prior lay-off experience are more likely to become unemployed across waves, and, among men, are also more likely to move into part-time employment.

Savings characteristics are another important determinant of employment patterns across waves. Pension coverage lowers part-time work and raises retirement among men, while uniformly encouraging employment among women. It seems that for women, pension status represents an aspect of job quality that encourages continued employment and discourages labor market exit across the board. Household savings encourage retirement for both men and women, and, for men, also discourage movement into unemployment.

Finally, there is tremendous continuity in employment status across waves, as indicated by the effect of previous-wave employment status on change over time. Those who are not working full-time in a given wave are significantly less likely to return to full-time employment across waves, and there is considerable movement across nonemployed categories. It is telling that unemployment in a previous wave makes movement out of the labor force particularly likely. Previous research has shown that this extremely disadvantaged pathway is more common among minority than among white unemployed workers (Couch 1998; Flippen and Tienda 2000).

Conclusions

Overall, these results confirm that blacks and Hispanics are more vulnerable than whites to involuntary job loss in the preretirement years. They are more likely to exit the labor force through pathways other than retirement, exhibiting higher rates of unemployment and nonparticipation in the cross-section and greater movement into unemployment and part-time work over time. Once unemployed, they are less likely to become reemployed and more likely either to experience protracted unemployment or to exit the labor force altogether (Flippen and Tienda 2000).

Race differences in employment status are greater among older men than older women, largely because mature black women have labor force histories that compare favorably to white women. However, this does not mean that black women are not disadvantaged relative to white men as they approach retirement age. On the contrary, both black and white women exhibit higher rates of unemployment and nonparticipation than white men at older ages.

Often neglected in studies of retirement, Hispanics are similar to blacks in their patterns of labor market exit. Hispanic men and women exhibit rates of unemployment comparable to those of blacks, and among women, Hispanics stand out as being particularly disadvantaged in the labor market. Clearly, more attention should be paid to older Hispanic workers, who are likely to face mounting labor market difficulties as greater numbers reach preretirement ages and as the returns to education remain high. Because Hispanics have very low education levels, on average, their market prospects at advanced ages remain particularly bleak. As this rapidly growing population ages, this issue will become an important policy concern.

The persistent racial and ethnic disparities in employment among statistically comparable mature adults testifies to the powerful influence of ascribed characteristics on labor force behavior throughout the life course. At a minimum, these findings support a status maintenance perspective on aging inequality. Groups that experience labor market difficulties during prime-aged working years, such as those employed in low-skill occupations, small firms, and industries vulnerable to downsizing during cyclical downturns, are also subject to job dislocation and involuntary pathways out of the labor market as they approach retirement age. Likewise, employment instability at younger ages is associated with decreased earnings and lower occupational mobility, and it heightens workers' vulnerability to employment disruptions and premature labor force withdrawal in the preretirement years. On balance, these results imply that as greater numbers of disadvantaged minority workers age, economic inequality among seniors is likely to increase. Preretirement labor force activity is clearly embedded in earlier work experiences, thus both ameliorative and preventive measures for groups that experienced labor market disadvantages during their prime working years are warranted.

These findings have important implications for the future well-being of elderly minorities, who are often motivated to bolster low retirement income and savings through prolonged labor force participation. Combined with secular trends toward independent living among elderly persons, the inability of many minority seniors to prolong market activity implies that large segments will continue to be at serious risk of poverty in old age. The income consequences of premature labor market withdrawal, especially in the absence of adequate pension supports, point to substantial race and ethnic economic inequality in the future as greater numbers of minorities reach retirement ages. The fact that the U.S. retirement welfare system is based largely on chronological age rather than ability to work (in that disability benefits are far less generous and more difficult to obtain than Social Security benefits) only exacerbates this problem.

Thus, these findings sound a warning to the many scholars and public policy planners who advocate measures to increase labor force participation among elderly persons as a means of prolonging Social Security solvency. Because such policies emphasize labor supply rather than labor demand, they neglect potentially adverse impacts on the economic well-being of elderly low-skill and minority workers, for whom the labor market often represents an inhospitable environment.

Moreover, these policies neglect the substantial impediment to increased labor supply posed by poor health and functional limitations, another factor that disproportionately affects minority workers. Any reduction in Social Security benefits achieved through delaying the standard retirement age will likely be at least partially offset by rising disability claims.

Notes

1. The analyses are restricted to age-eligible HRS respondents because their non-age-eligible spouses are not randomly selected and therefore not nationally representative. Analyses are further restricted to persons who had worked during the twenty years before the baseline interview in 1992 because employment pathways are not salient for those who had withdrawn from the market before that time.

2. Respondents in the HRS were asked if they had any difficulties performing a wide array of tasks, ranging from picking up a dime to climbing several flights of stairs. Respondents who experience difficulty getting out of bed, bathing, dressing, or feeding themselves are defined as having an ADL limitation. Mobility/large muscle limitations are defined as difficulty with at least one of the following: walking several blocks, walking across a room, climbing several flights of stairs, sitting for two hours, getting up after sitting for an extended period, stooping, kneeling, crouching, or pushing or pulling heavy objects.

3. Though mature black women fare relatively well compared to white women, they are still disadvantaged in the market relative to white men. Previous tabulations (Flippen and Tienda 2000) from a model testing for interaction effects among race, ethnicity, and sex showed that black women, like black men, are significantly more likely than statistically comparable white men to be unemployed, retired, and out of the labor force. White women are also more likely to be unemployed than their male counterparts, but these differences are on the margin of statistical significance. Thus, black women's historically high labor force participation rates may attenuate their economic marginalization at advanced ages, but the vestiges of disadvantage persist throughout the life course.

References

Belgrave, L. L. 1988. The effects of race differences in work history, work attitudes, economic resources, and health on women's retirement. *Research on Aging* 10:383–98.

Boaz, R. 1988. Early withdrawal from the labor force: A response only to pension pull or also to labor market push? *Research on Aging* 9:530–47.

Bound, J., M. Schoenbaum, and T. Waidman. 1995. Race and education differences in disability status and labor force attachment in the Health and Retirement Study. *Journal of Human Resources* 30:S227–67.

Burr, J. A., M. P. Massagli, J. E. Mutchler, and A. M. Pienta. 1996. Labor force transitions among older African American and white men. *Social Forces* 74:963–82.

Couch, K. A. 1998. Late life job displacement. *Gerontologist* 38:7–17.

DeViney, S., and A. M. O'Rand. 1988. Gender-cohort succession and retirement among older men and women, 1951 to 1984. *Sociological Quarterly* 29:525–40.

Diamond, P. A., and J. A. Hausman. 1984. The retirement and unemployment behavior of older men. In H. Aaron and G. Burtless, eds., *Retirement and Economic Behavior.* Washington, D.C.: Brookings Institute.

Doeringer, P. 1990. Economic security, labor market flexibility, and bridges to retirement. Pp. 3–19 in P. Doeringer, ed., *Bridges to Retirement*: I.L.P. Press.

Flippen, C. A., and M. Tienda. 2000. Pathways to retirement: patterns of labor force participation and labor market exit among the pre-retirement population by race, Hispanic origin and sex. *Journal of Gerontology-Social Sciences* 55B:S14–27.

Gibson, R. C. 1987. Reconceptualizing retirement for black Americans. *Gerontologist* 27:691–98.

Gibson, R. C. 1993. The black American retirement experience. Pp. 277–97 in J. S. Jackson, L. M. Chatters, and R. J. Taylor, eds., *Aging in Black America.* Thousand Oaks, Calif.: Sage.

Gohmann, S. F. 1990. Retirement differences among the respondents to the Retirement History Survey. *Journal of Gerontology* 45:S120–27.

Gustman, A., and T. Steinmeier. 1986. A disaggregated, structural analysis of retirement by race difficulty to work and health. *Review of Economics and Statistics* 68:509–13.

Hayward, M. D., and W. R. Grady. 1990. Work and retirement among a cohort of older men in the United States, 1966–1983. *Demography* 27:337–56.

Hayward, M. D., and M. Heron. 1999. Racial inequality in active life among adult Americans. *Demography* 36:77–91.

Hayward, M. D., S. Friedman, and H. Chen. 1996. Race inequities in men's retirement. *Journal of Gerontology: Social Sciences* 51B:S1–10.

Hayward, M. D., W. R. Grady, M. Hardy, and D. Sommers. 1989. Occupational influences on retirement, disability, and death. *Demography* 26:393–409.

Manton, K. G. and X. Gu. 2001. Changes in the Prevalence of Chronic Disability in the United States Black and Non-black Population above Age

65 from 1982 to 1999. Proceedings of the National Academy of Sciences 98:6354–59.

Manton, K. G., and E. Stallard. 1997. Health and disability differences among racial and ethnic groups. Pp. 43–105 in L. G. Martin and B. J. Soldo, eds., *Racial and Ethnic Differences in the Health of Older Americans*. Washington, D.C.: National Academy Press.

Martin, L. G., and B. J. Soldo, eds. 1997. *Racial and Ethnic Differences in the Health of Older Americans*. Washington, D.C.: National Academy Press.

Mitchell, O. S., P. B. Levine, and J. W. Phillips. 1999. The impact of pay inequality, occupational segregation, and lifetime work experience on the retirement income of women and minorities. *AARP Public Policy Institute Paper #9910*. Washington, D.C.: AARP.

Murphy, K. M., and F. Welch. 1993. Industrial change and the rising importance of skill. In S. Danziger and P. Gottschalk, eds., *Uneven Tides: Rising Inequality in America*. New York: Russell Sage Foundation.

Mutchler, J. E., J. A. Burr, M. P. Massagli, and A. Pienta. 1999. Work transitions and health in later life. *Journal of Gerontology-Social Sciences* 54B:S252–61.

O'Rand, A. M., and J. C. Henretta. 1999. *Age and Inequality: Diverse Pathways through Later Life*. Boulder, Colo.: Westview Press.

O'Rand, A. M., J. C. Henretta, and M. L. Krecker. 1992. Family pathways to retirement. Pp. 81–98 in M. Szinovacz et al., eds., *Family Retirement*. Thousand Oaks, Calif.: Sage.

Quinn, J. F. 1999. New paths to retirement. In B. Hammond, O. Mitchell, and A. Rappaport, eds., *Forecasting Retirement Needs and Retirement Wealth*. Philadelphia: University of Pennsylvania Press.

Quinn, J. F., and M. Kozy. 1996. The role of bridge jobs in the retirement transition: Gender, race and ethnicity. *Gerontologist* 36:363–72.

Ruhm, C. J. 1996. Gender differences in employment behavior during late middle life. *Journal of Gerontology* 51B:S11–17.

Santiago, A. M., and C. G. Muschkin. 1996. Disentangling the effects of disability status and gender on the labor supply of Anglo, Black and Latino older workers. *Gerontologist* 36:299–310.

Smith, J. P., and R. S. Kington. 1997. Race, socioeconomic status and health in late life. Pp. 106–62 in L. G. Martin and B. J. Soldo, eds., *Racial and Ethnic Differences in the Health of Older Americans*. Washington, D.C.: National Academy Press.

Waite, L. J. 1995. Does marriage matter? *Demography* 32:483–507.

Wray, L. A. 1996. The role of ethnicity in the disability and work experience of preretirement-age Americans. *Gerontologist* 36:287–98.

Wykle, M., and B. Kaskel. 1991. Increasing the longevity of minority older adults through improved health status. Pp. 24–31 in J. L. Angel and D. P. Hogan, eds., *Minority Elders: Longevity, Economics and Health*. Washington, D.C.: Gerontological Society of America.

Zsembik, B. A., and A. Singer. 1990. The problem of defining retirement among minorities: The Mexican Americans. *Gerontologist* 30:749–57.

8. The Oldest Old and a Long-Lived Society
Challenges for Public Policy
Judith G. Gonyea

The definition of old age as beginning at age 65 is a relatively recent phenomenon. It reflects the decision of European nations and the United States in the formation of their old-age social insurance programs in early part of the twentieth century to establish this chronological age as determining eligibility. With the passage of the 1935 Social Security Act, the United States instituted the age of 65 as the marker of "normal retirement" and the beginning of "old age." Increasing life expectancies, however, are causing us to rethink what we mean by "old." Today, we often do not think of a healthy, vigorous, and socially engaged person in his or her 60s or 70s as "elderly." In fact, one-third of Americans in their 70s perceive of themselves as "middle-aged" (National Council on Aging 2000).

Gains in life expectancy have resulted in members of the U.S. older population spanning four—even five—decades. Individuals in their 60s, 70s, 80s, 90s, and 100s are all found among the ranks of the elderly. The growing age diversity of the older population suggests increasing heterogeneity in members' health status, behavioral patterns, economic status, and social arrangements. The "democratization of aging"—that is, the new reality that the vast majority of Americans are attaining old age and even advanced old age—has led researchers, practitioners, and policymakers to differentiate between the "young old" and the "oldest old" (Neugarten 1974; Harris et al. 1978; Treas and Bengston 1982). In fact, the term "oldest old" was coined by Matilda White Riley and Richard Suzman in a presentation at the 1984 American Association for the Advancement of Science meeting in which they strove to draw the scientific community's attention to this emerging age population. As editors of a special issue of *Milbank Quarterly* devoted to the topic of the oldest old, Suzman and Riley wrote that it was "so new a phenomenon that there is little in historical experience that can help in interpreting it." Yet they also went on to predict that given their rising numbers, the oldest old would "no longer remain invisible" in the economy, the polity, and the health and social service systems (1985, p. 177). Reflecting the accuracy of their prophecy, the three age categories of: the young old (65 years to 74 years), the middle old (75 years to 84 years), and oldest old (85 years and older) are now often employed by demographers, economists, social, behavioral and health researchers, and policymakers to both describe and predict trends in the U.S. older population.

The significance of the aging of the older population—and the even faster growing very old population—has not been lost on the world of public policy. The public policy outlook of an aging United States has become increasingly dire, as referents have moved from "the graying of the federal budget" (Hudson 1978) to "a fiscal black hole" (Callaghan 1987) to nothing less than "apocalyptic demographic forecasts" (Robertson 1991). Concomitantly, the long-held view of older people as "deserving" has come into question. Older citizens are viewed as "greedy," and concerns are voiced about intergenerational justice and equity. The political power of elderly persons and their disproportionate use of public resources are viewed as restricting disadvantaged children's access to adequate nutrition, health care, and education (Preston 1984). Intergenerational conflict is at the heart of the *New York Times* columnist William Safire's May 15, 1995, op-ed piece in which he wrote that borrowing to fund the growing deficit is "no longer . . . a gift to our old but a theft from our young."

Concerns about the extent of public spending on older people are reflected in the current debates about privatization of Social Security and managed care as a mechanism to control the public health care costs of Medicare. Growing concerns about the increasing public costs of these programs are legitimate; nonetheless, they often ignore the significant gains in the older population's well-being that have directly resulted from federal expenditures. Social Security has been central to the threefold drop, over a thirty-year period, in poverty among the aged; Medicare has brought acute health care coverage to virtually the entire older population, literally twice what it was in 1965; and Medicaid has funded vast amounts of intensive long-term care services. These comments ignore, as well, the particular areas of vulnerability associated with the recent and continuous rise of the oldest old.

As the following discussion makes clear, the oldest old are diverse.

While they are the least likely to fit the new stereotype of the elderly described by Robert Binstock (1994) as "prosperous, hedonistic, selfish, and politically powerful"; neither are they inevitably poor, frail, and isolated. Still, as we will discuss, advanced old age is associated with a greater risk of experiencing economic hardship and disabling health conditions. Two key policy questions are: What will be the impact of an increasing number of oldest old members of the U.S. systems of care such as health care delivery and financing, informal caregiving, and public and private pensions? And how do we as a society respond to the challenges of an aging population to promote the economic well-being and health of our very oldest citizens? The policy test lies in identifying individuals who have disabilities or vulnerabilities associated with very advanced age and asking how policy responses can be better directed toward these needs and whether such responses should be based on advanced chronological age alone or on functional status and income measures, which may apply to populations of all ages.

Population Trends and the Oldest Old

Over the past century the number of older Americans has increased more than tenfold, to 35 million age 65 or older in 2000. Currently one in eight Americans is age 65 or older, and by 2030 demographers estimate that one in five Americans will be among the ranks of the elderly. Equally important, the older population is also aging as more persons are surviving to their 80s and 90s. The population age 85 and older is currently the fastest growing segment of the older population. In 2000, approximately 2 percent of the U.S. population or about 4 million Americans were age 85 and older; by 2050, the ranks of the oldest old is projected to increase to almost 5 percent of the U.S. population or almost 19 million Americans (see Fig. 8.1). Currently, there are about 65,000 individuals age 100 or older in the United States, and the number of centenarians is projected to reach 381,000 persons by 2030 (U.S. Bureau of the Census 2000). Many of these dramatic changes in the older population that will occur during the next four to five decades are, in fact, due to the baby boom cohort's arrival at old age. As reflected in Figure 8.1, the most rapid increase in the population 85 years and older will occur between 2030 and 2050 as the baby boom generation join the ranks of the very old. Based on increasing life expectancies, the Census Bureau's population projections suggest

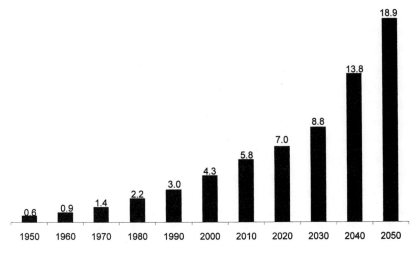

Fig. 8.1. U.S. population age 85 years and older, 1950 to 2050 (in millions).
Source: U.S. Bureau of the Census 1996

that by the middle of this century, more than 40 percent of adults age 65 and older can expect to live to at least age 90 (U.S. Bureau of the Census 2000).

It is immediately striking, however, that the oldest old are predominantly women. In 2000 there was a sex ratio of two men for every three women age 65 and older; however, this gap widens among the oldest-old. At ages 85 and older, the ratio is approximately 4 men for every 10 women. In fact, in recent years the sex ratio has narrowed as the gap between male and female life expectancy has decreased. In 2000 American women who reached age 65 could expect to live an additional 19 years, while American men could anticipate another 16 years. This narrowing of the gender gap in life expectancy is primarily due to declining male mortality rates in deaths due to heart disease. In the decades of the 1980s and 90s, the mortality rates for heart disease and stroke—two of the three leading killers of older Americans— declined by approximately one-third (Federal Interagency Forum on Aging-Related Statistics 2001). U.S. Census Bureau projections suggest that the sex ratio will continue to rise and level off to about 6 men for every 10 women for those age 85 and older by 2050 (U.S. Bureau of the Census 2000).

The nation's older population is becoming more racially and ethnically diverse, although not as rapidly as the total U.S. population. Currently the vast majority (86.7%) of Americans 85 and older identify as non-Hispanic white; however, the percentages of black and Hispanic-origin elders are projected to steadily increase throughout the next decades. By 2050, the proportion of blacks and Hispanics who are 80 years and older could increase to approximately one-third. Significant differences in life expectancies, however, do exist by race. For example, the life expectancy at birth is lower for blacks than for whites; and at most ages, the mortality rates of blacks are higher than for whites. In 2000, the life expectancy of white women exceeded that of black women by about five years. This black-white life expectancy gap narrows and falls to zero at age 85. This narrowing results from a "crossover" in the mortality rates for blacks and whites in advanced old age. After the age of 90, blacks have more years of additional life than do whites. There is debate about the meaning of the crossover phenomenon, with some suggesting it is an artifact of inaccurate birth dates (i.e., lack of birth records, overstatement of ages) and others offering sociobiological explanations of a select group surviving harsh conditions in early life (Elo and Preston 1994; Johnson 2000)

The Social World of the Oldest Old

Given that women both live longer than men and tend to marry men who are older than they are, it is not surprising that women are less likely to share their later years of life with a spouse (Fig. 8.2). Whereas 60 percent of men aged 85 and older are married, only 13 percent of their female counterparts have partners. More than three-quarters (79%) of women age 85 or older are widows, compared to 33 percent of men age 85-plus. Although few of the current cohort of oldest old are either divorced (3%) or never married (4%), these percentages will rise as future generations, such as the baby boomers, enter the ranks of this age group (U.S. Bureau of the Census 2002). These generational shifts in marital and divorce patterns may have a significant impact on the well-being of future cohorts of American elders, since marital status is correlated with a number of measures of economic, physical, and emotional well-being in later life. Older married individuals, on average, have higher household incomes, better physical health, lower rates of depression, and less risk of institutionalization as compared to their nonmarried counterparts. Indeed, spouses are the primary caregivers for frail and disabled partners.

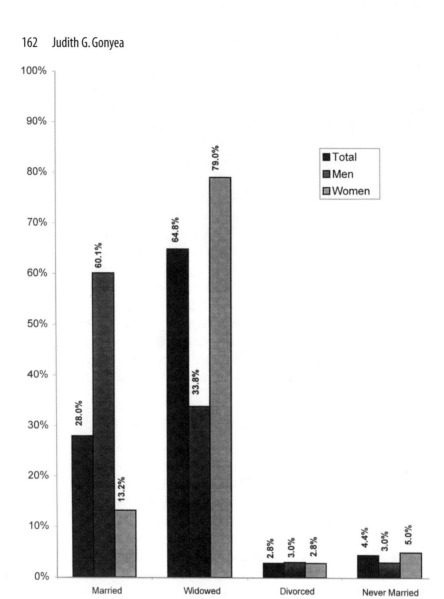

Fig. 8.2. Marital status of Americans age 85 and older, by gender, 2002.
Source: U.S. Bureau of the Census 2002

  The gender gap in spouse survivorship affects living arrangements
in later life. Older women are at least twice as likely as older men to
live alone. By age 85, six out of ten women live alone, compared to
only three out of ten men (National Center for Health Statistics 1999).
Older persons typically enter nursing homes when physical disabilities

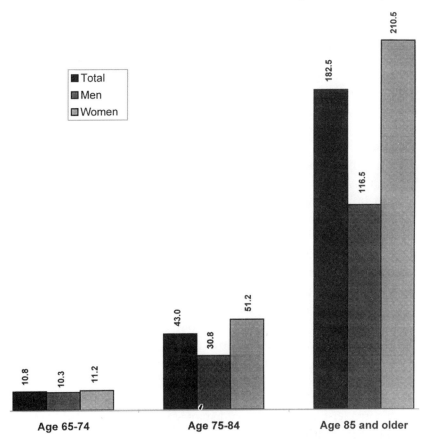

Fig. 8.3. Nursing home residence (residents per 1,000 population) for older Americans, by age and gender, 1999. Source: Federal Interagency Forum on Aging-Related Statistics 2001

and/or mental incapacity prevent them from living on their own or being cared for within the community. Although only a small proportion of the young old—approximately 1 percent of persons age 65 to 74 and 4.7 percent of persons age 75 to 84—resided in nursing homes in 2000, this figure rises dramatically to slightly more than one in five (22.2%) persons age 85 and older (National Center for Health Statistics 2002). Women have higher rates of nursing home residence than do men, and this gender difference increases with age (see Fig. 8.3). More than half of elderly residents in nursing homes are 85 years of age and older, and three-quarters are women. Nearly two-thirds of residents are widowed (Gabrel 2000).

Income and the Very Old

In recent decades, older Americans have experienced greater financial security as a result of the introduction of cost-of-living adjustments (COLAs) to Social Security benefits and the availability of health insurance through the Medicare and Medicaid programs. In 1959, 35 percent of persons age 65 and older were living in poverty—a figure that exceeded the percentage of poor children or working-age adults. Today, only 9.2 percent of adults age 65 to 74 and 11.2 percent of adults age 75 and older were among the ranks of the poor—a statistic that falls below the poverty rates for young children and adults (U.S. Bureau of Labor Statistics and Bureau of the Census 2002). Yet despite considerable economic gains, older women and persons of color are at much greater risk of facing poverty in old age than white men. Table 8.1 presents the percentages of the poor by age, gender, race, and Hispanic origin for the older population in 2001. The interactive effects of gender, race, and age on the experience of poverty are reflected in the fact that the poorest group of elderly people is black or African American women, followed by Hispanic women. Indeed, African American women are four times more likely than older white men to experience poverty in later life, 28 percent versus 7 percent (U.S. Bureau of Labor Statistics and Bureau of Census 2002).

This gender-based economic disparity in old age has led some to comment that although older men experience a mortality disadvantage, they do have a quality of life advantage—particularly older white men (Longino 1988; Barer 1994). As Thompson (1994, p. 10) suggests, "death may come sooner, but later life for older men presents fewer problems." Four factors contribute to the risk of poverty for both men and women in older life: living longer, being widowed, living alone, and a lifetime of working in the secondary sector of the labor force. Yet as noted above, each of these factors is more likely to occur in women's lives.

Health and the Oldest Old

Historically, the image of very old people has been one of frailty. Yet, as Camacho and colleagues (1993) note, whereas "this is an accurate picture for some of the oldest-old, we know that there are many oth-

Table 8.1 Percentage of older Americans living in poverty, by age, gender, race, and Hispanic origin, in 2001

Sex and Age	Total	White	Black	Hispanic Origin*
Both sexes				
65 to 74 years	9.2	7.8	20.2	21.8
75 and older	11.2	10.2	24.2	22.0
Males				
65 to 74 years	6.8	5.7	14.3	17.5
75 and older	7.3	6.4	18.1	19.4
Females				
65 to 74 years	11.2	9.6	24.5	25.0
75 and older	13.6	12.5	28.3	23.7

Source: U.S. Bureau of Labor Statistics and Bureau of the Census 2001, table 1
*Hispanics can be of any race.

ers who are able to maintain a high level of function at this age." In fact, the oldest-old's self-assessments of their health status suggest that the majority view their health positively. Although self-assessed health (rated as excellent, very good, good, fair, or poor) declines with age, approximately three-quarters (77%) of the young-old (65–74) and two-thirds (68%) of the older-older (75 years and older) rated their health as at least "good" in 2000. More self-rating of health as good to excellent is correlated with lower risk of mortality (National Center for Health Statistics 2002). There are, however, significant race and ethnic differences. Throughout the ranks of older adults and for both men and women, Hispanic and non-Hispanic black elders are less likely than non-Hispanic whites to offer a positive assessment of their own health. For example, only one in five African Americans 85 and older rated his or her health as "very good" or "excellent." These discrepancies reflect objective differences in health status and disability as well as cultural and class differences in health assessment (National Center for Health Statistics 1999).

Although noting that chronological age of older adults is not a good indicator of health status since interindividual variations in health are greatest in later life, Santos-Eggimann emphasizes that "from a public health perspective, young and old populations are undoubtedly different. With the emergence of large cohorts of individuals reaching and dying at, an advanced age, aging countries are experiencing an epidemiological transition characterized by changes in the main cause of death and morbidity profile" (2002, p. 287).

The current leading cause of death for persons age 65 and older in the United States is heart disease, followed by cancer, stroke, and chronic obstructive pulmonary diseases. Among adults age 85 and older, heart disease accounts for 40 percent of all deaths (National Center for Health Statistics 1999). These are diseases in which, as Santos-Eggimann (2002) emphasizes, a prolonged period of functional decline, disability, and high rates of heath services utilization typically precede death. Although other chronic diseases have lower fatality rates they also can significantly compromise the older adults' quality of life.

The most common chronic health conditions among the elderly are arthritis, hypertension, heart disease, cancer, diabetes, and stroke (Fig. 8.4). Among the 70 and older population, the majority—63 percent of women and 50 percent of men—report having arthritis, and hypertension affects almost one out of every two elders. Slightly more than one in every ten adults age 70 and older reports having diabetes (National Center for Health Statistics 1999). Again, the prevalence of certain chronic conditions varies by gender, race, and ethnicity. For example, among the elderly, Hispanic and non-Hispanic black women have diabetes prevalence rates that are twice as high as non-Hispanic women (National Center for Health Statistics 1999).

Chronic health conditions often restrict elders' ability to perform the activities of daily living (ADLs) such as dressing, bathing, and eating, and the instrumental activities of daily living (IADLs) such as meal preparation and housecleaning. Once again, the risk of disability increases dramatically with age. Whereas only about 3 percent of non-institutionalized Americans age 65–74 reported problems with ADLs in 2000, this figure rose to almost 10 percent of community-based Americans age 75 and older. Similarly, while only slightly more than 6 percent of community-based Americans age 65 to 74 cited having limitations in IADLs, almost one in five (19.3%) of Americans age 75 or older reported such restrictions (National Center for Health Statistics 2002).

Cognitive impairments, particularly Alzheimer disease and other dementias, also compromise dramatically the quality of life of both the affected elder and his or her family. And once again, the incidence of

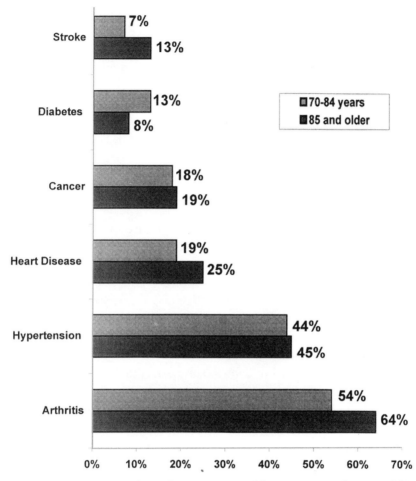

Fig. 8.4. Chronic health conditions among older Americans, by age, 1995.
Source: National Center for Health Statistics 1999

memory problems rises dramatically with age. Although only about 4 percent of adults aged 65 to 69 experience either moderate or severe memory loss, by age 85 one out of every three individuals was found to have at least a moderate memory problem (Federal Interagency Forum on Aging-Related Statistics 2001). Moreover, poor cognitive functioning is a significant risk factor for entering a nursing home. Higher rates of depressive symptoms—which are correlated with poorer physical health, greater functional limitation, and higher rates of health services utilization—are also found among the oldest-old.

While severe depressive symptoms are experienced by approximately 15 percent of adults ages 65 to 69, the incidence of severe symptoms of depressions reaches 23 percent among those 85 and older. Interestingly, while in earlier life stages women are more like to report depressive symptoms than men do, there is no gender difference among the oldest-old. In fact, the suicide rate for persons age 65 and older is higher than for any other age group—and the rate for elders age 85-plus is the highest of all—nearly twice the overall national average (National Center for Health Statistics 1999).

Age-Based Programs and the Oldest Old

As the above discussion makes clear, many of the economic, social, and health characteristics of the oldest old differ from those of the young old. Because of these described factors, the differential importance of public policy allocations for the oldest old, as compared to the young old, cannot be overstated. Receipt of Social Security has become almost universal among older U.S. citizens. In 2001, 91 percent of the aged received a Social Security benefit. Moreover, Social Security represents the largest share of income for older adults. Aggregate income for Americans in later life comes from: Social Security, 39 percent; earnings, 24 percent; pensions, 18 percent; asset income, 16 percent; and other sources, 3 percent (U.S. Social Security Administration 2001). Yet as reflected in Table 8.2, shares of income from each source differ greatly by income level. Older adults in the lowest quintile receive the largest share of their income from the Social Security benefit (82%), and public assistance provides the second largest share (9%). In contrast, for those older adults in the highest income quintile, earnings represent the largest share of income (36%), followed by assets (23%), followed by pensions (20%) and Social Security (19%) (U.S. Social Security Administration 2001). As the oldest age group has the highest poverty rate—among those 80 and older, 12 percent are "poor" and 8 percent are "near poor"—the relative importance of the Social Security benefit to this age population is apparent.

More than 96 percent of older Americans are covered by Medicare, which provides affordable coverage for most acute health care services. The importance of the Medicare Program for older Americans' physical and fiscal well-being cannot be overemphasized. Medicare provides access to such health services as inpatient hospital care, physi-

Table 8.2 Source of income among persons age 65 and older, by income quintile, 2001

Income Source	Lowest Quintile	Second Quintile	Third Quintile	Fourth Quintile	Fifth Quintile
Social Security	82.1%	81.4%	65.4%	45.8%	19.0%
Asset income	2.4	4.6	8.6	11.8	19.0
Pensions	3.2	7.1	14.9	23.2	19.8
Earnings	1.4	3.2	7.8	15.8	36.3
Public assistance	9.2	1.8	0.8	0.3	0.0
Other	1.7	1.8	2.5	3.1	2.3
Total	100.0	100.0	100.0	100.0	100.0

Source: U.S. Bureau of the Census 2002

cian care, outpatient care, home health care, and care at a skilled nursing facility. Although adults age 65 and older made up only 12 percent of the population, National Center for Health Care Statistics reveals that they comprised almost one-quarter (24.3%) of all physician visits—about 200.3 million contacts in 2000. Those 85 and older averaged 15 physician visits per year versus about 11 visits for those age 65 to 84 (O'Neill and Patrick 2002). The 75-plus age group is also much more like to have to have physician visits in the home (28.8%) than is the 65–74 age group (9.7) (National Center for Health Statistics 1999).

Despite Medicare coverage, older Americans still face significant out-of-pocket costs to meet their health care needs. In recent years, growing attention has focused on the lack of a Medicare benefit for prescription medications. Analysis of the 1995 Medicare Current Beneficiary Study revealed that prescribed medications have grown to account for more than one-third of older Americans' total out-of-pocket health care payments (Crystal et al. 2000). These data revealed that the sickest and poorest of older adults—the groups who must often most need health care and are the least able to afford it—face significant out-of-pocket medical expenses, particularly in regard to prescription drugs. Those elders age 85 and older were paying 22 percent of their income for out-of-pocket medical costs versus those age 65–74 who paid 17 percent in total out-of-pocket costs for health care. Although older adults in the highest-fifth income level devoted only 9 percent of their income to out-of-pocket health care costs, elderly Americans in the lowest-fifth income level spent almost a third of their

Table 8.3 Projections of national long-term care expenditures for elderly persons, 2000 (in billions of 2000 dollars)

Payer	Institutional	Home	Total
Medicare	12.3	17.1	29.4
Medicaid	36.2	7.1	43.3
Private long-term care insurance	<5	<5	5.0
Out-of-pocket	34.3	8.5	42.8
Other payer	<5	<5	<5
Total	85.8	37.2	123.1

Source: U.S. Congressional Budget Office 1999

income on health care costs (Crystal et al. 2000). This study underscores the potential impact that Medicare reform proposals, particularly around the creation of a subsidized prescription drug benefit, could have on the most physically and economically vulnerable of older Americans.

In fact, analysis of Medicare beneficiary data reveals significant differences in health care expenditures and types of services by different age groups within the older population. In 1999 the 85-plus age group's $16,596 average annual expenditure (both out-of-pocket costs and insurance costs) for health care was almost 2.5 times as great as the 65 to 69 age group's average expenditure of $6,711. For those entering old age—the 65 to 69 age group—the largest share of health care costs are for inpatient hospitalization (37.8%) and medical outpatient care (37.2%) followed by prescription drugs (13.3%). In contrast, for the oldest old—the 85-plus age group—the largest share of health care costs are for nursing home care (45.5%) followed by inpatient hospital care (22.2%), medical outpatient care (17.4%) and skilled nursing facility and home health care (9.2%) (Federal Interagency Forum on Aging-Related Statistics 2001).

Long-Term Care and the Oldest Old

The growing ranks of the oldest old has increasingly focused attention on the issue of long-term care, which includes an array of medical, social, personal care, and support services needed by people who have lost some capacity for self-care as a result of a chronic illness or disability. Because they are more likely to experience functional limitations, older adults are much more likely to require long-term care services than are younger adults. Adults age 65 and older currently account for almost three-quarters of all long-term care spending.

While before the 1970s and 1980s, families' role in caring for older dependent members was largely invisible and assumed to be nonexistent, today the central role that families play in the lives of frail elders is widely recognized, and the term "family caregiver" has entered American lexicon. According to the 1989 National Long Term Care Survey, more than 90 percent of community-dwelling elders with disabilities receive care informally from family, friends, and neighbors. Seventy percent of caregivers are women, typically either spouses, daughters, or daughters-in-law. Since the 1980s, however, the use of informal care as the exclusive source of help has declined from 74 percent in 1982 to 64 percent in 1994, while the use of combined informal and formal care has increased from 21 percent to 28 percent during the same time span. The percentage of elders who rely exclusively on formal supports has remained approximately 8 percent (National Center for Health Statistics 2000). Not surprisingly, the percent of paid caregivers increases with age. In 1995, among those receiving help, adults age 85 and older were 1.4 times as likely to have paid caregivers as those age 70 to 74 (1994 National Health Interview Survey, Second Supplement on Aging).

From 1990 to 1997 the use of home health services increased substantially in part due to the expansion of coverage criteria for the Medicare home health care benefit—from 2,141 home visits per 1,000 enrollees in 1990 to 8,227 visits per 1,000 enrollees in 1997. In 1998, as a result of changes in Medicare payment policies for home health care, the visits from Medicare claims declined to 5,058 visits per 1,000 enrollees (National Center for Health Statistics 1999). This change in Medicare payment policy greatly affected the oldest old, who are the heaviest consumers of home health care. In 1998 the 85-plus age group had 12,709 home health visits per 1,000 enrollees, which was approximately six times as many home health visits as the young old (65 to 74 years) and twice the number of home health visits for the middle old (75 to 84 years) age groups (National Center for Health Statistics 1999). As discussed earlier in this chapter, the very old are the heaviest users of skilled nursing facilities. Among Medicare beneficiaries age 85 and older, one out of every five faced an admission to a skilled nursing home facility in 1998.

Home health care represents an important option for elders who prefer to remain in the familiar surroundings of their home. Moreover, home health services (e.g., nursing care, physical therapy, homemaker services) often allow patients to be cared for at a lower cost than a nursing home or hospital. Indeed, the cost of institutional care is enormous. In 1996 the average health care expenditures among community-based Medicare beneficiaries was $6,360, whereas this figure was $38,906 for those Medicare beneficiaries who were institutionalized part or all of the year (National Center for Health Statistics 1999).

In fact, the rising public cost of long-term care has captured national attention. The Congressional Budget Office (CBO) estimates that expenditures on long-term care totaled more than $120 billion, with the federal government being the largest purchaser. In 1995 Medicare and Medicaid together accounted for approximately $50 billion, or 56 percent, of long-term care expenditures of older Americans. The CBO notes that although the Medicare pays primarily for acute medical services, beneficiaries may also receive long-term care coverage through the program's skilled nursing and home health care benefits. Indeed, Medicare is the largest purchaser of home health care. It is also important to note that the $120 billion figure does *not* include an estimate of the economic costs of the informal care provided by families.

The CBO estimates that total long-term care expenditures will increase at a rate of 2.6 percent a year above inflation over the next forty years, from $123 billion in 2000 to $346 billion by 2040 (in 2000 dollars). Although the CBO predicts some reduction in the age-specific prevalence of functional disability, this reduction will be offset by increasing demand as the baby boomer generation enters the ranks of the very old and the 85-plus population grows to more than three times its current size by 2040. As the CBO estimates reflected in Figure 8.5 suggest, the costs of long-term care are borne not only by the federal government but also by older adults in out-of-pocket costs. However, as revealed in Table 8.3, the burden of these out-of-pocket costs is most heavily felt by those who require nursing home or institutional care.

The U.S. system of long-term care is firmly planted in a residualist tradition wherein the government provides benefits only when the individual or family resources and market sources have failed. Indeed, Medicaid, a federal grant-in-aid program that helps states pay for medical assistance for individuals with low income and few resources, has

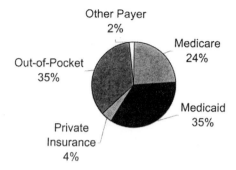

Fig. 8.5. Long-term care expenditures for elderly persons, by payer source, 2000 (total = $123 billion). Source: U.S. Congressional Budget Office 1999

emerged as a key payer of long-term care expenditures, particularly institutional care (see Table 8.3). In 2000, 84 percent of Medicaid funds were estimated to go toward institutional care, while only 13 percent were devoted to home or community-based care (U.S. Congressional Budget Office 1999). The disproportionate amount of funding for institutional care, as shown in Table 8.3, has been strongly criticized by a number of advocates for older adults. These critics argue that Medicaid's heavy emphasis on nursing home care means that many frail elders in the community go without services that could better support their independence in their own homes (Kane, Kane, and Ladd 1998). In many states a large portion of Medicaid dollars support poor elderly nursing home residents who had been middle class before their institutionalization. There is a growing public sentiment that individuals and families should not be forced to face impoverishment as a result of long-term care costs and that a financing mechanism that provides an alternative to means-tested Medicaid is needed.

Since the mid-1980s there has been considerable growth in the number of private insurance companies offering long-term care insurance. Yet from a public policy perspective, private insurance is unlikely to provide adequate funding for long-term care. Private insurance paid only 4 percent, or $5 billion, of the $123 billion of long-term care expenditures in 2000 (Table 8.3). For many Americans the cost of purchasing long-term care insurance is prohibitive. Moreover, economic models suggest that even by the year 2030 only 10 percent of elderly persons will be able to purchase long-term care insurance at a cost of less than 5 percent of their total income (Zedlewski and McBride 1992).

As an alternative to either public assistance Medicaid or the private market, the United States could offer families more complete protection against the catastrophic costs of long-term care by adopting a public insurance model. Despite our nation's historic residualist philosophy, social insurance models have been successfully implemented to avert two other potential economic catastrophes confronted by families: Social Security protects families from impoverishment caused by inadequate retirement income and savings, and Medicare protects individuals against poverty caused by a lack of acute medical care coverage in old age.

A clear advantage of a compulsory and universal public insurance model for protection against the cost of long-term care is that it allows the creation of large risk pools. By doing so, it avoids the adverse selection problem found in private market insurance, which ultimately drives the cost upward and makes policies unaffordable to most potential consumers. Yet as a number of policy analysts note, the current political, social, and economic climate does not make such an initiative likely (Howe 1999; Hudson 1999). Although there appears to be limited scope for extending private insurance in long-term care, there is also little interest in creating a social insurance pillar. Ironically, the success of past U.S. age-based policies (e.g., Social Security, Medicare), which has raised the aggregate well-being of the older population, coupled with a conservative ethos or political mood, has fueled recent discussions to partially privatize and individualized these programs (Hudson 1999).

Perhaps the best prospects for the challenges of developing and financing a public insurance model of long-term care that emphasizes community-based services lies in the building of coalitions of advocates for the aging and advocates for persons with disabilities. Such a strategy suggests that the social insurance must be functionally based and not population centered. Although the presence of chronic illnesses and disabilities is positively correlated with age, aging does not equal disability. In fact, 49.7 million, or almost one in every five noninstitutionalized Americans age 5 and older, has a disability as defined by being: 5 years and older and having a sensory, physical, mental, or self-care disability; 16 years and older and having difficulty going outside the home; or 16 to 64 years of age had having an employment disability. Based on this definition, 7 percent of boys and 4 percent of girls age 5 to 15 have disabilities, 20 percent of men and 18 percent of women ages 16 to 64 have disabilities, and 40 percent of men and 43 percent of women 65 years and older have disabilities (U.S. Bureau of the Census 2000). In fact, in the national health care debate that occurred during the Clinton administration, several of the proposed health care plan models included long-term care services for individuals of all ages based on a beneficiary's need for assistance in performing activities of daily living, severe cognitive impairment, or profound mental retardation. Despite the failure of these legislative proposals to move forward, they have clearly introduced the principle that any public insurance model for long-term care will be based on need-for-service rather than age-based criteria.

Conclusion

The importance of age-based programs for our nation's oldest old is beyond dispute. For the vast majority of individuals age 85 and older, Social Security is their largest source of income, and virtually all elderly persons gain access to health care coverage (physician and hospital services) through Medicare. To a large extent, the success of these programs lies in the decision to design them based on social insurance principles. Inherent in both programs is the concept of providing universal protection to older citizens for the loss of income in old age through compulsory participation in order to allow the pooling of resources and the sharing of risk. It has long been recognized that universal programs avoid the stigmatization and stereotyping that occurs with means-tested programs. Moreover, the decision to make these programs age-based makes sense in that, for the majority of Americans, income and access to health care insurance are connected to employment.

While these age-based programs have improved the aggregate well-being of older people, they do not adequately address the differences that exist within the aging U.S. population, including those of advanced old age. Clearly, a significant proportion of the oldest old is vulnerable. Relative to the young old, the oldest are both poorer and in worse physical health.

Riley, Kahn, and Foner (1994) offer the concept of "a structural lag" as a framework for understanding the mismatch between rapidly changing human lives, especially the phenomenon of longer and healthier lives, and social institutions. This concept is instructive in assessing the fit between population dynamics and policy design. For example, one of the basic assumptions at the enactment of the Social Security program—that only a small percentage of Americans would survive to old age and that those who did would receive benefits for only a brief period of time—is no longer true. Similarly, when Medicare was introduced in 1965, little attention was focused on the demographic implications of the oldest old. Nor was it originally envisioned that Medicaid, a program designed to finance acute health care for low-income people of all ages, would become the primary third-party payer for nursing home care for a large segment of the older U.S. population.

The aging of the baby boom generation has increasingly focused attention on meeting the long-term care needs of the future oldest U.S. citizens. Undoubtedly, the sheer size of the baby boom cohort as it enters advanced old age will have a major impact on the nation's health and social service systems. Yet predicting the precise impact of this demographic shift on individuals, families, and government is difficult because the effects may be lessened or exacerbated by a number of social, economic, and health trends. For example, optimistic forecasts suggest that advances in medical technologies, surgeries, pharmaceuticals, and prevention will lead to declining disability rates and compressed morbidity in the older population and thus reduce the economic burden of long-term care. More pessimistic forecasts, however, suggest that the dramatic growth of the oldest old, the most disabled segment of the aging population, will overwhelm the long-term care system and lead to a rapid increase in long-term care expenditures.

It is also important to underscore that even among these "elite survivors" to advanced old age, inequalities by gender, race, and social class exist (Crystal and Shea 1990; Thorsland and Lundberg 1994; Jeffereys 1996; Schoenbaum and Waidman 1997; Dunlop et al. 2000). These inequalities are derived from the fact that, although the United States does a better job than other industrialized countries in maintaining preretirement income in old age, it has one of the least egalitarian systems of income distribution before retirement (Myles 1988). Although medical advances are often touted as having a profound impact on late-life disability rates, in fact, the greatest gains in prevention of chronic diseases may be achieved through a focus on early life experiences. Childhood and young adulthood exposure to diseases, poverty, inadequate nutrition, and substandard housing are increasingly being linked to a number of morbidities in later life, including cancer, arthritis, and cardiovascular diseases (Blackwell, Hayward, and Crimmins 2001). Although future cohorts of the older U.S. population as a whole may be better off, a disproportionate share of older persons of color and women may be left behind.

Indeed, long-term care in later life is most often about women's lives. As the data presented in this chapter suggest, women are more likely to be the consumers and providers of long-term care services as a result of both their longer life expectancy and their greater likelihood of assuming the caregiver role. Thus, women are major stakeholders in the long-term care debate. With longer life expectancies, we might anticipate that the experiences and problems of the young old caring for the oldest old will become even more familiar in our society. Faced with their own diminishing physical strength and stamina, these older daughters and wives may face considerable challenges in caring for their frail family members.

The inadequacies of our nation's long-term care system, including the fragmentation of services, the lack of continuity of care, and a funding bias toward institutional care, have been well documented (Kane, Kane and Ladd 1998; Coleman 2002). Critics of the existing system emphasize the continuing dominance of a medical model of care in spite of considerable evidence supporting the importance of social and environmental approaches to the delivery of long-term care services. Yet despite widespread dissatisfaction with our current system, debate about long-term care policy seems to be primarily centered on short-term fixes to address specific hardships experienced by users and growing concerns about public cost.

The U.S. demographic shift toward becoming an older society, coupled with a cultural shift emphasizing the inclusion of persons with disabilities in all aspects of society, may, however, offer an opportunity to bring structural reform to our nation's long-term care system. Recent legislation such as the Americans with Disabilities Act and the Olmstead Decision increasingly mandate that services, programs, and facilities promote independence, inclusion, and consumer empowerment for individuals of all ages with disabling conditions. As this chapter emphasizes, age is associated with, but not defined by, disability. More than half of people with chronic disabilities living in the community are under 65, and almost all Americans are unprotected against the catastrophic health care costs associated with a chronic and severe disabling condition. While the oldest old have much to gain through a shift toward a social insurance model of long-term care, I have suggested that the best way to achieve this policy objective may be through a functionally based or disability-based program rather than an age-based program. This social insurance approach, rather than fueling the fires of a "generational equity debate," emphasizes a lifelong, intergenerational sharing of, and paying for, costs of long-term care.

References

Barer, B. 1994. Men and women age differently. *International Journal of Aging and Human Development* 38:29–40.

Binstock, R. 1994. Changing criteria in old-age programs: The introduction of economic status and need for services. *Gerontologist* 34:726–30.

Blackwell, D. L., M. D. Hayward, and E. M. Crimmins. 2001. Does childhood health affect chronic morbidity in later life? *Social Science and Medicine* 52:1269–84.

Callahan, D. 1987. *Setting Limits: Medical Goals in an Aging Society.* New York: Simon and Schuster.

Camacho, T., W. Strawbridge, R. Cohen, and G. Kaplan. 1993. Functional ability in the oldest old. *Journal of Aging and Health* 5:439–54.

Coleman, E. A. 2002. Challenges of systems of care for frail older persons: The United States of America experience. *Aging Clinical and Experimental Research* 14:233–38.

Crystal, S., R. W. Johnson, J. Harman, U. Sambamoorthi, and R. Kumar. 2000. Out-of-pocket health care costs among older Americans. *Journal of Gerontology—Psychological and Social Sciences* 55:S51–62.

Crystal, S., and D. Shea. 1990. Cumulative advantage, cumulative disadvantage, and inequality among elderly people. *Gerontologist* 30:437–43.

Dunlop, D. D., L. M. Manheim, J. Song, and R. W. Chang 2002. Gender and ethnic/racial disparities in health care utilization among older adults. *Journal of Gerontology—Psychological and Social Sciences* 57:S221–33.

Elo, I. T., and S. H. Preston. 1994. Estimating African-American mortality from inaccurate data. *Demography* 31:427–58.

Federal Interagency Forum on Aging Related Statistics. 2001. *Older Americans 2000: Key Indicators of Well-Being.* Washington, D.C.: Author.

Gabrel, C. S. 2000, April 25. Characteristics of elderly nursing home current residents and discharges: Data from the 1997 National Nursing Home Survey, *Advance Data* 312, National Center for Health Statistics.

Harris, T. M., R. Kovar, R. Suzman, J. Kleinman, and J. Feldman. 1978. Longitudinal study of physical ability in the oldest-old. *American Journal of Public Health* 79:698–702.

Howe, A. L. 1999. Extending the pillars of social policy financing to aged care. *Social Policy and Administration* 33:534–51.

Hudson, R. B. 1978. The "graying" of the federal budget and its consequences for old age policy. *Gerontologist* 18:428–40.

Hudson, R. B. 1999. Conflict in today's aging politics: New population encounters old ideology. *Social Service Review* 73:358–79.

Jefferys, M. 1996. Social inequalities in health: Do they diminish with age? *American Journal of Public Health* 86:474–75.

Johnson, N. E. 2000. The racial crossover in comorbidity, disability and mortality. *Demography* 37:267–83.

Kane, R. A, R. L. Kane, and R. C. Ladd. 1998. *The Heart of Long-Term Care*. New York: Oxford University Press.

Longino, C., Jr. 1988. A population profile of very old men and women in the United States. *Sociology Quarterly* 29:559–64.

Myles, J. 1988. Postwar capitalism and the extension of Social Security into the retirement wage. In M. Weir, A. Orloff, and T. Skocpol, eds., *The Politics of Social Policy in the United States*. Princeton, N.J.: Princeton University Press.

National Center for Health Statistics. 1999. *Health and Aging Chartbook* (PHS 99-1232-1). Washington, D.C.: Government Printing Office.

National Center for Health Statistics. 2002. *Health, United States, 2002* (PHS 2002-1232). Washington, D.C.: Government Printing Office.

National Council on Aging. 2000. *Myths and Realities 2000 Survey Results*. Washington, D.C.: Author.

Neugarten, B. 1974. Age groups in American society and the rise of the young-old. In F. Eisele, ed., *Political Consequences of Aging*. Philadelphia: American Academy of Political and Social Sciences.

O'Neill, G., and M. Patrick. 2002. *The State of Aging and Health in America*. Washington, D.C.: Merck Institute of Aging and Health and Gerontological Society of America.

Preston S. H. 1984. Children and the elderly in the U.S. *Scientific American* 251(6):44–49.

Riley, M. W., R. Kahn, and A. Foner, eds. 1994. *Age and Structural Lag*. New York: Wiley.

Robertson, A. 1991. The politics of Alzheimer's disease: A case study of apocalyptic demography. In M. Minkler and C. Estes, eds., *Critical Perspectives on Aging: The Political and Moral Economy of Growing Old*. New York: Baywood.

Santos-Eggimann, B. 2002. Evolution of the needs of older persons. *Aging Clinical and Experimental Research* 14:287–92.

Schoenbaum, M., and T. Waidman. 1997. Race, socioeconomic status, and health: Accounting for race differences in health. *Journal of Gerontology-Series B* 52:61–73.

Suzman, R, and Riley, M. W. 1985. Introducing the "oldest old." *Milbank Quarterly* 63:177–86.

Thompson, E., Jr. 1994. Older men as invisible men in contemporary society. In E. Thompson Jr., ed., *Older Men's Lives.* Thousand Oaks, Calif.: Sage.

Thorsland, M., and O. Lundberg. 1994. Health and inequalities among the oldest old. *Journal of Aging and Health* 6:51–69.

Treas, J., and V. Bengston. 1982. The demography of mid- and late-life transitions. *Annals of the American Academy of Political and Social Science* 461:11–21.

U.S. Bureau of the Census. 1996. *Current Population Reports: Special Studies* P23-190. Washington, D.C.: Author.

U.S. Bureau of the Census. 2000, January. *Projections of the Resident Population by Age, Sex, Race, and Hispanic Origin, 1999–2100.* Washington, D.C.: Author.

U.S. Bureau of the Census. 2001. *Census 2000 Demographic Profile.* Washington, D.C.: Author.

U.S. Bureau of the Census. 2002. *Current Population Survey Annual Social, and Economic Supplement.* Washington, D.C.: Author.

U.S. Bureau of Labor Statistics and Bureau of the Census. 2001, March. *Current Population Series, Annual Demographic Survey,* Supplement. Washington, D.C.: Author. (http://ferret.bls.census.gov/macro/032002/pov/new01_001/htm)

U.S. Bureau of Labor and Bureau of the Census. 2002. *Current Population Survey, Annual Demographic Survey, March Supplement.* Washington, D.C.: Author.

U.S. Congressional Budget Office. 1999, March. *Projections of Expenditures for Long-term Care Services for the Elderly.* Washington, D.C.: Author.

U.S. Social Security Administration. 2001. *Income of the Aged Chartbook, 2001.* Washington, D.C.: Author.

Zedlewski, S., and T. McBride. 1992. The changing profile of the elderly: Effects on future long-term care needs and financing. *Milbank Quarterly* 70:247–76.

III. Aged-Based Public Policies

9. Reframing Social Security
Cures Worse than the Disease

Pamela Herd and Eric R. Kingson

The politics of Social Security is forever changed. While it is open to a broader range of policy choices, it is also ideologically driven and more contentious. It is less bounded by the traditions of compromise and incremental change that have guided Social Security reform for decades. Policy options such as privatization and means testing, heretofore considered outside the parameters of political reality, have been legitimized during the past decade by being seen as requiring serious discussion.

This chapter reviews the emergence of the changed politics of Social Security and discusses its implications. We dispute claims that Social Security is "broken," as some say, and we discuss why individual accounts are not a panacea for Social Security's financial and equity problems. In particular, we make the case that richer Americans are the most likely to benefit from partial privatization proposals, while those struggling to make ends meet will see little benefit. We question whether partial privatization is a realistic market solution based on libertarian principles, suggesting that it more closely resembles a thinly disguised vehicle for benefiting "the Dow."

Budgetary crises and partial privatization proposals shape the current debate and stifle other approaches to modernizing the program, and the proponents of privatization have been very successful at framing the debate in a way that calls for dramatic reforms. But Social Security's actual problems are far less dramatic and thus require far less dramatic solutions. Consequently, in the conclusion, we note alternative solutions to Social Security's financing problems that do not violate its guiding values and principles or the protections that it provides.

The Values, Principles, and Structure of Social Security

Knowledge of program benefits and of the values and principles that structure Social Security is an important prerequisite to understanding the state of the current policy debate. Most Americans understand that the program provides cash benefits to retirees, severely disabled workers and survivors, and some spouses and young dependents—about 45 million people, including 23 million retirees, 9 millions spouses, 5 million disabled workers, 165,000 spouses of disabled workers, 5 million surviving parents of young children and aged widow(er)s and parents, 3.8 million children, and a few other groups (Social Security Administration 2001). But few recognize that Social Security is the foundation of most families' retirement, disability, and life insurance protection. Six out of ten private sector workers have no other pension protection. On average, more than two-thirds of all the income going to the bottom 60 percent of elderly households (65 and over), comes from Social Security. For a young family with two small children, Social Security is, on average, the equivalent of a $400,000 term life insurance policy.

Social Security is based on the principle that providing widespread and basic protections against risks related to retirement, disability, and survivorship is in the interest of the nation and its citizenry. Hence, as Reinhart Hohaus, an actuary and executive of Metropolitan Life Insurance Company observed many years ago, concerns for providing "adequate" benefits must drive a social insurance program (Hohaus 1938; 1960). In turn, "individual equity"—the principle that benefits paid should directly reflect the size of premium payments—structures benefit payments from private insurance. Consequently, the Social Security benefit formula is structured to assure that people who work consistently at low and modest wage levels receive a substantially larger rate of return on their payroll tax payments than those with substantially higher earnings—roughly twice the size. Similarly, the annual cost-of-living-adjustment (the "COLA") assures that Social Security benefits maintain their purchasing power no matter how long a beneficiary lives. To do otherwise would undermine income adequacy for many among the nation's most vulnerable elderly and disabled persons—those living into advanced old age. Individual equity is honored as a secondary goal by the provision of generally larger benefits amounts for persons who make larger Old Age and Survivors and Disability Insurance (OASDI) tax payments.

The public has begun to understand that Social Security is funded primarily on a "pay-as-you-go" basis, meaning that there is only modest advance-funding of the program and that the Social Security Administration does not deposit payroll tax contributions into an account earmarked with the name of each worker. Current generations of beneficiaries are supported primarily by taxes on the current workforce. Taxes received from treating a portion of Social Security payments as taxable income also go into the OASDI trust funds as do the interest payments made by the federal treasury on the nearly $1.4 trillion that the federal treasury has borrowed from the trust funds.

But the public does not have much of a grasp of the politics that constrain future congresses and presidential administrations to meet their obligations to the American public. Unlike private pensions and private life insurance, a social insurance system does not need to be advanced funded to be financially viable. The taxing power of the federal government, the stability of the nation, and the political survival instincts of elected politicians guarantee that benefits will be available for today's and tomorrow's workforce. In other words, the promises made to today's workers are backed in essentially the same manner as the nation's currency—by the full faith and credit of the U.S. government. This does not mean that there is not a financing problem, only that—assuming the continuity of the U.S. government into the future—it is inconceivable that future congresses and presidential administrations would not act to assure the timely payment of benefits. Benefit amounts might be larger or smaller than anticipated in 2003, and the age of eligibility for full benefits might be ratcheted up and/or taxes increased. But—in spite of sensational claims of "impending bankruptcy"—barring the complete collapse of the United States economy and government, there is virtually no possibility that Social Security will not be there for today's and tomorrow's workforces.

So what has happened in the politics of Social Security that has enabled opponents of the traditional Social Security program considerable success in framing the future of Social Security as a choice between partial privatization and system bankruptcy?

The Changing Politics of Social Security

There was nothing foreordained about Social Security's becoming the dominant source of income security for aged, disabled, and surviving family members. Initially, the welfare program, Old Age Assistance (OAA), enacted in 1935 along with what we now call Social Security (initially called "Old Age Benefits" and then "Old Age Insurance"), was more popular (Berkowitz 1997). Social Security collected taxes in the midst of the Great Depression without paying its first benefits until 1942. OAA provided immediate relief through matching federal grants-in-aid to cash-strapped states that gave cash benefits to poor elders. Through the 1940s, the value of OAA benefits closely rivaled that of Social Security.

The enactment of the 1950 Amendments expanded coverage and substantially increased monthly benefit amounts for current and future beneficiaries. With these amendments, Social Security became the preeminent source of income protection for the old and survivors; and later, with the enactment of the 1956 Amendments, for long-term, severely disabled workers. The pattern of incremental expansion and liberalization of benefits that began with the 1939 amendments that added survivors and dependents benefits continued through the early 1970s. Early retirement options were added in 1956 and 1981, eligibility for disability benefits were liberalized in the 1960s, benefit levels substantially increased in from 1965 through 1972, and an annual Cost of Living Adjustment was implemented in 1974.

From its enactment in 1935, conservatives resented Social Security. Calling for repeal of Social Security, the 1936 Republican presidential nominee, Alf Landon, termed the payroll tax a "cruel hoax," part of an "unjust, unworkable, stupidly drafted and wastefully financed" program. With the 1937 Supreme Court decision (7-2) upholding the constitutionality of the Social Security Act and its social insurance features, frontal attacks by major political figures on the idea of Social Insurance became rare (Derthick 1979; Ball 2000). Republican nominee Barry Goldwater's suggestion that participation in Social Security be made "voluntary" became a source of ridicule, a symbol of his "radical conservatism" (Derthick 1979, p. 187) and contributed to his landslide loss to Lyndon Johnson in the 1964 election.

But until relatively recently, mainstream conservative opposition did not seek to undo or dramatically restructure Social Security. Conservatives sought to "hold the line wherever the line might be at the moment." The effect of this was primarily "to delay or restrict officially sponsored expansion, but not to defeat it—at least not for a very long, anyway—in favor of a fundamentally different alternative" (Derthick 1979, p. 132).

Hence, from the early 1950s through the early 1970s a strong favorable consensus facilitated the incremental expansion of the program. The popularity of the program combined with Barry Goldwater's experience and politicians' reticence to risk being seen as challenging the growing voice of elder advocacy organizations led to Social Security being viewed as "the third rail of politics." Touch it and risk political death! Few dared.

Even during the mid-1970s and early 1980s when projected financing shortfalls needed to be addressed, radical reform was off the table, as were large benefit cuts. When the Reagan administration sent up a trial balloon in 1981 that would have addressed the projected shortfall through substantial benefit reductions, public outcry quickly forced the administration to retreat, setting up a commission primarily to provide political cover for Republicans until after the 1982 midterm Congressional elections. This bipartisan commission enunciated first and unanimously that its members rejected means-testing and voluntary approaches and recommended that Congress "should not alter the fundamental structure of the Social Security program or undermine its fundamental principles" (National Commission on Social Security Reform 1983). Ultimately, President Reagan agreed to accept a legislative package that contained a balance of revenue increases (e.g., taxation of benefits, acceleration of pre-existing payroll tax increases, changed tax treatment of the self-employed, and expansion of coverage to new federal employees) and benefit reductions (e.g., a six-month permanent delay in the COLA, gradual increase in the age of eligibility for full benefits).

But by the 2000 presidential election, three presidents and twenty years later, the third rail of politics became touchable, and the politics of Social Security were forever changed. Concerns about chronic federal deficits, population aging, rising health care costs, and projected shortfalls in Social Security underlay new calls for reform. Throughout the 1990s an increasing flurry of newspaper and magazine headlines declared that Social Security was bankrupt, leading to a gradual undermining of American faith in the program, especially among young adults (Kingson and Quadagno 1995; Quadagno 1996). Millions believed they would not receive benefits in retirement. George

W. Bush seized on these concerns in the presidential election and proposed his solution to the problem.

Picking up on proposals put forth and skillfully disseminated by conservatives for over a decade, he argued that a portion of payroll taxes should be diverted to individual investment accounts. Conservatives had come to realize that the elimination of Social Security, and consequently of payroll taxes, was unlikely. So they switched strategies. "Partial privatization" would be better than "no privatization," and some hoped it might serve as the "camel's nose under the tent" on the way to a fully privatized system. The alternative was to sell a market approach as a "solution" to Social Security's financing troubles. Individual accounts would not only cure Social Security's bankruptcy blues but would also allow Americans more choice, increased savings, and bigger returns on their retirement investments—all while making the program more equitable for women and minorities.

But how much, if any of this, is true? Not much, as we suggest in the sections that follow.

Framing the Problem: Is Social Security Really Broken?

One of the most contentious areas of debate regarding Social Security reform is the scope of the program's financing problems. Few experts disagree on the existence of a financing problem. But there is disagreement on the extent and on whether the shortfall represents a "manageable problem" or "a crisis" (Kingson and Quadagno 1995; Quadagno 1996). Media coverage has been largely one-sided, reinforcing the "crisis" image of a weak, financially unstable Social Security system. In an op ed column that appeared in the *Boston Globe,* Jacoby (1994) draws on the conservative image of Social Security as an elaborate Ponzi scheme that will gradually bankrupt young Americans. And the cover of *Time* presented "The Case for Killing Social Security," which emphasized the program's financing woes (Church and Lacayo 1995).

The broadest critique of Social Security is that young Americans cannot financially support the growing number of elderly Americans. At the beginning of the twentieth century, the ratio of workers to retirees was about 12 to 1. By 1990 it had dropped to 5 to 1. And by 2020 it is projected to be about 3 to 1 (Harrington Meyer and Herd 2001). Fewer young Americans will be forced to support more and more elderly Americans, taxing their incomes and resources. But this is only half the story. Those under age 18 are also supported (even more so than the elderly) by working-age adults. And because of a falling fertility rate, the overall number of dependents, both children and the elderly, on working Americans has remained and will remain relatively stable through 2050 (Harrington Meyer and Herd 2001).

Another way to sort out the extent of Social Security's financial problems is to examine population aging in other countries. Most European countries and Japan have even greater proportions of their population aged 65 and over and will experience an even faster growth of their aging population (Kalish and Tetsuya 1999; Kingson 1999). The percentage of GDP spent on public pensions is expected to rise from 5 to 7 percent from 2000 to 2040 in the United States. In comparison, it is expected to rise from 12 to 20 percent in France, 11 to 14 percent in Germany, and 11 to 16 percent in Japan (Bosworth and Burtless 1997). Furthermore, the per capita income in the United States is among the highest in the world and the tax rate is two-thirds to one-half of most other Western industrialized nations (Kingson 1999). Thus, increased tax rates to support the elderly would fall much easier on Americans. Relative to most Western nations, our public pension financial problems are relatively small.

Nonetheless, even though fewer numbers of dependent children and comparisons to other Western nations shed a different light on the magnitude of Social Security's problems, it does not make them nonexistent. Ultimately, there *are* fewer working Americans to contribute for an increasing number of older Americans receiving Social Security benefits. The most recent Social Security trustee report shows that by 2018 outgoing benefits for current retirees will exceed incoming revenues from current workers' payroll taxes. A $2.3 trillion trust fund will make up the difference until 2042, when it is projected to be exhausted (Board of Trustees 2003).

The emptying of the trust fund in 2042 is part of the rationale for describing Social Security as bankrupt. The trustee report states, however, that 73 percent of benefits could still be paid out, given no change in current policy. Furthermore, implementing a 1.92 percent increase in the payroll tax—.96 percent each on employer and employee—would define away this shortfall, although there would still be need to make adjustments to address the larger annual deficits projected past 2042. Crisis proponents rarely include these figures in their commentary.

How certain are these projections in the first place? Trust fund depletion is projected to take place nearly forty years from now. Depending on the extent to which actual demographic and economic change conforms to the Social Security's actuarial assumptions, the deficit may be larger or smaller than anticipated. That demographic and economic actuarial assumptions are changed on an annual basis as new information comes to light is a strength, not a weakness. The Social Security Board of Trustees—the secretaries of the Treasury, Labor, and Health and Human Services; the Commissioner of Social Security; and two publicly appointed trustees—use the projections provided by Social Security's Office of the Actuary to provide a reasonable basis for assessing the financial status of the program. The projections serve as an early warning system, providing lead time for changes that need to be made from time to time.

It is important to remember, however, that seventy-five-year projections are not fact. Making assumptions about what the world will look like that far into the future is tricky. Consequently, the trustees actually project three different estimates—a low cost, a medium cost, and a high cost estimate. These estimates vary based on differing assumptions about economic growth, how many children the average family will have, and how long they expect the average American to live. The medium cost projection, which is the one most reported, estimates that trust fund assets will run out in 2042. The high cost projection is that it will run out in 2031. But the low cost estimate indicates it will remain in the black as far the trustees project, out to 2080. These parameters, both the negative and positive, must be kept in mind when evaluating the general health of the program as well as any reforms.

A further bone of contention between crisis yea-sayers and nay-sayers has been over the trust fund. Those who promote the crisis perspective argue that the trust fund is not real. An American Enterprise Institute article argues that the government bonds that make up the trust fund are "vaporware, pieces of paper. The IOUs [bonds] have to be converted to cash, and only the Treasury can do that. How? Either by increasing taxes, cutting federal spending, or borrowing" (Glassman 2001).

But the "vaporware" trust fund argument has significant problems. Assets started building in the trust fund in 1983 to help offset future shortfalls due to demographic changes in the age composition of the population. Payroll taxes were increased with the knowledge that more revenue would come in than benefits would go out for many years into the future. While the extra revenue could have been used to buy stocks or private bonds, it was used to buy U.S. government debt instead. Every dollar that the government borrowed from itself meant a dollar that it did not have to borrow from outside sources, thus improving cash flow. And current U.S. government debt totals put out by the Department of the Treasury already account for money owed to Social Security beneficiaries through the trust fund. The trust fund monies would simply be transferred from one column (intergovernmental debt) to another (privately held debt). Social Security surpluses allowed the government to hold off from borrowing from private sources for many additional years. And each year, the Treasury makes interest payments—$80 billion dollars in calendar year 2003 alone—to the OASDI trust funds.

The most egregious part of the "fantasy trust fund" argument regards the resulting policy recommendation that benefits would need to be cut or payroll taxes raised even more than the trustee report states (Feldstein 1999). Arguing for cuts in benefits or increases in the payroll tax to offset "imaginary" assets in the trust fund requires the assumption that there is no difference between payroll and regular income taxes. Payroll taxes are regressive. Low-income people pay higher percentages of their income in payroll taxes than do those with high incomes. Income taxes, on the other hand, are progressive. Higher-income people pay higher percentages of their income to taxes than low-income individuals. Income taxes are used to pay for everything from defense spending to public programs like Head Start. Regressive payroll taxes are justified because eventually individuals receive progressive Social Security benefits. The trust fund is made up of payroll tax dollars, not income tax dollars. Arguing that future beneficiaries should not be able to draw on those trust fund dollars for their benefits means that they would not see all the regressive tax dollars they paid into the system come back out in their benefits. Instead, their payroll taxes would have been spent on tax cuts for the wealthy, among other budgetary items.

To make the issue more intuitive, imagine a low-income worker who paid payroll taxes from 1982 through 2020. For all those years she paid additional payroll taxes, outside what was needed to fund current beneficiaries, which were spent on everything from building roads to reducing tax rates for well-off Americans. But in retirement, she receives a dramatic benefit reduction because policymakers decide that the trust fund wasn't real after all. The result is that the money spent on roads and tax reductions came out of the regressive payroll taxes that she paid, as opposed to the progressive income taxes that are supposed to fund that kind of spending. The alternative, raising payroll taxes, would be relatively equivalent because it would demand that her daughter's payroll taxes fund initiatives that should be covered by progressive income taxes.

Another problematic outcome of arguments that the trust fund is imaginary concerns Americans' faith and trust in government. As previously noted, the trust fund is a promise to future beneficiaries that the government must keep. The U.S. government would never default on debt owed to the private sector, so why should it be able to default on debt owed to the American people? Paul Krugman provides an analogy in a 2001 *New York Times* op ed column (2001). He tells the story of a man who loans his retirement savings to his nephew. When he asks for the money back now that he is retiring, the nephew tells him he won't pay because "the only way I could honor that promise is by earning more or spending less money on myself. And you can't ask me to do that." Americans' ability to trust the U.S. government would be considerably undermined if policymakers chose to behave like that naughty nephew.

Is the Cure Worse than the Disease?

As criticism of Social Security mounted throughout the 1990s, proposals such as large benefit cuts and means testing came onto the agenda. Limited enthusiasm for these types of reforms, however, eventually pushed them off again. But the mounting—and often alarmist and inaccurate—criticisms of Social Security's overall financial health began to take its toll on the public's perception of the country's largest social welfare program (Quadagno 1996). While support for the program remained strong, by the late 1990s, millions of Americans voiced a belief that they would not receive Social Security checks in retirement. Criticism also came from scholars and activists who argued that Social Security was unfair to women and minorities. At the same time, the stock market was reaching unprecedented heights, garnering large returns in many retirement savings accounts. In this context, conservatives began to argue for partial privatization, claiming it could be a market cure for a failed government program. They claimed it would be the panacea for all of Social Security's problems, from financial to equity issues. George W. Bush agreed and made the creation of individual accounts a centerpiece of his presidential campaign. In the following section, we will examine whether partial privation will live up to the expectations of the reform's strongest proponents.

The Cure for Systemic Financial Problems?

The calls for individual accounts were premised first and foremost on Social Security's financial problems. The strongest critique privatization proponents made was that pay-as-you-go financing, where current worker taxes pay the benefits for current retirees, was the root cause of the program's financial problems. The contrasting approach is a prefunded system: we save for our own retirement, as opposed to our children funding it. A prefunded system would not be vulnerable to financing problems induced by demographic change. Initial suggestions to prefund by investing the Social Security trust fund in private stocks and bonds as opposed to government bonds were quickly and effectively shoved off the table by those who feared government intervention in the market. Instead, conservatives swiftly backed individual account proposals. A portion of each American's Social Security taxes would be diverted to individual accounts to fund their own retirement.

Whether one favors or opposes partial privatization proposals, there is no question that prefunding through individual accounts would actually worsen Social Security's financial problems. Transfer costs spoil the "perfect panacea scenario." If current workers diverted a portion of their payroll taxes to individual accounts, these dollars could not be devoted to current retiree's benefits. The shortfall that results dramatically alters Social Security's financial health, emptying the trust fund by 2024 rather than 2028. And the payroll tax increase required to bring the system in balance would rise from less than 1.9 percent to 3.9 percent (Orszag and Greenstein 2001). In other words, shifting 2 percent of payroll from Social Security to private accounts essentially doubles the financing problem of the program. And if it is done in the manner that President Bush advocated during his campaign—without reducing the benefits of current retirees or older workers and without raising taxes—then it will require a roughly 45 percent reduction, on average, in the anticipated Social Security benefits of today's young workers.

Improving Benefits?

Along with fixing Social Security's financing, partial privatization proponents argued Americans would receive larger benefits if a portion of their taxes were invested in the stock market. There are four reasons why this is not as clear as privatization proponents claim (Aaron et al. 2001). First, the transfer costs would dramatically offset increases in rates of return (Geanakoplos, Mitchell, and Zeldes 1999). Current workers will have to pay for the system transfer, either through benefit cuts or through higher tax rates. The partial privatization plans put forth by the Presidential Commission to Strengthen Social Security provide a good example of this. To fund individual accounts as well as cope with long-term Social Security imbalances, the Commission relied on between $2 and $3 trillion in general revenue transfer as well as substantial benefit cuts. This general revenue transfer would have made up for a minimum of two-thirds of Social Security's projected shortfall. But because of transfer costs to instate the individual accounts, the Commission also instituted large benefit cuts. A low-income two-earner couple would face a 10 to 20 percent reduction in scheduled benefits, depending on the specific plan. And medium- and high-earner two-earner couples would face 20 to 30 percent in benefit reductions, depending on the specific plan (Diamond and Orszag 2002).[1]

The second factor working against larger returns, particularly for low-income beneficiaries, regards administrative costs. The cost of administering accounts eats away at their value. And the more choices individuals have, the higher are those costs (Diamond and Orszag 2002). Consequently, decentralized systems are the most expensive. For example, in the United Kingdom, administrative costs consume up to 40 percent of account assets over an individual's lifetime. Proposals put forth by the Social Security Commission were based on a centralized system, which would be more efficient and less costly. The Commission assumed administrative costs would swallow 0.3 percent of the account's value. This value, however, does not include the cost of setting the account up, the financial education costs (the government will be primarily responsible for dispensing information), the additional investment options for the larger accounts, and the possible reduction in restriction on asset choices over time, which would increase costs.

Dramatic fluctuations in the stock market are the third reason why claims that individual accounts would improve benefits are questionable. The most recent market crash was a stern reminder of the issue. The historical average rate of return in the stock market is 5.5 percent for the kind of portfolio that would make up individual accounts. The projected annual return on the Social Security reserves now invested in government bonds is 3 percent. The problem with the 5.5 percent average return is precisely that it is an average. The higher return comes at the price of increased risk borne by the individual investor. The consequence is illustrated by what would happen to comparable beneficiaries who retired just before and just after a major drop in the market. Someone retiring in March 2001 would receive a benefit one-third smaller than a similar individual retiring in March of 2000 (Aaron et al. 2001).

Another critical factor in determining the rate of return is based on the old adage that it takes money to make money. Rates of return depend on the degree of risk an individual investor is willing to make. Those with more money are able to take more risks and thus make more money. For example, retirees could choose a variable- or an inflation-adjusted annuity. The variable-adjusted annuity produces the greater average return. However, the year to year payout from it varies, depending on the strength of the market. For an individual with large assets, this kind of risk is reasonable. For a low-income beneficiary largely relying on Social Security for income, large benefit fluctuations from year to year would not be feasible.

Improving Social Security for Women and People of Color?

Proponents of partial privatization argue that individual accounts will improve Social Security for women and people of color. Ironically, they have drawn on longstanding liberal critiques of the program to do so. They have not, however, adequately established that individual accounts would actually improve the program for these groups.

The first critique is that Social Security is unfair to African Americans because they do not live as long. One Republican interest group (Gopac) in Kansas City aired a radio ad that compared Social Security benefits to "reverse reparations"—except blacks were paying them to whites (*Milwaukee Sentinel* 2002). The ad stated, "You've heard about reparations, you know, where whites compensate blacks for enslaving us. Well, guess what we've got now: Reverse reparations" (Marquis 2002). African Americans often contribute but then die before receiving their retirement benefits or receive those benefits for a shorter period of time than white beneficiaries. The assets in the individual accounts, in contrast, would be passed on to other family members.

African Americans, however, have some distinct advantages under the current Social Security structure. First, and most importantly, the progressive benefit formula provides a substantially larger rate of return for low-wage workers, a group in which African Americans are overrepresented. Second, they are disproportionately more likely to receive disability benefits, which help offset their higher rates of chronic illnesses that lead to an earlier death. Third, when Social Security beneficiaries die, widows and children often receive benefits based on the deceased worker's record. In a different fashion than assets in individual accounts, those contributions are eventually received by other family members. Moreover, partial privatization plans put forth by the Presidential Commission on Social Security would dramatically reduce disability benefits (Aaron et al. 2001). While it is likely that this flaw would be fixed in the actual legislation, it provides evidence that concerns about equity issues are not at the forefront in the minds of those promoting individual accounts.

Partial privatization proponents have also picked up on liberal critiques that Social Security is unfair to women. Women are a cause for concern, given their higher poverty rates and lower Social Security benefits in old age (Smeeding, Estes, and Glasse 1999). There are three specific critiques. First, Social Security does not compensate women for raising their children. Most mothers have considerably lower lifetime earnings, and eventually benefits, as a result of reduced labor force participation due to their child rearing responsibilities. Second, spousal and widow benefits (98 percent of which are received by women) undermine the program's progressiveness. These benefits require no contributions. Consequently, a woman who does no paid work and has no children but is married to a wealthy man would likely get a higher spouse benefit, and eventually widow benefit, than a low-income working woman with children. Third, the program does not adequately protect divorced women. Eligibility for the spousal benefit, which is 50 percent of the primary worker benefit, requires a minimum ten-year marriage. And even if a divorced woman had a ten-year marriage, she would receive a benefit only half the size of her ex-husband's.

While all of the claims above are valid, the pertinent question is whether partial privatization can fix these problems. Individual accounts will neither offset women's lower benefits that result from raising children nor will it improve the program's redistributive nature, because individual accounts will reduce the program's progressive benefit. Under the current program, individuals with low earnings receive a benefit that is a higher percentage of their average lifetime earnings than do high-income individuals. While currently all tax dollars spent on Social Security are subject to the progressive benefit formula, under partial privatization plans a portion of those dollars would now be diverted to individual accounts, where they would not be subject to the progressive benefit formula.

Individual accounts by themselves will not improve benefits for divorced women. In fact, they could reduce them, depending on their structure. The Presidential Commission on Social Security, however, proposed an individual account structure, which required that in a divorce, the assets in the account accrued during a marriage would be split. If this measure were not in place, however, many divorced women would take a reduction in their benefit.

Social Security has also been criticized for not adequately protecting very-low-income elderly Americans. Will partial privation improve the lot of low-income elderly Americans? The Presidential Commission on Social Security's proposals did include measures to improve the portion of the traditional benefit for low-income beneficiaries. But it is not at all clear that low-income Americans would substantially benefit from the individual accounts.

One of the most consistent claims of privatization proponents is that individual accounts would create assets that could be passed on to family members. This is particularly vital for low-income Americans, most of whom are asset poor. This ignores, however, the way the current program, in essence, passes on resources to family members. Widows, children, and even spouses of Social Security beneficiaries can receive benefits based on the primary claimants' records. For example, many widows of low-income workers in the WTC catastrophe received Social Security survivor benefits.

Furthermore, it is not actually clear that individual accounts would actually improve the assets of low-income Americans. The issue is evident in the report by the President's Commission on Social Security Reform. All of their benefit analyses were based on the assumption that the full amount in the individual account was applied to an annuity in retirement. At the same time, they emphasized that personal accounts would improve "inheritable assets," particularly for those in the middle and lower quintiles of the wealth distribution, so that "the increase in bequests should help to reduce wealth inequality" (p. 29). The problem, as Peter Diamond and Peter Orszag maintain, is that the commission tries to have it both ways. If beneficiaries want to pass on assets to their children, they must reduce the benefits they receive in retirement. Given that low-income beneficiaries are already taking a 10 to 20 percent reduction in their scheduled benefits under the commission's plans, it seems odd to conclude that these beneficiaries would be able to take a further reduction in their benefits so that they could pass along assets to their children.

A Market Solution?

One significant irony to the privatization debate is that many of the actual individual account proposals are not as much of a market solution as their promoters claim. Ironically, they really do not offer much choice. In an effort to claim individual accounts can be as safe as the current program, most proposals have put heavy restrictions on where individuals can invest their money. And it will take a year for contributions to be invested. Individuals also cannot withdraw money from their accounts until they retire. And beneficiaries will face restrictions on withdrawals from the account in retirement. To ensure that beneficiaries have an adequate income until they die, there are restrictions on how much of the account must be annuitized versus withdrawn as a lump sum.

Moreover, individual accounts will mean a bigger government. The administrative state will grow to help oversee these accounts. For example, to protect beneficiaries as the current structure does, the Presidential Commission on Social Security required that the government be primarily responsible for deciding where individuals can invest their money and for educating them on how to do it. The heavy government involvement and limitations on choice reflect lessons learned from other nations' experiences with privatization. The United Kingdom's numerous problems with its almost fully privatized system made it clear that most people did not fare well with a lot of choice and little government intervention (Orszag 1999).

Ultimately, partial privatization proposals are more pro-business than they are free market. The reaction of the business community largely reflects this. They have been generally quite supportive of partial privatization, recognizing that billions of new dollars could flow into their coffers. New lobbying groups have popped up over the past couple of years. For example, the Coalition for American Financial Security, which was founded by executives from investment firms like the Frank Russell Company, State Street Global Advisors, Mellon Institutional Asset Management, and Brinson Partners, is raising money to help advertise and promote Bush's partial privatization plan. The administrative costs associated with millions of new individual accounts could swell profits for many investment firms. Though there is a group of investment firms that have been less supportive of partial privatization, their rationale is also profit driven. They worry about very limited profit potential from accounts. One issue is that many of the accounts will be quite small, limiting the administrative fees that investment firms could reap. Another issue that concerns investment firms is that the government will cap fees, also reducing their potential gain (Przybyla 2001).

Other lobbying groups have been formed by the larger business community that will generally benefit by having billions funneled into many publicly traded companies. For example, the Alliance for Worker Retirement Security (now COMPASS—Coalition for Modernization and Protection of America's Social Security), which is backed by the National Association of Manufacturers, the U.S. Chamber of Commerce, and other business groups, is hiring new employees to gear up its lobbying. The group's director, Charles Blahous, left the organization to be staff director for the Presidential Commission on Social Security Reform (Stevenson 2001).

In the end, the government would face a conflict between protecting beneficiaries and supporting business. The Presidential Commission's individual account proposals reflect this conflict. For example, it will take over a year for workers' money to actually be deposited into their accounts. This choice was made because business would have to do additional paperwork, leading to new costs, for contributions to be immediately credited. The interests of business won out in this conflict. And there will be many more choices for the government to make if these accounts are created, both at their inception and in gradual reforms that occur even after their creation.

Reframing the Solutions

Social Security's actual problems are far less dramatic than its critics imply and thus require far less dramatic solutions than they have proposed. Moreover, the recent bear market has opened a new opportunity for those who oppose privatization to highlight the importance of the existing Social Security program and, concurrently, to advance other solutions to its problems.

The security of the existing benefit structure in sharp contrast to the dramatic drops in the stock market has fostered doubt about privatization as many retirement investment portfolios were decimated. More than three in four Americans between the ages of 50 and 70 who own stock or other investments have self-reported losses in their accounts over the past two years. About one-quarter of this group have delayed their retirement, returned to work in retirement, started to look for work, or are considering one of these steps (Brown 2002). The 2002 elections reflected these changed circumstances: many politicians seeking elected office shrank back from any semblance of support for partial privatization. Moreover, the Republican National Committee formally recommended that Republicans seeking election should use the term "individual account" instead of "privatization." Thus, many claimed they were opposed to privatization in their campaigns, while in the small print claiming they were for individual accounts. President Bush, however, has maintained that he will continue to seek partial privatization. But they have not stated what is the most obvious—that the foundation of retirement, disability, and survivorship security should not be subjected to the vagaries of financial markets.

Importantly, there are alternative incremental solutions to Social Security's financing problems that are superior to the large cuts proposed by the privatizers. The current shortfall is 1.92 percent of taxable payroll. Thus, the simplest alternative is to raise the payroll tax by 1.92 percent divided between employees and employers, though of course it would still be necessary to address the structural shortfalls in the out years. While a large payroll tax increase is neither feasible nor necessarily desirable, modest increases (e.g., 0.25 percent on employer and employee) placed 20 or 40 years in the future might easily be a part of a solution. Given that many Americans have been told it would take 8 to 14 percent increases, this might seem like small and absorbable change.

Proposals to raise the maximum taxable income ceiling ($87,000 in 2003) could address a substantial portion of the shortfall. One could argue that an increased burden should be placed on firms offering disproportionately high salaries by subjecting 100 percent of the employer's payroll to FICA taxation. This could address about half of the financing problem. The widening income gap in the United States—the upper-income quintile's share having risen from 45.1 percent in 1983 to 48.3 percent ten years later—could be viewed as providing the rationale to do so. Leaving the employee share capped would eliminate the need to give excessively large benefits in the future to the highest-income workers. A more modest proposal would restore and maintain the proportion of wages covered by the payroll tax— now at 88 percent and projected to drop to 85.5 percent in ten years— to the 90 percent level. This would address about 14 percent of the projected financing problem.

In place of these proposals, there are a plethora of moderate reform alternatives. The retirement age could be increased from 67 to 68. The last bend point could be reduced, thus slightly reducing benefits for very high earners. Or a portion of fringe benefits could be treated as taxable. The point is that financing problems can be resolved without dramatic programmatic change or dramatic benefit decreases.

Finally, the most flexible alternative to the financing problem would allow for unanticipated changes in the economy and the program's fiscal health. Assuming modest economic growth (1.3 to 2 percent of real GDP) over the next thirty to sixty years, future workers will not face extraordinary burdens in financing benefits for future retirees. If the economy grows at a slower rate, however, reforms could be implemented in 2027 when we expect to start drawing on the trust funds reserves. Another set of changes could be scheduled fifteen years later, to capture the greatest savings in the out years when the gap between anticipated income and costs is expected to be largest. Even if such adjustments were scheduled, we should expect that we will return to Social Security financing many times before 2070 and make changes as future experience proves better or worse than currently anticipated.

Conclusion

Budgetary crises and partial privatization proposals have shaped the current politics of Social Security reform and stifled other approaches to improving the program. Drastically cutting benefits or targeting through means testing has not gained popular momentum. Given the failure of proposals to dramatically reduce benefits, proponents of partial privatization argued that individual accounts would save Social Security, all while improving benefits. But individual accounts are just a new twist on an old agenda. The core principle of privatization is that individuals should solely bear the economic risks associated with retirement. Accordingly, a perfectly privatized Social Security would entail its elimination. Partial privatization moves closer to this goal.

But the very reason for Social Security's existence serves as a reminder of the importance of the program's goal to ensure income security in retirement. Before its creation, individuals bore the economic risks associated with retirement solitarily. However, the Great Depression, spawned by the 1929 market crash, provided clear evidence that the government would need to bear a portion of the risk. The program's goal was very clear. Social Security would be the government-guaranteed leg of the three-legged stool, of which the other parts were savings and pensions. The danger of partial privatization, however, is that shortening the government's leg will make the stool unstable. And those most at risk from being hurt by partial privatization are the ones who can least afford it.

A more quiescent and less ideologically driven politics holds greater promise of addressing the projected shortfalls and of advancing the values that inform the program—concern to assure that every American has basic protection against risks related to retirement, disability, and survivorship. It remains to be seen whether the next national election will enhance or foreclose the possibility of a more sober and productive politics of Social Security.

Notes

1. These figures are based on an inflation-adjusted annuity that does not fluctuate from year to year. An alternative approach is to use a variable-adjusted annuity, which would produce higher returns. But using a variable-adjusted annuity would mean that retirees' benefits would fluctuate from year to year depending on the market. This would be a risky way to set up retirement income.

References

Aaron, H. J., A. Blinder, A. Munnell, and P. Orszag. 2001. "Perspectives on the Draft Interim Report of the President's Commission to Strengthen Social Security." Center on Budget and Policy Priorities. www.cbpp.org.

Ball, R. M. 2000. *Ensuring the Essentials: Bob Ball on Social Security.* New York: The Century Fund.

Berkowitz, E. D. 1997. The historical development of Social Security in the United States. Pp. 22–38 in E. R. Kingson and J. H. Schulz, eds., *Social Security in the Twenty-first Century.* New York: Oxford University Press.

Board of Trustees. 2003. *2003 Annual Report of the Trustees of the Federal Old-Age and Survivors Insurance and Disability Insurance Trust Funds.* Washington, D.C.: Government Printing Office.

Bosworth, B., and G. Burtless. 1997. Budget: Population aging. *Brookings Review* 15(3):17–21.

Brown, S. K. 2002. *Impact of Stock Market Decline on 50–70 Year Old Investors.* Washington, D.C.: AARP.

Church, G., and R. Lacayo. 1995. Social Security: The numbers don't add up—and the politicians won't own up. *Time,* March 20.

Derthick, M. 1979. *Policymaking for Social Security.* Washington, D.C.: Brookings Institution.

Diamond, P., and P. Orszag. 2002. *Reducing Benefits and Subsidizing Individual Accounts: An Analysis of the Plans Proposed by the President's Commission to Strengthen Social Security.* New York: The Century Fund.

Feldstein, M. 1999. America's golden opportunity. *Economist,* 13 March, 41–43.

Geanakoplos, J., O. Mitchell, and S. Zeldes. 1999. Social Security's Money's Worth. In O. Mitchell, R. Myers, and H. Young, *Prospects for Social Security Reform.* Philadelphia: University of Pennsylvania Press.

Glassman, J. K. 2001. "Welfare State Enthusiasts Desperately Fight Social Security Reform." The American Enterprise Institute. www.aei.org.

Harrington Meyer, M., and P. Herd. 2001. Aging and aging policy in the U.S. Pp. 375–88 in J. Blau, ed., *Blackwell Companion to Sociology.* Oxford, UK: Blackwell Publishers.

Hohaus, R. A. 1938. Factors in old age security. *Record of the American Institute of Actuaries* (June): 84.

Hohaus, R. A. 1960. Equity, adequacy, and related factors in old age security. In W. Haber and W. J. Cohen, eds., *Social Security Programs, Problems and Policies,* R. D. Irwin, Inc: Homewood, Ill.

Jacoby, J. 1994. The Social Security scam. *Boston Globe,* 20 December.

Kalish, D. W., and A. Tetsuya. 1999. "Retirement Income Systems: The Reform Process Across OECD Countries." Paris, France: Organization for Economic Cooperation and Development.

Kingson, E. R. 1999. Invited testimony for "Hearing on Social Security Reform Lessons Learned in Other Countries," before the U.S. House of Representatives, Committee on Ways and Means, Washington, D.C., February 11, 1999.

Kingson, E. R., and J. Quadagno. 1995. Social Security: Marketing radical reform. *Generations* 19(3):43–49.

Krugman, P. 2001. Sins of commission. *New York Times,* 25 July.

Marquis, C. 2002. Parties criticized for ads citing Social Security. *New York Times,* 13 September.

Milwaukee Sentinel. 2002. Republicans withdraw Social Security ad. 13 September 13.

National Commission on Social Security Reform. 1983. *Report of the National Commission on Social Security Reform.* Washington, D.C.

Orszag, P. 1999. "Administrative Costs in Individual Accounts in the United Kingdom." Center on Budget and Policy Priorities. www.cbpp.org.

Orszag, P., and R. Greenstein. 2001. "Voluntary Individual Accounts for Social Security: What are the Costs?" Center on Budget and Policy Priorities. www.cbpp.org.

President's Commission to Strengthen Social Security. 2001. *Strengthening Social Security and Creating Personal Wealth for all Americans.* www.css.gov.

Przybyla, H. 2001. Funds cool to retirement reform. *Seattle Times,* 29 June.

Quadagno, J. 1996. Social Security and the myth of the entitlement crisis. *Gerontologist* 36(3):391–99.

Smeeding, T., C. Estes, and L. Glasse. 1999. "Social Security Reform and Older Women: Improving the System." Center for Policy Research Income Security Policy Series Paper No. 22, The Maxwell School. Syracuse, N.Y.: Syracuse University.

Stevenson, R. 2001. Two sides tally to shape Social Security discussion. *New York Times,* 17 June.

U.S. Social Security Administration. 2001. *Social Security Supplement.* www.ssa.gov.

10. Sustaining Medicare as an Age-Related Program

Marilyn Moon

Medicare, like Social Security, is a program in which the bulk of benefits go to older Americans. By design, the majority of beneficiaries of the Medicare program are persons aged 65 and older who qualify for some type of Social Security benefit. By most accounts, Medicare consistently ranks among the most popular of federal programs, offering health insurance to groups of the population that have largely been spurned by the private insurance market. It is a consciously age-based program, meeting the particular needs of older (and disabled) individuals.

Medicare will likely continue as an age-based program (in addition to its coverage of persons with disabilities) because the basic rationale (covering a population largely spurned by the private sector) still remains. While there is some interest by the private sector in serving parts of this population, that role is contingent on requirements for guaranteed issue and renewal that preclude private insurers from serving only high-risk individuals—the situation that now shelters any private insurance participation for Medicare beneficiaries. Medicare also plays an important redistributive role within and across generations. All individuals are eligible for the same benefit package regardless of what they pay in. And across-generation subsidies occur as health care costs increase through time. Moreover, the presence of Medicare likely protects the rest of the insurance market from having to absorb very-high-risk individuals.

Yet in this era of antigovernment sentiment even a popular program is not immune from scrutiny for ways to slow the growth in spending. The 1980s and 90s focus on limiting the size of government led to numerous efforts to hold down the costs of the program over time. Debates over comprehensive changes have continued into this new century. One policy change that has already been proposed and that will likely continue to be debated is raising the eligibility age for Medicare. For those focused on cost issues, the goal would likely be to raise the eligibility age from its current 65 to age 68 or 70, for example. Alternatively, some proponents of incremental expansion in public programs would like to see the age of eligibility lowered so that younger retirees and persons with no labor force attachment could get Medicare coverage. In that case, the eligibility age is often proposed to be 60 or 62.

Moreover, legitimate concerns about the future of our entitlement programs and somewhat more gratuitous warnings about intergenerational warfare also dictate the need to carefully reexamine Medicare. It is in this context that a frank discussion about age-related programs is raised. The broadest issue arises over the relevance of the program— is it still needed? And even if it is, what changes are likely to be considered, and how do they relate to the age of beneficiaries?

Context Matters

Raising the question about the need for a separate age-related health care program in the midst of a serious debate about providing universal health insurance coverage for all Americans is quite different from raising the issue in the context of a discussion of what programs to eliminate or scale back.

When the context was achieving a program in which health insurance would be available to everyone, then questions about varying needs of populations of different ages were key. Are there practical reasons for keeping older Americans in a separate program? When it was first passed, Medicare was considered by many to be the first step toward national health insurance. In that way, it was to have ceased being an age-based program over time as the program was expanded. But the arguments for Medicare were made in the context of high rates of poverty of a group largely outside the labor force—and hence with little ability to attain reasonable health insurance coverage. It has survived for more than thirty-five years as an entitlement limited to only certain groups of the population; though over a lifetime, it is an entitlement in which nearly every American can participate.

Today, however, moving away from age-based policy would mean not expansion but rather elimination of Medicare. That is, the debate over national health insurance has subsided substantially since

1994–95, and today most discussions of expanded public policy in the area of health insurance rely on incremental changes directed at groups defined by age or income. In a world of scarce resources, which are the most deserving groups? Since the collapse of serious debate on universal coverage in 1994, Medicare's future has generally been discussed in this latter context. Improvements in coverage of children through Medicaid expansions and the State Children's Health Insurance Program (SCHIP) have taken off some, but not all, of the pressures regarding whether older Americans' needs should be placed above those of children. As the baby boom generation moves inexorably toward retirement age and the inevitable increases in Medicare spending necessary to meet those needs occur, the rhetoric over holding down costs will undoubtedly escalate further.

A brief respite in these efforts occurred at the beginning of the new century as consensus on a need to add prescription drugs to the benefit package and a brief flirtation with a balanced budget made some expansion appear possible. Although the Medicare Prescription Drug, Improvement, and Modernization Act of 2003 has finally established a prescription drug benefit to begin in 2006, it is not only less than what many beneficiaries expected, but it also includes a number of changes in Medicare presumably designed to slow the growth of spending over time.

The Need for an Aged-Based Health Care Program

Medicare's treatment of older Americans addresses several important needs. It is in most ways as relevant today as it was in 1965.

Medicare as a Tool to Address Market Failure

First, to understand the appropriate role of Medicare, it is important to examine it as a retirement program as well as an age-related one. In that sense, age is largely a proxy for retirement, and Medicare effectively extends insurance to people who are, in large part, out of the labor force and for whom group insurance is therefore difficult to obtain. Most Americans get their health care benefits through their employer or the employer of a family member. Such coverage is at least partially subsidized by the employer (and by taxpayers through employers' deductions). Just as important, people obtain "group" insurance, which is more efficient to provide and considerably less expensive than individually based policies. Historically, few insurance companies wanted to offer individual policies to people over age 65. Not only were there expenses in marketing to individuals, but also older Americans were considered an undesirable risk group in the 1950s and early 1960s. While younger families were increasingly obtaining insurance, the elderly were left behind. The health care "have nots" were increasingly older Americans. In large measure, government took on the task because of a failure of the market to offer such services.

One of Medicare's strengths is its sharing of risks across a large group of the population. With about 41 million beneficiaries, Medicare is essentially the largest risk group for health insurance in the United States. Implicitly, costs for 85-year-olds with health problems are averaged in with costs for healthy 70-year-olds, making insurance less expensive than if these 85-year-olds were seeking insurance in the private market from a company that covered a much smaller number of people. The private market does not have risk pooling on its agenda in the same way. Private profit-making firms naturally seek to hold down their costs, and the easiest way to do so is to preclude high-risk enrollees. Thus, without substantial regulatory intervention, the market fails to provide universal coverage, especially for this age group.

While some private insurers are now willing to provide supplemental insurance or even full benefits as an option (Medicare+Choice) under Medicare, this happens in the context of protected competition where risks are lower than they would otherwise be. That is, Medigap (supplemental) insurers face relatively limited liability, and after an initial enrollment period, they can exclude enrollees. HMO plans that have operated under Medicare+Choice have been able to "cream skim" the market and thus reduce the risks they face by limiting enrollment to healthier beneficiaries. A number of studies indicate that major problems with Medicare+Choice call into question the ability of the private sector to do a good job in covering all seniors and persons with disabilities (Brown et al. 1993; U.S. GAO 2000; Gold 2001). Furthermore, health maintenance organizations (HMOs) that are allowed to enroll Medicare beneficiaries have never covered more than a minority of older beneficiaries. HMOs have steadily withdrawn from this market since 1997 when legislation attempted to reduce the implicit subsidies arising from risk selection.

At the same time, many employers who have been offering subsidies for insurance before their retirees become Medicare-eligible and for Medicare supplemental benefits are now beginning to reduce their commitments. Although this has not yet had a major impact on the portion of individuals served by former employers, it certainly seems that retiree coverage has peaked (Kaiser HRET 2002).

In the 1990s and early 2000s, private insurers became increasingly unwilling to cover persons in their early sixties in individual policies. Even good health may be no guarantee of finding an affordable policy. Thus, Medicare's contribution to guaranteeing insurance remains relevant in 2003, and problems may extend below Medicare's current eligibility age.

Differences in Insurance Needs by Age

Age also plays another role in insurance. Even under private coverage, people of different ages are recognized as having different needs and different levels of expenditures. For example, people over 65 in the United States spend on average over four times as much as younger persons, and in other industrialized countries that ratio is even greater (Reinhardt 2000). Thus, to some extent age distinctions may be a natural way to subdivide the population by risk group. Among those under age 65, for example, insurance companies often set premiums based on age, and states that establish rules for acceptable variations in insurance usually include age as a legitimate factor.

Medicare effectively groups together a population of those most expensive to insure. In fact, even during the debate over national health insurance in 1992–94, Medicare was to be kept intact and separate from coverage for younger families. Otherwise, adding this population to the general risk pool for such younger families would significantly raise the average costs of insurance to them. Full community rating—that is, setting only one price for health insurance—is essentially a very redistributive system at any one point in time. Because older people tend to require more health care, establishing a single insurance premium in a given area would require most young people to pay much more than the costs of their own care for their coverage. Older persons, on the other hand, would pay much less. And because younger families tend to be less well off, such impacts raise equity issues.

In our fragmented health care system, such community rating poses a number of problems. While there is some pressure to reform insurance so that it is priced on the basis of at least a modified community-rated system, it would become much more difficult to do so if the elderly and disabled were included as well as people from birth to age 64. For example, employers would be less likely to offer insurance to all workers if their rates were subsidizing the oldest-old in our society as well. This would immediately raise the costs of insurance for such employers. (And there are practical difficulties of applying full-community rating in the United States because, for example, employers can serve as their own insurers and restrict their risks to their own pool of workers.) Thus, for practical reasons it makes sense to retain an age-related health insurance scheme for older people when there is no feasible way to deal with the redistributional questions that community rating raises in a decentralized insurance world. Such age relating protects both the old and the young.

Medicare as a Redistributive Tool

When Medicare was enacted in 1965, one of the justifications for focusing on seniors was that almost no one over the age of 65 could afford private insurance; they were simply too poor (Marmor 1970). While that was never true for all of those over 65, the low-income population was a much greater proportion of all the elderly than it is today. The average rate of poverty has declined from 28.5 percent in 1966 to 10.4 percent in 2002 (Federal Interagency Forum 2000; U.S. Bureau of the Census 2003).

The greater average affluence of older Americans has caused some policymakers to question the need for Medicare as it currently stands. However, health care costs have grown faster than the incomes of the over-65 population, resulting in higher per capita spending on health as a share of income than in 1965. Whereas seniors devoted about 19 percent of their incomes to acute health care spending in 1965, it reached over 22 percent in 2000 (Moon and Storeygard 2002b). Nonetheless, Medicare beneficiaries are now more heterogeneous than in the past. A large number still would need subsidies before they could purchase insurance, but at least some older couples are now quite well off, thus complicating the issue of the need for subsidies.

One of the challenging issues for financing health care for older Americans is how best to recognize this heterogeneity in economic status. For some, the answer is simple: means-test the program and limit its availability to those who are unable to afford insurance on their own, or at least require higher-income individuals to pay greater premiums. But often missed in such a discussion is the fact that Medicare is a re-distributive program. The payroll tax for Medicare has no upper limit, so persons with very high incomes pay a lot into the system. Further-more, three-quarters of revenues for Part B (Physicians' services) come from general revenues—where higher income persons also pay more.

Without Medicare, many middle-income seniors would have great difficulty paying for their care. One solution that is sometimes sug-gested is for individuals to create savings accounts to meet their future needs. But it is difficult at age 40, for example, to predict health care needs into the future. For the most part, costs of health care grow faster than the incomes of persons 65 and over. As a result, Medicare has been redistributive across generations as well. In general, this has worked well, ensuring that older Americans are able to get mainstream care.

Who Should Pay for Medicare?

An important implication for an age-related public program is the vis-ibility it brings to the issue of who should pay for such a program. When enacted, both Social Security and Medicare were often presented as contributory programs into which individuals would pay during their working lives to ensure protection in old age (or after becoming disabled).But in practice, these programs have been redistributive from one generation to the next. In part this reflects our unwillingness as a society to delay paying benefits until individuals contribute across all their working lives. This would mean a 35-year start-up period. Thus, subsidies were used to speed up the process. Moreover, as each gener-ation has become better off than the last, these mechanisms have helped to share that well-being with seniors.

The aging of society has caused some people to question whether we can continue that practice, however. And indeed, combined with large federal deficits and resistance to increased taxes, Medicare, like other programs, has been subjected to budget-cutting efforts over time. Al-though age of eligibility has occasionally been raised as an issue, it has never gathered much attention. But changing the age of eligibility is likely to become a more important issue as the share of seniors rises relative to the rest of the population.

Raising the Age of Eligibility

The rationale for increasing eligibility age is quite straightforward: life expectancy is increasing, and the age of normal retirement benefits for Social Security is rising under current policy. So why not Medicare? Life expectancy has increased by more than three years since Medicare's passage in 1965, offering one justification for delaying eligibility (National Center for Health Statistics 2002). The higher costs of the resulting additional years of coverage need to be paid for in some way, and when these are combined with pressures that will arise from the aging of the baby boom generation, some changes will need to be made. In the eyes of many, that means delaying eligibility by raising the age at which people qualify for Medicare. A slow phase-in of that change would coincide with the rising burdens that demography will pose. And if people begin to work longer, delaying their retirement, this option becomes more viable.

Indeed, the arguments posed by supporters of this approach often draw analogies to Social Security, where the normal age of retirement began rising in the year 2000. It will eventually reach 67, and future policy changes in this program may take that even higher. But several things are quite different for Medicare. First, while the normal age of eligibility would rise for Social Security, under current law, people could still choose to draw benefits at age 62. They would simply receive a smaller benefit. Medicare, on the other hand, as now constituted does not offer an early eligibility option.

Raising the age of eligibility would seem to retain benefits for those most in need. But in fact, age is not a very good proxy for need. The health status of people 65 and above varies substantially within each age group (Helbing 1993), and spending also varies more within each age group as compared to across-group variation. For example, although the oldest old do use more health care than other age groups among the elderly, the differential is not nearly as dramatic as many believe. In 1999, Medicare's fee-for-service beneficiaries over age 85 represented 13 percent of enrollees and accounted for just 16 percent of total spending. Compare this to the fact that the top 15 percent of Medicare beneficiaries in terms of spending accounted for nearly 75 percent of Medicare expenditures (U.S. HCFA 2003).

In addition, ability to afford to insure against ill health also varies substantially within age groups. While younger members of the Medicare-eligible population tend to have higher incomes than their counterparts who are, for example, over the age of 80, averages hide a great deal of diversity within this population. If the justification is to focus more on ability to pay, then an income or means test is certainly a more direct way to do so. But many supporters of Medicare do not want to see it make major distinctions in eligibility by income. The popularity of the program arises in part because of its universality, prompting some to argue that universality should simply begin a little later. However, if done to serve as a proxy for targeting Medicare by ability to pay, this is a very crude mechanism.

Raising the eligibility age would also create other disadvantages. Without private insurance reform, those out of the labor force might find it difficult to obtain insurance. Employers will face higher insurance costs if they provide retiree benefits to fill in the gaps of a rising age of eligibility. Alternatively, they might cut back on coverage, increasing the numbers of persons who would have to pay on their own or go uninsured. As a consequence, if the number of uninsured rises, placing burdens on public hospitals, if the costs of producing goods and services rise to pay greater retiree health benefits, if the number of young families supporting their older relatives increases, we will be just as burdened as a society. Thus, we will not have solved anything, although the balance on the federal government's ledgers will improve.

Finally, raising the age of eligibility for Medicare would not result in substantial savings if it is done appropriately. About 5 percent of Medicare beneficiaries are aged 65 and 66. If the age of eligibility were increased to 67, however, savings would be substantially less than 5 percent—likely in the range of 2 to 3 percent of Medicare's overall spending—because persons in these age groups have lower Medicare costs than other beneficiaries. This is particularly the case because those aged 65 and 66 who became eligible as disabled beneficiaries would stay on the Medicare roles (Waidmann 1998).

Despite these potential problems, it seems likely that increasing the age of eligibility for Medicare will continue to be debated over time. Moreover, as part of a broader package of budget savings, this change in Medicare may be preferred to more stringent means testing or other types of changes such as moving Medicare to a voucher-type system.

One way to soften the blow of an increase in the age of eligibility for Medicare might be to create a new standard for qualifying for disability above a certain age and to eliminate the current two-year waiting period before obtaining eligibility. In that case, at least those who were not able to work longer because of health problems could still get Medicare as disabled beneficiaries even if they did not yet qualify on the basis of the new age criteria. Similarly, eligibility for Medicaid could be expanded somewhat for those who might be disenfranchised by a higher age of receipt for Medicare. Finally, absent broad insurance reform, it would be crucial to allow older Americans to buy into the program, because they otherwise might not be able to attain insurance at any price.

What about raising the age of eligibility but then using some of the savings to expand help for the chronically ill and the disabled? Expansions in Medicare's benefit package to better cover chronic care could be justified if the program were targeted on those aged 75 and older, for example. A modified package of benefits could be extended to the old-old (at 70 or 75, for example) and the disabled, while offering a more basic plan with higher personal contributions for those below the new eligibility age. And this lower tier might be extended even further down the age scale to aid early retirees and perhaps even unburden some employers who now face high subsidy costs. This type of change could improve on basic proposals to raise the age of eligibility for Medicare. But it is hard to imagine how to design such a package that would not raise overall costs.

Other Options

Certainly raising the age of eligibility is not the only option available for addressing the cost of Medicare over time. A whole range of cost-saving measures have been considered for Medicare, including means-testing eligibility for the program, reducing benefits, raising the Part B premium, and increasing reliance on the private sector. Most of these involve serious trade-offs in terms of reductions in access to care or eligibility in exchange for lower costs. Greater reliance on the private sector falls into this category if it means turning Medicare into a defined-contribution rather than defined-benefit program. That effectively shifts the risks of greater costs over time onto the beneficiaries themselves. Proponents of such an approach often argue, however, that reliance on private insurers will itself result in lower costs for the same benefits. Yet despite these claims, the evidence largely points in the opposite direction: Medicare is not less efficient than the private sector, and under the Medicare+Choice program in which private plans were allowed to serve beneficiaries, they were largely able to do so only by avoiding high-risk patients (U.S. GAO 2000; Boccuti and Moon 2003).

A different approach would be to increase funding for the Medicare program. It is simply not feasible to expect that a benefit whose costs grow each year with the overall costs of health care and with the increasing number of persons eligible for the program could succeed over time without an infusion of new resources. Cost-cutting efforts can go only so far. Opponents of higher taxes stress the "unsupportable" higher costs that would have to be absorbed. But with even modest increases in productivity over time, younger persons will have sufficient resources not only to meet all the needs from Medicare but also to substantially raise their standard of living at the same time (Moon and Storeygard 2002a). Intergenerational redistribution is feasible without unduly penalizing the young.

In considering whether to increase the age of eligibility for Medicare, it will be important to weigh the costs and benefits of these and other options. In some cases an increase in eligibility age may be a fairer approach than other proposals—even from the standpoint of protecting older Americans. For example, turning the program over to private insurers will disproportionately disadvantage the sickest and oldest beneficiaries. In that context, requiring higher contributions from younger beneficiaries or changing eligibility age may do a better job of protecting the most vulnerable than privatization for all beneficiaries.

It is also important to consider interactions among options. For example, proposals to fully or partially rely on private plans to cover Medicare beneficiaries, creating a "defined-contribution" approach, become even more problematic if the age of eligibility is raised. When plans can charge additional premiums (as is now allowed to a limited degree under the HMO option and would be the case for changes offered in the House of Representatives Medicare legislation of 2003), they could begin to influence even more dramatically who will enroll. For example, some might use high premiums to concentrate on a higher-income market. This would implicitly discriminate against older beneficiaries who tend to have lower incomes. Moreover, by choosing what additional benefits to offer, plans may also discourage those beneficiaries who need home health care, for example, versus health club memberships. An age-related issue arises because of the disproportionate number of chronic health care needs among the older population. The ability of insurers to game the system is greater for this population. This suggests another reason for partitioning health insurance by age. What works for the young may not always work for older persons.

Conclusion

It would be difficult to overstate how much the tenor of debate regarding health care has changed since May 1994, when national health insurance seemed possible. Prospects for expanding coverage under Medicare along with a minimal expansion of long-term care services seemed to be plausible early in the 1990s. But by the beginning of 1995, the discussion shifted to how much could be wrung out of the Medicare program to help balance the federal budget. Legislation in 1997 did just that—cutting back on payments to providers of care and shifting greater costs onto beneficiaries. Only the addition of a limited prescription drug benefit has proven possible in the current environment. And as the baby boom generation begins to retire at the end of this decade, it is likely that concerns will once again focus on how to hold the line on spending if the current attitudes about government and taxation remain (Moon and Storeygard 2002a).

With substantial reductions in federal spending on the horizon for the Medicare program, some new ways of thinking about Medicare are needed. Rather than rejecting a proposal such as raising the age of eligibility as undesirable, it must be viewed in the context of what other changes are likely. How does such a proposal measure up to means-testing the program or converting it to a voucher system? These and other proposals for change have both crude and subtle impacts on Americans of different ages. Vouchers, for example, are likely to be harder on the oldest old, while means testing eliminates higher-income persons of any age. But how do we weigh these alternatives in the context of an individual's lifetime? Careful debate ought to go into any choices among these alternatives.

Thus, we are likely to retain Medicare as an age-related program, although the ages affected may change over time. Age is a simple criterion to measure and enforce—as compared to economic resources or levels of disability, for example. A higher eligibility age can also be viewed as consistent with the expanding life expectancies of older Americans, so that Medicare continues to cover people for an average fixed number of years at the end of life. Despite its disadvantages, these basic factors may make this a policy that is preferable to other changes that could undermine the principles and viability of a key health care program.

There are also legitimate insurance reasons to maintain some age distinctions. To keep insurance more affordable for younger people, it is appropriate to have a separate program like Medicare. This also affords the opportunity to fine-tune coverage—although that is an area where Medicare has lagged and that may now be too expensive to change, at least in the current political climate.

But if raising the age of eligibility for Medicare is the direction in which we move, it will be critical to push other parts of society to develop consistent policies and attitudes. First, Social Security and Medicare need to be closely coordinated. If reductions in benefits occur for both, for example by raising the age of eligibility, those who must retire early will find it very expensive to both subsist on reduced Social Security benefits and seek their own health insurance. But even more important, private pensions, work opportunities for older workers, rules for private insurance, and general attitudes of society must also change if higher age criteria are to be successful and not simply result in lower standards of living over time.

References

Boccuti, C., and M. Moon. 2003. Comparing Medicare and private insurers: Growth rates in spending over three decades. *Health Affairs* 22 (March/April): 230–37.

Brown, R., D. Clement, J. Hill, S. Rettchin, and J. Bergeron. 1993. Do health maintenance organizations work for Medicare? *Health Care Financing Review* 15 (Fall): 7–23.

Federal Interagency Forum on Aging Related Statistics. 2000. *Older Americans 2000: Key Indicators of Well-Being.* Washington, D.C.: Government Printing Office.

Gold, M. 2001. Medicare+Choice: An interim report card. *Health Affairs* 20 (July/August): 120–38.

Helbing, C. 1993. Medicare program expenditures. Pp. 55–96 in *Health Care Financing Review: Annual Statistical Supplement 1992.* Washington, D.C.: Government Printing Office.

Kaiser Family Foundation and Health Research and Educational Trust. 2002. *Employer Health Benefits 2002 Annual Survey.* Menlo Park, Calif.: Kaiser Family Foundation.

Marmor, T. R. 1970. *The Politics of Medicare.* Chicago: Aldine.

Moon, M. 1996. *Medicare Now and in the Future,* second edition. Washington, D.C.: Urban Institute Press.

Moon, M., with P. Herd. 2002. *A Place at the Table: Women's Needs and Medicare Reform.* New York: Century Foundation Press.

Moon, M., and M. Storeygard. 2002a. Solvency or Affordability? Ways to Measure Medicare's Financial Health. Henry J. Kaiser Family Foundation Discussion Paper, March.

Moon, M., and M. Storeygard. 2002b. Stretching Federal Dollars: Policy Trade-Offs in Designing a Medicare Drug Benefit with Limited Resources. Commonwealth Fund Policy Brief.

National Center for Health Statistics. 2002. *Health, United States, 2002 With Chartbook on Trends in the Health of Americans.* Hyattsville, Md.: NCHS.

Reinhardt, U. E. 2000. Health care for the aging baby boom: Lessons from abroad. *Journal of Economic Perspectives* 14 (Spring): 71–83.

U.S. Bureau of the Census. 2003. *Consumer Income Series, P60-222.* Washington, D.C.: GAO.

U.S. General Accounting Office. 2000. *Medicare+Choice: Payments Exceed Cost of Fee-For-Service Benefits, Adding Billions to Spending,* no. GAO/HEHS-00-161, Washington, D.C.: GAO.

U.S. Health Care Financing Administration. 2003. *Health Care Financing Review: Medicare and Medicaid Statistical Supplement, 2001.* Baltimore: U.S. Department of Health and Human Services.

Waidmann, T. 1998. Potential effects of raising Medicare's eligibility age. *Health Affairs* 17 (March/April): 156–64.

11. The Politics of Aging within Medicaid

Colleen M. Grogan

Health care in the United States is often characterized as a "two-tiered" system in which the tiers are separate and unequal. Medicare, our universal health insurance program for elderly persons, defines the upper tier where recipients qualify for benefits without having to satisfy a means test. Medicare is governed by uniform national standards, has strong public support, and is politically stable. Medicaid, our health care program for "the poor" defines the lower tier. Medicaid is a targeted, means-tested program that is often considered to be stigmatizing, institutionally fragmented, and politically vulnerable (Rosenberry 1982; Brown 1988; Kuttner 1988; Grogan and Patashnik 2003a).

Given the saliency of this two-tiered image, one would predict, under a "veil of ignorance"[1]—that is, knowing nothing about the political history of these two programs—that benefits under Medicare have substantially expanded under an arena of strong public support and political stability since its enactment in 1965, whereas Medicaid has suffered repeated periods of policy retrenchment under its stigmatizing, politically vulnerable umbrella. Although one can find specific policy examples that fit this prediction, the general trend in both programs (at least since the mid-1980s) has been the reverse. While the recipient pool for Medicaid has in many ways exploded since the 1980s, the recipient pool for Medicare and the benefits they have access to have remained largely constant (Oberlander 2003). The reasons behind this political puzzle are complex and are the subject of a much longer manuscript currently in preparation by the author. I raise it here, however, because acknowledgment of this trend reversal throws into question the usefulness of the two-tiered image for understanding the political evolution of these two programs.

One fundamental problem with the two-tiered image is that it fails to recognize that these programs—as do most social welfare programs—typically contain contradictions in goals and purposes (Marmor, Mashaw, and Harvey 1990; Grogan and Patashnik 2003a). For example, the targeted Medicaid program often fails to serve those in greatest need and yet extends its reach to the middle class, while the universal Medicare program often provides extra benefits to low-income recipients. In thinking more generally about universal welfare state programs, Theda Skocpol labels the latter phenomenon "targeting within universalism." She points to Social Security as the leading modern example: while it benefits politically from being a universal program that provides a basic social entitlement to the middle class, it is also the nation's most effective antipoverty program, offering proportionately more generous pensions to retirees with a history of low earnings (Skocpol 1995, pp. 263–64).[2]

Grogan and Patashnik (2003a) invert Skocpol's analysis and label the former phenomenon—extending benefits to a relatively large middle-class constituency within the context of a means-tested design—as "universalism within targeting." They note that middle-class participation in targeted programs is most likely when the programs involve the delivery of very expensive goods and services, such as education or health care. As a result, the targeted program's threshold of means-tested income is set high enough that a significant number of people from mainstream backgrounds qualify (also see Gilbert 2001). Medicaid's incorporation of middle-class senior citizens in nursing homes is a good example of universalism within targeting (Grogan and Patashnik 2003a).

Another reason for elderly middle-class participation in the targeted Medicaid program likely has to do with a positive social construction of the elderly. Schneider and Ingram (1997) argue that the political vulnerability associated with certain targeted programs is not inherent to means testing per se, but rather stems from the provision of benefits to groups that are perceived to be undeserving. Thus, following this logic, it is likely that the political possibility of incorporating the middle class within Medicaid also stems from the social construction of the targeted group—in this case, a group perceived to be socially deserving.

In this chapter, I analyze the politics of Medicaid's incorporation of the middle class by examining the social construction of elderly persons within the Medicaid context. Understanding Medicaid's middle-class incorporation among the elderly is important for two reasons. First, examining Medicaid's middle-class incorporation and its associated politics opens the door to reexamining the political evolution (and possibilities) of targeted programs in general (not just Medicaid) as something other than pure policy retrenchment. Because the enactment of targeted programs is much more usual than the creation of universal programs in the United States, this reexamination seems worthwhile. Second, documenting the evolving social construction of elderly persons within Medicaid allows us to consider whether various framings of social deservingness give rise to new political possibilities. In particular, despite repeated advocacy for long-term care expansions within Medicare, elderly middle-class incorporation may give rise to universal long-term care within Medicaid. This notion is not so far-fetched, especially if one considers that most universal programs in other countries began as targeted programs with middle-class incorporation.

The framing of Medicaid's middle-class incorporation in the United States, however, is complex. Although the generally positive social construction of elderly persons as socially deserving allowed universalism within targeting to occur under Medicaid, the enactment of Medicare alongside Medicaid and the incorporation of other needy groups within Medicaid has created multiple and conflicting frames of elderly deservingness. In particular, three distinct social constructions of elderly persons are apparent simultaneously and at different points during Medicaid's political evolution.

The first section of this chapter reviews Medicaid's legislative origins to explicate how this means-tested program expanded to incorporate elderly middle-class Americans.[3] The second section elaborates on the three distinct frames of elderly deservingness within Medicaid and discusses how various frames have been more salient at different times. In each of these sections I discuss how the Medicaid program changed in ways that influenced the salience of the frame. Finally, I conclude by considering the potential of any one frame to dominate under the politics of Medicaid's universalism within targeting, and the implications of various frames for Medicaid's future policy and political possibilities.

Medicaid's Political Origins and Development

Medicaid's adoption in 1965 must be understood in the context of the long struggle to adopt universal health insurance in the United States.

By the late 1950s, liberal proponents of health care reform focused their attention on senior citizens, a clientele group that was viewed sympathetically and was already tied to the state through the Social Security system. In 1964, most informed observers thought Congress would adopt one of three alternative approaches to improve access to health care for elderly persons: (1) a universal hospital insurance program based on Social Security (the King-Anderson bills of 1963 and 1964); (2) a voluntary physician services program supported by beneficiary premiums; or (3) an expansion of the means-tested Kerr-Mills program, which offered a wide range of health care benefits to the low-income elderly. Under the influence of Ways and Means Committee Chairman Wilbur Mills, the Social Security Amendments of 1965 combined all of these approaches into a single package. By all accounts, the creation of this massive "three-layer cake" took nearly everyone by surprise (Marmor 1973; Stevens and Stevens 1974). The first layer was Medicare Part A, a hospital insurance program based on the Social Security contributory model. The second layer was Medicare Part B, a voluntary supplementary medical insurance program funded through beneficiary premiums and federal general revenues. The third and final layer was the Medicaid program (originally called Part C), which broadened the protections offered to the poor under Kerr-Mills. The Kerr-Mills means test was liberalized in order to cover additional elderly citizens, and eligibility among the indigent was broadened to include the blind, the permanently disabled, and adults in (largely) single-headed families and their dependent children.

Medicaid carried over two crucial provisions from Kerr-Mills that would profoundly influence its subsequent policy evolution: the concept of medical indigency and comprehensive benefits. Kerr-Mills had originally been drafted in 1959 as an alternative to the Forand bill, which proposed universal coverage for elderly persons with a restricted benefit package (Marmor 1973). Proponents of the Kerr-Mills approach argued that a means-tested program would be more efficient than a universal program because it offered help to the most needy. They also argued that this approach offered the truly needy more security than the Forand bill because it provided comprehensive benefits—covering hospital, physician, and nursing home services. Although Kerr-Mills was a targeted program, it was designed to be distinct from welfare. Eligibility for benefits under Kerr-Mills was restricted to the "medically indigent." These were older persons who needed assistance when they became sick because they had large medical expenses relative to their current income. Proponents emphasized that the "medically indigent should not be equated with the totally indigent" (Fein 1998). The latter term refers in this case to those who receive cash assistance. The moral argument behind this expansion reasoned that the sick elderly should not have to become completely impoverished. Indeed, medical indigency was put in place with the idea that sickness should not cause impoverishment. Both policy concepts—comprehensive benefits and medical indigency—were carried over from Kerr-Mills and enacted under the Medicaid program in 1965.

As mentioned above, the adoption of Kerr-Mills in combination with Medicare Part A and B was completely unexpected, in part because means-tested Kerr-Mills (presented in 1964 bills as Eldercare) and universal Medicare offered fundamentally competing notions of social provision.[4] The concept of medical indigency was strategically included under Kerr-Mills, and subsequently under Eldercare bills, as an alternative to universalism. As a result, in light of universal Medicare, the medical indigency concept often confused policymakers. Yet by keeping it in place, the seeds of middle-class reliance on Medicaid were planted.

Because Medicare covered only hospital and physician care services, Medicaid emerged as the most significant payer of nursing home care. As early as 1970, Medicaid was the dominant governmental purchaser in the nursing home market (Table 11.1). In 1980, Medicaid spending on nursing home care ($8.8 billion) not only surpassed all other public sources combined ($0.7 billion) but also slightly exceeded out-of-pocket payments for nursing home care ($7.4 billion). Medicaid nursing home expenditures rose rapidly during the 1990s. By 1997, Medicaid nursing home expenditures ($39.4 billion) greatly exceeded out-of-pocket payments for nursing home care ($25.7 billion). In that year, Medicaid picked up almost half (47 percent) of the $83 billion spent on nursing homes in the United States.

Not surprisingly, given demand and spend-down provisions under Medicaid, many senior citizens who receive Medicaid do not have a history of poverty before entering a nursing home. Indeed, a summary of the literature on nursing home use indicates that approximately 60 percent of people residing in nursing homes have Medicaid as a payment source on any given day. Somewhere between 33 and 40 percent

Table 11.1 Nursing home care expenditure in billions of dollars, by source of funds, 1970–97

Year	Total	Private			Public	
		Out of Pocket	Private Health Insurance	Other Private Funds	Medicaid	All Other Public Sources
1970	4.2	2.3	0.0	0.2	0.9	0.8
	(100)	(54)	(0)	(5)	(21)	(19)
1980	17.6	7.4	0.2	0.5	8.8	0.7
	(100)	(42)	(1)	(3)	(50)	(4)
1990	50.9	21.9	2.1	0.9	23.1	2.8
	(100)	(43)	(4)	(2)	(45)	(6)
1997	82.8	25.7	4.0	1.6	39.4	12.0
	(100)	(31)	(5)	(2)	(47)	(14)

Source: Health Care Financing Administration, Office of the Actuary (also in Grogan and Patashnik 2003a)
Note: Percentages (shown in parentheses) may not add up to 100 due to rounding.

of nursing home residents are eligible for Medicaid on admission. Only about one-third of those who do not have Medicaid as a payment source at admission remain private payers throughout their stay. Two-thirds of such individuals eventually spend down their savings to Medicaid levels (Cohen, Kumar, and Wallack 1993).

The significance of middle-class reliance on Medicaid raises an important question: Why haven't elderly Americans claimed the Medicaid program as "their own?" Why haven't they lobbied more persistently for Medicaid to be the United States' long-term care program? The answer to this question lies in the simultaneous creation of Medicare and Medicaid. Elderly Americans have always advocated for a Medicare expansion approach because Medicare is perceived to be "their program" and because it is perceived to be more politically acceptable than Medicaid. Indeed, notions of elderly deservingness within Medicaid have been strongly influenced by perspectives of possibilities for expansions within Medicare. As the prospects for Medicare expansions have changed over time, and elderly fortunes have changed over time, and Medicaid continues to expand over time, multiple frames of elderly deservingness within Medicaid have emerged.

Competing Frames of Elderly Deservingness within Medicaid

Three distinct social constructions of elderly persons are apparent simultaneously and at different points in time during Medicaid's political evolution: elderly Americans as too deserving for a stigmatized means-tested program such as Medicaid; elderly Americans as too well off relative to other needy groups and therefore undeserving of Medicaid as a targeted program for the poor; and elderly Americans as deserving of Medicaid's social entitlement. Note that these various frames of elderly deservingness under Medicaid depend not only on the social construction of elderly persons, but also on political constructions of the Medicaid program itself. Thus, in my attempt to show that notions of elderly deservingness in relation to the program have changed over time, I document in each section below how political constructions of the Medicaid program have changed as well—from a program that was universally described as "residual" or as "stigmatized welfare" to a program that is consistently invoked today as a "crucial safety net for the needy" and sometimes as a "core social entitlement" on par with Medicare.

Elderly Persons as Too Deserving for Stigmatized Medicaid

Because the passage of both Medicare and Medicaid were unexpected and policymakers did not give much thought to the ramifications of medical indigency, policymakers viewed Medicaid as a relatively minor piece of the 1965 Social Security legislation and of much less significance than Medicare. Government estimates of Medicaid's future budgetary costs assumed that the program would not lead to a dramatic expansion of health care coverage (Stevens and Stevens 1974). For example, even assuming that all fifty states would implement the new program, the federal government projected Medicaid expenditures to be no more than $238 million per year above what was currently then being spent on medical welfare programs. As it turned out, this expenditure level was reached after only six states had implemented their Medicaid programs. By 1967, thirty-seven states were implementing Medicaid programs, and spending was rising by 57 percent per year (Congressional Research Service 1993, p. 30).

A key factor that explains Medicaid's early expenditure growth was the establishment of generous eligibility standards under various state

"Medically Needy" programs. Known as Kerr-Mill (medical indigency) extensions, the Medically Needy programs allowed states to extend Medicaid eligibility to persons with income levels above the regular Medicaid income eligibility established in each state. A number of states initially set quite generous Medically Needy eligibility levels. For example, under New York's Medically Needy enrollment standards, almost half of the state's population in 1966 could potentially have qualified for Medicaid's comprehensive medical coverage, including access to prescription drugs and long-term care facilities (Stevens and Stevens 1974).

New York state policymakers seem to have envisioned Medicaid as the stepping-stone to universal health care for its residents, which created a major branching point in U.S. health care policy. The federal government had to decide whether it should embrace this expansive vision of Medicaid, or instead restrict program eligibility to a narrow clientele. The government chose the latter course, clamping down hard on New York's attempted liberalization. In 1967, only a year after the New York expansion began, Congress passed legislation lowering the medically needy eligibility level to 133⅓ percent of a state's AFDC means-tested level.[5]

In halting New York's attempted liberalization in 1967, federal policymakers made a conscious decision to define Medicaid as a restricted welfare program, off-limits to the employed. "The House is moving toward a program where you provide medical care to those who can't pay, and expect people to pay it if they are working and can earn income," stated one conservative senator in floor debate (U.S. Senate Committee on Finance 1967). Although elderly persons—especially those in need of long-term care—are exempt from popular notions of a work requirement, this legislation did put strict limits on the generosity of medically needy programs, which in turn affected elderly persons.

Perhaps more important, this policy retrenchment solidified an image of Medicaid as a stingy welfare program not worthy of elderly Americans. Indeed, we see this framing quite clearly in hearings where Medicaid is discussed throughout the 1970s and into the 1980s. In hearings during the 1970s and 1980s where long-term care is the topic under consideration or health issues of concern to elderly persons more generally (e.g., Alzheimer disease) are discussed, Medicaid is not mentioned, is disregarded as inappropriate for elderly persons, or is quickly dismissed as a residual program unfit to meet the needs of elderly persons. For example, in a 1970 Senate hearing on the "Sources of Community Support for Federal Programs Serving Older Americans," among the four witnesses who discussed concerns about nursing home coverage, only one witness mentioned Medicaid and then only in passing. After describing the details of Medicare nursing home coverage (or lack thereof), he said, "These shortcomings apply equally to Medicaid situations." Although by 1970 Medicaid was already the primary public payer of nursing home care, the other three witnesses similarly focused on limitations in nursing home coverage under Medicare. Senator Long's statement in 1967 provides some insight into the emergence of this view: "We were warned for many years if we didn't pass Medicare that the cost of the Kerr-Mills program, which is Medicaid, as I understand it, that was the genesis of it, was going to skyrocket. Now we have Medicare and we also have this Medicaid program. As I understand the House bill tried to hold the cost of the Medicaid program down" (H.R. 12080, 1/20/67, P. 1547). Despite the fact that nursing home care was clearly not covered under Medicare and, indeed, extended to medically needy persons under Medicaid, there was a popular conception—against programmatic reality—that Medicare was for elderly persons and should therefore suffice to take care of elderly needs.

In a 1981 hearing on "The Impact of Alzheimer's Disease on the Nation's Elderly," several witnesses discussed the problem that nursing homes often reject patients with dementia due to lack of mental health coverage. Although this was clearly a limitation in Medicaid policy, almost all the policy recommendations focused on amending Medicare policy.

In another hearing that dealt with the "Impact of Federal Budget Cuts on the Elderly" in 1982, longtime advocate for elderly persons and chairman of the committee Representative Claude Pepper began his opening remarks by stating the premier deservingness of elderly persons across the board. However, in turning to discuss the "less-fortunate" elderly, he noted: "In spite of Social Security, one-sixth, over 16 percent, of the elderly live below the poverty line. . . . They lack decent housing. Medicare only pays 38% of their medical costs. They live under fear of serious disease when they would not have the aid of Medicare. They wouldn't be eligible for Medicaid because if you have anything at all to speak of, you are not eligible for Medicaid" (House Hrg.: 82-H141-22).

Although there were valid concerns about elderly persons having to impoverish themselves to become eligible for Medicaid long-term care services, and no spousal protections were in place at this time, by 1982 Medicaid nursing home expenditures greatly exceeded out-of-pocket payments for nursing home care. Nonetheless, the Medicaid program was generally dismissed out-of-hand as too stingy and stigmatizing to be an acceptable reform strategy for elderly persons. There is very little discussion about Medicaid reform under this framing; instead, Medicare is viewed as the appropriate program to devote advocacy efforts.

This framing of Medicaid applied when policymakers considered health care expansions to the nonelderly middle class as well. We see this in health care reform proposals during this period, where Medicaid is similarly invoked as a residual program. For example, under the National Health Plan Act (H.R. 5400 / S. 1812) presented in 1980, proposed revisions to Medicaid are summarized as follows: "Services available to low-income individuals under HealthCare would no longer be covered under Title XIX. Title XIX would continue as a residual program covering those services not under HealthCare." Under The Health Care for All Americans Act (H.R. 5191 / S. 1720), "the bill would make certain changes in the Medicare program. . . . Medicaid would remain as a residual program." Indeed, Medicaid was referred to as a "residual program" in every health reform bill presented in 1980.

Despite the persistence of this residual frame, the Medicaid program experienced significant changes during the 1980s that were difficult to ignore. These changes allowed policymakers to view both the program and elderly Americans' relationship to the program in a different light.

Elderly Persons as Too Well Off
for Medicaid's Needed Safety Net

In contrast to Medicaid's policy retrenchment era during the 1970s, the program experienced an expansionary period during the 1980s. In particular, there were two main expansionary policies: (1) expanded coverage for children and pregnant women, and (2) coverage expansions for low-income elderly financed by Medicaid. The cumulative force of these expansionary policies over the 1980s created a new framing of the Medicaid program by the early 1990s. By this time, very few described the program as residual. Instead, twenty-plus years after enactment, the program was recognized as a crucial safety-net for many diverse needy groups. Under this new understanding of the program and a relatively new emerging rhetoric of elderly as politically privileged to the detriment of younger generations, elderly middle-class inclusion in Medicaid was often discussed as problematic. Elderly persons were portrayed as too well off for the crucially needed and limited resources provided under means-tested Medicaid. I will first describe the two expansionary developments during the 1980s[6] and then document the emergence of this new frame.

Expanded Coverage for Children and Pregnant Women. The federal government enacted incremental Medicaid expansions for children or pregnant women and infants in every year between 1984 and 1990 (Tanenbaum 1995). By the end of this period, approximately 5 million children and half a million pregnant women had gained Medicaid eligibility (Rosenbaum 1993, pp. 45–82).

The targeted expansions for pregnant women and children emphasized a message that Medicaid served the "deserving poor," not just people on welfare (or more accurately on cash assistance). Yet advocates for these Medicaid expansions also argued that extending Medicaid coverage to pregnant women and children was cost-effective (Tanenbaum 1995). Health care costs associated with low-birth-weight babies rose dramatically during the 1980s in part because technological improvements were allowing more and more babies of lower and lower birth weight to be saved. Advocates argued that increasing access to prenatal care through Medicaid would yield significant economic savings through higher birth weights and better infant outcomes. A similar pragmatic argument was made for expanded coverage of children: inexpensive immunizations and well-child care were portrayed as prudent investments for a healthy population and strong future workforce (Sardell 1991, pp. 17–53).

Expansions for Low-Income Elderly Persons. Although the adoption of Medicare in 1965 successfully brought the aged into the mainstream of American medicine, serious gaps in coverage remained twenty years later. As mentioned, Medicare did not (and still does not) cover most long-term care needs, nor did the program cover prescription drug expenses. In addition, the out-of-pocket costs associated with Medicare's co-payments and deductibles could reach catastrophic proportions for many elderly people with serious medical conditions.

Low-income seniors not covered under Medicaid spent on average one-quarter of their annual income on medical bills (Rosenbaum 1993).

Given the Medicaid program's longstanding role in the long-term care sector, health reform advocates might have been expected to use it as the institutional vehicle for adopting catastrophic health care coverage. Instead, advocates for long-term care coverage primarily lobbied for Medicare expansions. The Medicare Catastrophic Care Act (MCCA) of 1988 was the federal government's response to this advocacy. The act expanded coverage to include outpatient prescription drug benefits and long-term hospital care. This represented the largest expansion to the Medicare program since its inception in 1965. To finance MCCA, however, the government made a sharp break from Medicare's social insurance tradition and required Medicare beneficiaries, rather than current workers, to shoulder the financial burden. In particular, Medicare beneficiaries were asked to pay special premiums according to family income to cover the cost of expanded benefits under MCCA. Controversy over this new financing scheme (and several other reasons)[7] ultimately led to MCCA's repeal just one year later. The irony of MCCA's repeal lies in two major expansionary policies that remained intact within the Medicaid program. The first expansion provided protections against spousal impoverishment by increasing the amount of money that seniors in the community can retain when their institutionalized spouses receive Medicaid benefits. The second expansion that was not repealed under MCCA was the creation of the Qualified Medicare Beneficiary (QMB) program. This program requires the Medicaid program to buy into the Medicare program for low-income seniors and persons with disabilities. Specifically, since 1989, Medicaid has been required to pay Medicare Part B premiums and cover any deductibles or cost-sharing expenses for elderly persons with incomes under 100 percent of poverty (in 1990 premium support was expanded to elderly persons with incomes up to 120% of poverty).

While budget constraints and a relatively large federal deficit were significant motivating factors behind MCCA's passage and its intragenerational financing scheme, a new rhetoric of intergenerational equity also contributed to its support in Congress. This new rhetoric emphasized two points: (1) relatively few resources were devoted to children in need because of large public costs imposed by elderly persons; and (2) families were financially burdened due to transfers from young to old to support large expensive federal programs (e.g., Social Security and Medicare) (Cook 1994). Several scholars have documented the emergence of the intergenerational equity theme during the 1980s around discussions about the elderly more generally and its particular importance for the passage and repeal of MCCA (Quadagno 1989; Cook 1994; Pierson and Smith 1994). Not surprisingly, given the significant expansions that remained for elderly persons within the Medicaid program after the MCCA repeal, this intergenerational equity discourse became infused into Medicaid's political discourse as well.

New Framing: Elderly as Too Well-off and Overburdening Medicaid. Intergenerational equity concerns probably emerged first among state actors. Indeed, it has long been the case that while elderly persons comprise less than 15 percent of Medicaid recipients, they account for more than 30 percent of the program's costs, in large part because of their nursing home care (Rosenbaum 1993). In light of these statistics, some advocates for poor children began in the 1980s to argue that it was inappropriate for a disproportionate share of Medicaid dollars to support elderly persons while younger people were struggling to pay for their health care (Benjamin, Newacheck, and Wolfe 1991). With federal mandates in the 1980s that expanded benefits to both "cost-effective" pregnant women and children and the "expensive" elderly, representatives from the states started to voice concerns that they could not legitimately finance expansions to both groups that difficult choices needed to be made or expanding long-term care costs would result in fewer services for poor families. For example, a representative from the State Medicaid Directors' Association made the following remarks in her testimony before the Subcommittee on Health and the Environment for a 1987 hearing titled "Medicare and Medicaid Catastrophic Protection":

> Obviously, for the private payer, the spousal protections . . . are very desirable and very needed. As you reduce their share of the cost, you are again passing those increases onto the Medicaid program. I'm not suggesting that you not do it, only to keep in mind that those Medicaid budgets are being consumed by long-term care expenditures. Because state revenues and local revenues are not limitless, again choices have to be made. What we are seeing in effect is Medicaid by default becoming a long-term care budget and not being able to cover more of the primary health care needs of women, children and families. (U.S. Congress 1988, 100-74, Matula, May 28, 1987, p. 433)

This intergenerational concern within Medicaid became even more heated as the elderly expansions were implemented at the state level in the early 1990s. For example, in a federal hearing titled "Medicaid Program Investigation," testimony from a state congressman from Michigan not only emphasized the disproportionate share of the Medicaid budget consumed by elderly persons but also suggested that such expenses were used inappropriately for expensive care during the last year of life:

> Congressman, two-thirds of our health care dollars are spent in the last year of life, and two-thirds of those are spent in the last 90 days. This is the fastest-growing part of our population. We have a dramatically aging society spending more and more on health care. The health care share of our budget in Michigan has gone from 20 percent of the budget in 1980, to 26.8 percent in 1990. Medicaid is one of the major problems and you will hear across the country, Medicaid is eating up State budgets. (U.S. Congress 1991, 102-91, Hollister, Oct. 2, 1991, pp. 272–73).

These quotes illustrate concerns emerging from the states in federal discourse over the Medicaid program. In all the hearings discussing Medicaid during the early 1990s and continuing throughout the decade, representatives from the states discussed the explosive costs of long-term care and how these costs forced them to choose between needy population groups. For example, many often mentioned the "truly" needy groups that Medicaid should cover but cannot, due to expensive long-term care costs, such as working families without insured. In North Carolina, the Medicaid director's attempt to simplify the complexity of the Medicaid program by presenting the following symbolic image sums up the way policy makers viewed the intergenerational tension within the program:

> The Medicaid program is up a creek. . . . In the creek are two islands. They are filled with people who need help with their medical bills.
> One island contains infants, children, teenagers, their parents. This island threatens to sink just by the sheer weight of the numbers of the people on the island, twice as many as occupy the second island.
> The second island has fewer people, but they are all severely disabled or elderly. The weight of their problems is twice as great as those on the first island. This island, too, is sinking fast, but, ironically, there is a boat docked here at the second island named Medicare, the good ship Medicare. It should be carrying the elderly and disabled to shore, but it

is so filled with holes it is of little use to the would-be patients. It does not go where the patients want to go.

The Medicaid program is the only available boat in the river, and its course is not clearly charted. Should it head toward the island and save the children and their parents or should it head in the opposite direction, tow Medicare's boat and bring those patients aboard? The answer is it must do both. Its seating capacity is unlimited by law. (U.S. Congress 1991, 102-91, Matula, September 10, 1991, p. 303)

Note that in addition to emphasizing a dichotomous choice between taking care of children versus elderly persons that is facing the states, this image also points to Medicare as the culprit in creating this tension within Medicaid and concludes by arguing that Medicaid has no choice—it must take care of both populations. The conclusion leads the reader to ask how Medicaid can possibly do both and to therefore to grapple with the question of how the program might be restructured. Should Medicaid remain a means-tested program and therefore make hard choices between needy groups, or should Medicaid become something else to accommodate the diverse needs of program recipients as well as other groups that need help? Indeed, this dilemma foreshadows the third frame that began to emerge around this time and became most pronounced during the 1995 debate about the Republican proposal to restructure the Medicaid program into a block grant. This frame emphasizes Medicaid as a core social entitlement that appropriately includes middle-class elderly persons who need long-term care. In contrast, the intergenerational equity frame implicitly paints Medicaid as a means-tested program that must choose between needy groups.

Elderly Persons as Deserving of Medicaid's Core Social Entitlement

At the same time that the intergenerational equity frame was emerging from the states, another frame was emerging that recognized the Medicaid program as a major social welfare program that—far from its rhetorical beginnings that defined it as a residual program—reaches into the middle class. For example, in a 1990 hearing titled "Medicaid Budget Initiatives," Chairman Henry Waxman highlighted the middle-class aspect of Medicaid in his opening statement.

Most people who need nursing home care eventually find themselves dependent on Medicaid. . . . It is absurd, and it is unacceptable that an individual could work hard for their entire life, set aside a fund for his or her retirement, then become—then have to be impoverished and go on welfare in order to take advantage of facilities and services and aids that flow from the Medicaid system. With the passage of Representative Kennelly's bill, my state and nine others are proposing to offer an alternative. (U.S. Congress 1991, 101-206, Waxman, Sept. 10, 1990, p. 2)

Rep. Kennelly's bill called for demonstration projects to develop private/public partnerships to encourage middle-class elderly to purchase long-term care insurance. Under this bill, "if and when an individual exhausts his or her insurance and applied for Medicaid, each dollar that the insurance policy has paid out in accord with state guidelines will be subtracted from the assets Medicaid considers in determining eligibility. In other words, coverage of long-term care expenses by private insurance would count as asset spend-down for the purpose of Medicaid eligibility" (U.S. Congress 1991, 101-206, Kennelly, Sept. 10, 1990, p. 23). Although Rep. Waxman, as chairman of the Subcommittee on Health and the Environment expressed general support for Kennelly's bill in his opening remarks, he raised concerns about whether this bill would create a new category of Medicaid eligibility— one that expanded eligibility to middle-class (or even upper-income) elderly by allowing Medicaid to be used to protect assets and to finance the transfer of wealth.[8] Kennelly's response to Waxman's concerns puts at the forefront the issue of whether Medicaid is still a truly means-tested program or has expanded to something beyond that:

First let me say that I think part of the reason you and I have different perspectives on this issue [whether her bill creates a new category of Medicaid eligibility] is that we start from very different points. You seem to see Medicaid solely as a means-tested entitlement for the poor. While I agree, I also see Medicaid as a program where, at least based on Connecticut figures, over 40 percent of those who receive Medicaid long-term care services did not start out poor.

I hear of financial planners teaching seniors how to transfer their assets and access Medicaid benefits and I feel there ought to be a better way. . . . Our society has changed markedly in the 25 years since the enactment of the Medicaid program to the point where many of those receiving Medicaid are not included in our traditional definition of "poor."

The current Medicaid long-term care program is a means-tested program in name only. The major asset most seniors possess is a house, which is typically protected by Medicaid. . . . Given the political pressures associated with the aging of the population, we are likely to see even more proposals to further increase the amount of assets exempted from Medicaid.

In that context, my proposal . . . may be the *only* proposal that has the potential of actually protecting Medicaid against further erosion of its means-tested origin. (U.S. Congress 1991, 101–206, Kennelly, Sept. 10, 1990, p. 23)

This quote is important for two reasons: first, as mentioned above, it shows that by 1990 Medicaid's means-tested origins were openly questioned; and second, it shows how intergenerational concerns fed into redefining the program. Kennelly explicitly acknowledges the political power of elderly Americans in support of her bill requiring middle-class elderly persons to purchase private long-term care insurance with Medicaid as a type of stop-gap coverage. However, her statement that Rep. Waxman views the Medicaid program as "solely a means-tested entitlement for the poor" is ironic, given that Waxman championed the Medicaid expansions for pregnant women and children throughout the 1980s. Waxman clearly envisioned Medicaid as a vehicle for expanding coverage to the uninsured, including working "middle-class" families. Indeed, this is pure conjecture, but his knowledge of Medicaid's expansionary tendencies might explain why he was concerned about creating yet another eligibility expansion, in this case to potentially well-off elderly who might receive benefits at the expense of other groups he cared about. Indeed, Waxman's expansive view of Medicaid as a core social entitlement is stated quite clearly in a 1991 hearing investigating the Medicaid program:

Medicaid is an enormously important and enormously complex program. It is the major source of health care reform for the poor in this country, covering more than 28 million poor people, roughly half of whom are children. It is the single largest payer for maternity care. . . . It is the single largest payer for nursing home care. . . . It is the single largest payer for residential services for individuals with mental retardation. . . . [The] program has been asked to solve almost every major problem facing this society, from infant mortality to substance abuse to AIDS to the need for long-term care. . . . Despite all of the current interest in health care reform, nothing will be enacted tomorrow, . . . [and] the poor in this country, mothers and children, the disabled, the elderly will continue to rely on Medicaid for access to basic health care. (U.S. Congress 1991, 102-91, Waxman, pp. 3–4)

Rep. Waxman's last statement about Medicaid's role in discussions about national health care reform is noteworthy. In sharp contrast to health care reform proposals offered in the early 1980s (discussed above) where Medicaid was easily dismissed as a residual program, most health care reform bills in the early 1990s proposed expanding Medicaid to cover the uninsured (e.g., using Medicaid 1115 waivers) or expanding access to private insurance and leaving the Medicaid program intact. Very few bills proposed eliminating the Medicaid program altogether.

Indeed, even during hearings about transforming the Medicaid program in 1995, Republican legislators in favor of block granting Medicaid went to great pains to stress that their goal was to strengthen and not to dismantle the program. For example, in Chairman Bilirakis's opening statement he said: "We all have very personal and compelling views about Medicaid. No one involved in this reform effort sees our objective as dismantling a program that is essential to millions of low-income Americans. In fact, we are motivated in this effort by the conviction that what we are doing will strengthen and preserve the Medicaid program for years to come, and that's our goal" (U.S. Congress 1996, 104-108, Aug. 1, 1995, p. 164). Liberals (or Democrats) might discard the sincerity of such statements as pure rhetoric, but it is important to note that the program had changed significantly enough that conservative Republicans felt compelled to frame their argument in this way.

While Republicans moved from a residual frame to a frame that supported the necessity of the Medicaid program, Democrats and advocates of the program went a step further during the 1995 debate. For example, the executive director of the Kaiser Commission on the Future of Medicaid concluded her written testimony presented at a 1995 hearing with the following summary of Medicaid's transformation over time:

Since its enactment in 1965, Medicaid has improved access to health care for the poor, pioneered innovations in health care delivery and community-based long-term care services, and stood along as the primary source of financial assistance for long-term care. In implementing solutions to meet the crises of today, it is important not to undo the progress Medicaid has made in providing health and long-term care for tens of millions of low-income and elderly and disabled Americans. (U.S. Congress 1996, 104-108, Aug. 1, 1995, Rowland, p. 177)

Even President Clinton recast Medicaid under this new frame as a middle-class entitlement during the 1995 debates. It was not surprising that President Clinton sought to rally public opinion against the GOP budget package by arguing that it would entail huge cuts in spending for Medicare, education, and environmental protection—three federal programs with obvious appeal for middle-class voters. However, quite startling was Clinton's explicit support for *Medicaid* on par with these other universal (i.e., middle-class) programs (Grogan and Patashnik 2003a). In explaining why protecting Medicaid was so vital, Clinton emphasized that Medicaid was a key support for senior citizens residing in nursing homes, that many of these seniors were middle class before they depleted their resources, and that they had middle-class children and grandchildren. Stated Clinton in one address:

Now, think about this—what about the Medicaid program? You hardly hear anything about Medicaid. People say, oh, that's that welfare program. One-third of Medicaid does go to help poor women and their poor children on Medicaid. Over two-thirds of it goes to the elderly and the disabled. All of you know that as well. [Commenting on Republican proposals] You think about how many middle-class working people are not going to be able to save to send their kids to college because now they'll have to be taking care of their parents who would have been eligible for public assistance. (U.S. Newswire, 15 September 1995)

Note the huge political significance of this frame: by 1995, Medicaid's long-term care role and financial protection policies were sufficiently recognized that is was acceptable for the president in a major public address to explain Medicare and Medicaid as comprising a health care *package* for the mainstream elderly (Grogan and Patashnik 2003a). In sum, Clinton sought to cast Medicaid as a broad social entitlement that incorporated the middle class.

Emphasizing elderly middle-class incorporation is an important aspect of the core social entitlement frame. All advocates for elderly persons mentioned this middle-class incorporation in Medicaid during the 1995 hearings. For example, a representative from the American Association of Retired Persons (AARP) began her testimony by saying

"[I] testify today on behalf of the almost 5 million older Americans who rely on Medicaid." She then went on to say, "Many who need long-term care start off as taxpaying middle class Americans. They worked hard and saved" (U.S. Congress 1996, 104-108, Aug. 1, 1995, Braun, p. 288–89). Note the change in discussion about elderly middle-class Americans in Medicaid. In 1990, Representative Kennelly recognized the importance of Medicaid for elderly middle-class Americans and offered a bill to keep them out of the program and preserve Medicaid's means-tested origins. In 1995, advocates, congressional members, and the president mentioned elderly middle-class Americans in Medicaid as a central reason why the program should be viewed as a core social entitlement.

This strategic recasting also found expression in the 1996 Democratic Party platform document. The platform stated that securing both Medicare and Medicaid was a "duty for our parents, so they can live their lives in dignity" and prominently pledged to protect Medicaid in particular from devastating cuts that "would jeopardize the health care of children and seniors." Inspection of Democratic Party platforms from 1984, 1988, and 1992 reveals that the platforms either did not mention Medicaid (1984 and 1988) or discussed the program only in the context of welfare reform and encouraging work.

Also important in the 1996 Democratic platform is the effort to mention the importance of Medicaid to both children and elderly persons—specifically downplaying the intergenerational tension. In contrast to the intergenerational frame that emphasized children, disabled persons, and elderly persons as separate competing groups, many advocates presenting a core entitlement frame discussed these groups as a coalition coming together under Medicaid, all needing important and necessary health care services. For example, the senior vice president for public policy of the Alzheimer's Association began his remarks in the 1995 Medicaid transformation hearing with the following point:

You have assembled this panel to talk about Medicaid and the elderly. But before doing that, I want to make a broader point. Distinctions among 'categories' of Medicaid beneficiaries are arbitrary and potentially dangerous. The elderly need long term care because of their disabilities; people with disabilities are aging; disabling illnesses like Alzheimer's and Parkinson's—generally considered diseases of aging—are striking younger people as well. That is why the Alzheimer's Association has always approached the long term care issue as part of a coalition of aging, disability, and children's organizations that make up the Long Term Care Campaign. (U.S. Congress 1996, 104-108, Aug. 1, 1995, McConnell, p. 261)

This testimony from the representative from the Alzheimer's Association is also important because it illustrates how far the program's frame in relation to elderly persons has shifted over time. In sharp contrast to the 1981 hearing on elderly persons and Alzheimer's disease, in which representatives dismissed Medicaid out of hand, the representative in 1995 said, "My testimony will focus on Medicaid as a vital lifeline to long term care, because that is what brings families dealing with Alzheimer's disease into the system."

Conclusion

In this chapter, I have documented how the various frames of elderly deservingness under Medicaid depend not only on the social construction of elderly persons but also on political constructions of the Medicaid program itself. Medicaid has clearly evolved away from its political frame as a residual program to a program that is either portrayed as a crucial means-tested program for many needy groups or as a core social entitlement that helps the needy and appropriately extends its reach into the middle class. Indeed, this is the crucial question about Medicaid today: Should we preserve its means-tested origins, or should we let (or encourage) the program to evolve into something more universal?

As Medicare continues to be stuck in gear, and the enactment of targeted programs (rather than the creation of universal programs) continues to be the norm in the United States, it is important to reexamination Medicaid's possibilities. While the factors that lead to passage or failure of a particular bill are always more complex than simply analyzing elite discourse can tell you, it is noteworthy that the framing of Medicaid as a core social entitlement that emphasized elderly middle-class incorporation was successful in fighting back Republican efforts to block grant the program in 1995 (which advocates viewed as a major policy retrenchment). This suggests that targeted programs, rather than suffering from an unchangeable stigmatized rhetoric, can change and be recast in more politically acceptable ways. It also suggests that targeted programs can evolve from a negative frame to a more positive frame over time, and with this new frame can perhaps become acceptable to middle-class groups. Despite repeated advocacy for long-term care expansions within Medicare, it is Medicaid that has changed most significantly in this regard over time. Indeed, elderly middle-class incorporation may give rise to universal long-term care within Medicaid. As mentioned above, this notion is not so farfetched if one considers that most universal programs in other countries began first as targeted programs with middle-class incorporation.

The framing of Medicaid's middle-class incorporation in the United States, however, is complex. Although the generally positive social construction of elderly persons as socially deserving allowed universalism within targeting to occur under Medicaid, the enactment of Medicare alongside Medicaid and the incorporation of other needy groups within Medicaid has created multiple and conflicting frames of elderly deservingness, as the above analysis shows. The three distinct social constructions of elderly persons presented above are salient at different points during Medicaid's political evolution, but they also appear simultaneously. While the residual frame is largely absent from political discourse about elderly Americans and Medicaid today, one can still find traces of it. When discussing the spend-down process, for example, policy elites often emphasize Medicaid as a stingy, inadequate program in which elderly persons must lose their dignity to become eligible. Moreover, despite the good intentions of diverse advocacy groups (representing children, elderly, and disabled) to present a united front, when budgets get tight at the state level, the intergenerational equity frame often rears its ugly head. Real reform efforts often need a consistent and common frame (or theme). The social entitlement frame, if presented in a consistent united manner, might allow Medicaid to act as a stepping-stone to universal long-term care coverage or universal health care coverage more generally for the currently uninsured. Unfortunately for reform advocates, however, such consistency is often difficult to maintain throughout the ebb and flow of budgetary politics.

Notes

1. I use John Rawls's phrase from *A Theory of Justice* (1971) here.
2. This essay was originally published in *The Urban Underclass*, edited by C. Jencks and P. E. Peterson (Washington, D.C.: Brookings Institution, 1991, 1988).

3. This section draws heavily from two articles by Grogan and Patash-nik (2003a; 2003b).

4. While unexpected, the adoption of both in hindsight makes sense given the incentives of key political actors at the time (for further explanation, see Grogan and Patashnik [forthcoming]).

5. This bizarre fractional percentage to determine eligibility is a testament to Medicaid's complexity.

6. For more detail on these expansions, see Grogan and Patashnik (forthcoming).

7. For a book-length discussion that explains MCCA's passage and repeal, see Himmelfarb (1995).

8. This is taken from Kennelly's testimony and prepared statement for the record, where she responds to Chairman Waxman's questions and concerns about her bill.

References

Benjamin, A. E., P. W. Newacheck, and H. Wolfe. 1991. Intergenerational equity and public spending. *Pediatrics* 88(1): 75–83.

Brown, M. K. 1988. The segmented welfare state: Distributive conflict and retrenchment in the United States, 1968–1984. Pp. 182–210 in his *Remaking the Welfare State: Retrenchment and Social Policy in America and Europe*. Philadelphia: Temple University Press.

Cohen, M. A., N. Kumar, and S. S. Wallack. 1993. Simulating the fiscal and distributional impacts of Medicaid eligibility reforms. *Health Care Financing Review* 14(4):133–50.

Congressional Research Service. 1993. *Medicaid Source Book: Background Data and Analysis (A 1993 Update)*. Washington, D.C.: Government Printing Office.

Cook, F. L. 1994. The salience of intergenerational equity in Canada and the United States. Pp. 90–129 in T. R. Marmor, T. M. Smeeding, and V. L. Greene, eds., *Economic Security and Intergenerational Justice: A Look at North America*. Washington, D.C.: Urban Institute Press.

Fein, S. 1998. The Kerr-Mills Act: Medical care for the indigent in Michigan, 1960–1965. *Journal of the History of Medicine* 53 (July): 285–316.

Gilbert, N., ed. 2001. *Targeting Social Benefits*. New Brunswick, N.J.: Transaction Publishers.

Grogan, C. M., and E. M. Patashnik. 2003a. Universalism within targeting: Nursing home care, the middle class, and the politics of the Medicaid program. *Social Service Review* 77:51–71.

Grogan, C. M., and E. M. Patashnik. 2003b. Between welfare medicine and mainstream entitlement: Medicaid at the political crossroads. *Journal of Health Politics, Policy and Law* 28(5):821–58.

242 Colleen M. Grogan

Himmelfarb, R. 1995. *Catastrophic Politics: The Rise and Fall of the Medicare Catastrophic Coverage Act of 1988*. University Park: Pennsylvania State University Press.

Kuttner, R. 1988. Reaganism, liberalism, and the Democrats. Pp. 99–134 in S. Blumenthal and T. B. Edsall, eds., *The Reagan Legacy*. New York: Pantheon.

Marmor, T. R. 1973. *The Politics of Medicare*. New York: Aldine.

Marmor, T. R., J. L. Mashaw, and P. L. Harvey. 1990. *America's Misunderstood Welfare State*. New York: Basic Books.

Oberlander, J. 2003. The *Political Life of Medicare*. Chicago: University of Chicago Press.

Pierson, P., and M. Smith. 1994. Shifting fortunes of the elderly: The comparative politics of retrenchment. Pp. 21–59 in T. R. Marmor, T. M. Smeeding, and V. L. Greene, eds., *Economic Security and Intergenerational Justice: A Look at North America*. Washington, D.C.: Urban Institute Press.

Quadagno, J. 1989. Generational equity and the politics of the welfare state. *Politics and Society* 17(3):353–76.

Rosenbaum, S. 1993. Medicaid expansions and access to health care. Pp. 45–82 in D. Rowland, J. Feder, and A. Salganicoff, eds., *Medicaid Financing Crisis: Balancing Responsibilities, Priorities, and Dollars*. Washington, D.C.: AAAS Press.

Rosenberry, S. A. 1982. Social insurance, distributive criteria and the welfare backlash: A comparative analysis. *British Journal of Political Science* 12(4):421–47.

Sardell, A. 1991. Child health policy in the U.S.: The paradox of consensus. Pp. 17–53 in L. D. Brown, ed., *Health Policy and the Disadvantaged*. Durham, N.C.: Duke University Press.

Schneider, A. L., and H. Ingram. 1997. *Policy Design for Democracy*. Lawrence: University Press of Kansas.

Skocpol, T. 1995. Targeting within universalism: Politically viable policies to combat poverty in the United States. Pp. 263–64 in her *Social Policy in the United States*. Princeton, N.J.: Princeton University Press.

Stevens, R. B., and R. Stevens. 1974. *Welfare Medicine in America: A Case Study of Medicaid*. New York: Free Press.

Tanenbaum, S. J. 1995. Medicaid eligibility policy in the 1980s: Medical utilitarianism and the 'deserving' poor. *Journal of Health Politics, Policy, and Law* 20(4):533–53.

U.S. Congress. 1988. *Medicare and Medicaid Catastrophic Protection*. Subcommittee on Health and the Environment of the Committee on Energy and Commerce. Hrg., House of Representatives, Serial No. 100-74, May 21, 27, 28; June 2, 1987. Washington, D.C.: Government Printing Office.

U.S. Congress. 1991. *Medicaid Budget Initiatives.* Subcommittee on Health and the Environment of the Committee on Energy and Commerce. Hrg., House of Representatives, Serial No. 101-206, September 10, 14, 1990. Washington, D.C.: Government Printing Office.

U.S. Congress. 1996. *Transformation of the Medicaid Program—Part 3.* Subcommittee on Health and the Environment of the Committee on Commerce. Hrg., House of Representatives, Serial No. 104-108, July 26, Aug 1, 1995. Washington, D.C.: Government Printing Office.

U.S. Senate Committee on Finance. 1967. Social Security Amendments of 1967, Part 3. 09th Cong., 1st sess., 20–22 and 26 September.

12. The Changing Face of Senior Housing

Jon Pynoos and Christy M. Nishita

In the 1960s and 1970s, policymakers and the general public viewed elderly persons as needy and deserving of housing assistance. In turn, U.S. housing policy responded by creating several programs for older persons. The success of those efforts has led critics to question whether elderly persons are now receiving more than their fair share of housing resources and whether senior housing still has a legitimate role to play. This chapter will demonstrate that there is a need and purpose for senior housing, in particular because housing policy has shifted toward supportive housing that meets the needs of frail older adults. This change reflects the view that age is no longer the primary criterion for senior housing; age has been replaced by age plus need. At the same time, changes in living arrangements, such as the rise in grandparents raising grandchildren, require flexibility in thinking about senior housing models and eligibility requirements. In the future, housing policy is likely to emphasize aging in place, including proposals to encourage homeowners to use their equity to defray costs for long-term care and the development of new types of housing based on principles of universal design. Such changes are driven by demographic trends, political forces, and public policy.

The History of Senior Housing: Elderly Persons as Deserving

In the first half of the twentieth century, elderly persons were seen both as financially needy and as desirable tenants, and therefore in need of housing assistance. When elderly persons became eligible for public housing in the late 1950s, projects were oriented to the active, well elderly. At this time, the federal government had a "bricks and mortar" approach to housing policy. Housing and services were treated as separate domains, each with its own set of policies, programs, regulations, and funding sources (Pynoos 1992). While housing projects included some special features for older people, such as emergency call buttons, few services were tied to the complexes. When services were provided, they had to be paid for through nonhousing sources. The primary role of the manager was caring for the property and rent collection.

In 1959, Section 202, a special housing program for elderly and handicapped persons, was created as part of the National Housing Act, further indicating that there was a need for elderly-specific housing. The program provides capital advances and project-based rental assistance to nonprofit sponsors for the development of supportive housing projects. The designers of the program did not want Section 202 housing to function as a nursing home or even as a home for the aged. Consequently, projects were built for ambulatory, independent elderly persons, although several features to prevent accidents (e.g., emergency call buttons and grab bars) were included, and space for services and common activities was allowed. Approximately 10 percent of the units were made accessible for persons with disabilities. Services such as meals, however, were not guaranteed, and residents and/or sponsors were responsible for paying for them when they were offered. The federal government's Department of Housing and Urban Development (HUD) continued its "bricks and mortar" approach.

Serious concerns were raised about the impact of elderly housing. The majority of critics contended that segregated living arrangements isolate the old from the rest of society. The formation of friendships would be restricted to those in the housing complex. Older persons would not be able to share their wisdom with the young, and this would ultimately lead to low morale and feelings of uselessness (Golant 1987). In particular, those with severe physical and mental impairments would not be able to leave their residential units. Even proponents were apprehensive that it might lead to isolation, depression, and ghettoization. There was a tremendous relief when early studies indicated that, in fact, the opposite was true (Carp 1987). The majority of elderly persons have numerous links to the "outside world" through clubs and organizations, visits by families and friends, and communication via phone and mail. For the most part, older residents were highly satisfied with the new housing. The new communities seemed to promote friendship, activities, and support. Living among same-aged peers offered opportunities to provide understanding and support with common age-related issues such as poor health or retirement (Golant 1987). Age-segregated housing also provided higher levels of security against crime than had many of the residents' former homes and apartments.

Currently, the Section 202 program, sponsored by nonprofit organizations, houses more than 381,000 older persons in more than 9,000 facilities (Commission on Affordable Housing 2002). Residents of Section 202 housing, one of the government's best programs, have their own private apartments, and rents do not exceed 30 percent of tenant incomes. The buildings are generally well maintained, and residents are highly satisfied with their accommodations (Golant 1992). Such federally subsidized housing for elderly persons benefits a disproportionate number of low-income older women who live alone, including a high percentage of minorities; these residents cannot afford other housing options.

Despite the popularity of Section 202 housing, construction of new units has dwindled. Section 202 is one of the few remaining production programs. HUD has shifted from supply-type housing to demand-oriented programs. Current production of 5,000 to 6,000 Section 202 units per year is far below the 20,000 units per year in the late 1970s (Commission on Affordable Housing 2002). At the same time, there is a large gap between the number of wait-listed applicants and the number of housing units available. Approximately nine applicants were waiting for each Section 202 unit that became available in 1999 (Heumann, Winter-Nelson, and Anderson 2001). It is common for applicants to wait more than four years for Section 202 housing (Pynoos et al. 1995).

The 2002 Commission on Affordable Housing and Health Facilities Needs for Seniors in the 21st Century (also known as the Senior Commission) was created by Congress to analyze current housing and health needs of older Americans and to make policy and legislation recommendations for increasing the availability of housing and services. It recognized that the loss of subsidized housing as a serious problem. The Senior Commission acknowledged the need not only to preserve the existing housing stock, but also to renovate and refinance Section 202 projects. An encouraging step in the right direction was $683 million authorized by HUD to Section 202 housing production in FY 2003, an increase of $4 million over the previous year.

Are Elderly Persons Receiving More than Their Fair Share?

The popularity of, and resident satisfaction with, the Section 202 program led some critics to argue that older persons have received more than their fair share of housing resources. Competition among groups representing elderly persons, persons with disabilities, and families with children emerged as they fought for a limited amount of subsidized housing. This criticism and competition are part of a larger trend in which elderly persons are seen as receiving a disproportionate amount of government benefits. However, such intergeneration tension is not as prevalent as portrayed in the media. In a survey, only 18 percent of respondents agreed with the statement that elderly persons receive more than their fair share of government benefits. If respondents perceived elderly persons to be better off, they were more likely to believe that the group was inequitably benefiting from government programs (Schlesinger and Kronebusch 1994).

Critics argued that elderly persons were benefiting from housing programs at the expense of families with children. Some argued that elderly households were less likely to experience excessive housing costs than nonelderly households (Golant and La Greca 1995) and that families were more likely to have multiple housing problems, often living in inadequate housing, overcrowded conditions, or paying more than 50 percent of income for rent (Khadduri and Nelson 1992). Furthermore, elderly persons have benefited from federal rental housing assistance at high rates. They are major beneficiaries of direct housing subsidies: more than 1 million elderly households receive housing assistance in the form of such programs as public housing, Section 202 housing, Section 221d3 housing, and Section 8 certificates and vouchers (HUD 1999).

Other analysts, however, pointed out that the overall picture of older adults masks the serious housing-related problems of specific subgroups. For example, some segments of the elderly population, such as minority groups, women, and very old persons, face poverty and physically deficient dwellings at similar rates as other low-income groups (Pynoos and Golant 1995). Older adults, however, are at a particular disadvantage in that their poverty status is often permanent, while among younger households it is more temporary. Moreover, older adults tend to have higher medical costs related to expenses such as prescription drugs than younger people, but because of living on a fixed income, they have limited ability to increase their ability to pay for them. The oldest-old, in particular, tend to have few assets and few sources of informal support (Pynoos and Redfoot 1995).

Older persons are also vulnerable to deficient housing environments. For example, as illustrated by the heat waves in Chicago and Paris during the last five years, a lack of air conditioning can be deadly to elderly persons; similarly, insufficient heating can lead to hypothermia in the winter (Klinenberg 2002). In addition, conventional housing may contain barriers and hazards that increase the risk of falls or other injury. It also usually lacks supportive features such as grab bars that can make tasks easier and promote independence.

Critics also argue that seniors have had an advantage because it is easier to get communities to approve elderly housing developments as opposed to family housing. However, even senior housing developments have recently faced considerable opposition from neighborhood groups. Overall, however, the arguments concerning whether seniors receive their fair share of subsidized housing suffer from too narrow a perspective. The basic problem is that housing itself is not an entitlement, and groups are fighting over a small and shrinking piece of the pie. Moreover, senior housing should be more broadly framed as an intergenerational issue that benefits persons of all ages. Senior housing offers a sense of security not only to elderly beneficiaries but also to families with older relatives. Affordable and suitable housing will lessen the strain on families, especially low-income families, to provide caregiving and economic support for older relatives. Furthermore, an adequate supply of senior housing will ensure a secure old age for all individuals.

Legislation Sanctioning Elderly Housing

Although the housing needs of certain elderly subgroups is significant, some groups have lobbied against elderly housing because it has kept out younger persons, especially families with children, who also have a great need for affordable and decent housing. This issue came to a head at the time of passage of the Fair Housing Amendments Act (FHAA) of 1988, which proved to be very contentious. The FHAA prohibits discrimination in housing but makes an exception for senior housing with certain stipulations. It precludes discrimination in the sale or rental of housing based on familial status; property owners cannot prevent occupancy of families with children. The FHAA also follows Title VIII of the Civil Rights Act of 1968, which prohibits discrimination in the sale, rental, or financing of dwellings based on color, religion, sex, or national origin. The FHAA expands this law to prohibit discrimination based on handicap. The term "handicap" is defined as "a physical or mental impairment which substantially limits one or more such person's major life activities; a record of having such an impairment; or being regarded as having such an impairment" (*Federal Register,* Vol. 54, No. 13, p. 3245). This rule applies to all types of dwellings, including apartments, condominiums, cooperatives, and mobile homes.

At the same time, the FHAA grants a nondiscriminatory exemption if senior housing meets certain requirements. It allows for elderly-only housing owing to the special health and social needs of older adults. This exemption in the FHAA was the result of long and laborious negotiations in Congress. Advocates for older adults insisted that some housing should be reserved to accommodate older adults' special needs and preferences for an age-homogenous environment (Morales 1990). The result was that landlords may qualify for senior housing if three conditions are met: (1) the housing is subsidized and is specifically designed and operated for elderly persons; (2) all residents are 63 years of age and older; or (3) 80 percent of the households have at least one person who is 55 years of age or older. Along with the third circumstance, the housing must also provide "significant facilities and services specifically designed to meet the physical or social needs of older persons" (42 U.S.C. §3607(b)(2)(C)(i)). The third circumstance is used most often by landlords because of its lower age limitation and greater flexibility in requiring only 80 percent of the households to meet this requirement.

At the same time, there has been much confusion because neither the statute nor the regulations define what constitutes "significant facilities and services." The statute merely states that these amenities must be "specifically designed to meet the physical or social needs of older persons." Such amenities include social and recreational programs, continuing education, information and counseling, homemaker, accessible physical environment, emergency and preventative health care programs, congregate dining facilities, and transportation. However, the regulations then state that the "housing facility need not have all of these features to qualify for the exemption" (24 C.F.R. §11.304 (b)(1)).

Overall, the housing provider must demonstrate that the structures and amenities have been designed, constructed, or adapted to meet the particular needs of older persons. The "significant facilities and services requirement" is based on the premise that older persons tend to suffer from health problems to a greater degree than younger persons and that older persons have more leisure time than younger persons. Disability advocates disputed the broad and vague regulations surrounding the "significant facilities and services" requirement. Managers could claim to operate "senior housing" without providing the needed supportive services to elderly residents.

A similar contentious battle occurred around housing younger persons with disabilities in Section 202 federally subsidized housing complexes for elderly Americans. In the late 1980s and early 1990s, an expansion of the definition of "handicapped" led to an increasing number of younger persons with mental disabilities and substance abuse problems moving into these housing projects, partly because of limited housing options. By 1993, approximately 50 percent of public housing projects for elderly Americans contained younger persons with disabilities. The "mixed housing" issue rose to prominence on the federal government's agenda due to: (1) media accounts of disturbances in public housing, (2) public housing managers' reports of problems, and (3) government studies suggesting difficulties integrating two populations (Pynoos and Parrott 1996). Advocates representing elderly persons fought to preserve age-specific housing, while advocates for persons with disabilities fought to maintain entry to these housing projects. Ultimately, it was a victory for elderly Americans because the Housing and Community Development Act of 1992 permitted Public Housing Authorities the option of designating public housing sites as elderly-only, disabled-only, or mixed housing.

The issue of senior-only housing has taken a new twist with the growing trend of grandparents raising grandchildren. This issue has resulted in a reexamination of existing legislation that sanctions senior housing. During the 1990s the number of grandparent-headed households increased due to drug abuse, AIDS, and incarceration. According to the U.S. Census, a significant proportion are single grandmothers, low-income, and in poor health. These grandparents face many economic, health, and legal problems, but an additional challenge faces grandparents living in senior housing. In public housing, proof of legal guardianship is needed to prevent eviction, whereas grandparents living in senior housing can be evicted for taking in their grandchildren (Minkler and Odierna 2001). Grandparents without legal custody do not qualify as "family" and therefore do not meet Section 8 eligibility requirements. The FHAA also prohibits using preference in designating housing specifically to grandparents raising grandchildren. Therefore, the Living Equitably—Grandparents Aiding Children and Youth (LEGACY) Act was introduced in the Senate and House in 2003 to overcome these barriers. This bill would create demonstration programs that determine the feasibility of providing Section 8 rental assistance to grandparents and of replicating Grandfamilies, a Boston housing project built specifically for grandparents raising grandchildren, within certain Section 202 projects. The bill also calls for the removal of barriers in the definition of family in order for grandparents to qualify for the Section 8 Family Unification Program. The legislation recognizes the difficulties facing grandparents raising grandchildren and the need for further legal exemptions for these grandparents in senior housing.

A Shift in Housing Policy toward Supportive Housing

The debates over the legitimacy of senior housing ignore the need for supportive housing, residential living arrangements that include special design features and the presence or provision of services (Pynoos and Golant 1995). The focus of senior housing in the government and private sector has increasingly focused on accommodating frail elderly persons. The transition from age-specific housing for independent elderly persons to needs-based housing for frail elderly persons has resulted from several trends.

During the late 1970s, some older residents who had moved into public and Section 202 housing in the early years of the programs were now in their late 70s or 80s. The average age of residents increased from 72 years in 1983 to 75 years in 1999. Housing project managers indicated that 30 percent of residents were aged 80 and older (Heumann, Winter-Nelson, and Anderson 2001). In addition, a large proportion of residents are frail. Housing project managers indicated that 22 percent of residents were frail in 1999, an increase from 13 percent in 1988 (Heumann, Winter-Nelson, and Anderson 2001). Housing that worked for them at younger ages did not have physically supportive environments, available services, or management trained to address their needs as they aged. Frail older persons, especially those with low incomes, had few residential options available to them when it became inefficient or too difficult to stay in their residences. Consequently, many older persons unnecessarily moved to more institutional settings such as nursing homes or board-and-care homes in spite of their desires to age in place.

A similar trend was also occurring in the private sector. Conventional single-family homes and apartments in the private sector were developed for independent persons. Little thought was given to the eventual suitability of this housing for persons who became frail (Pynoos 1993). Private apartments, like their counterparts in the public sector, rarely included spaces for services or employed managers trained in meeting the needs of elderly persons. Moreover, an increasing amount of housing was built in suburban areas where it was difficult to access public transportation and services.

Along with the aging of the residential population, a second trend, the deinstitutionalization movement of the 1960s and 1970s, has created an additional need for supportive housing. This movement was based on the assumption that persons with mental health problems could be better cared for in the community. The emphasis on community-based care led to the growth of special needs housing for persons with developmental disabilities, AIDS, substance abuse, and a variety of mental health problems. However, programs and new housing alternatives expected to help those who were deinstitutionalized have been limited by funding and neighborhood opposition.

Aging in Place in Section 202 Housing

As mentioned above, the increased age and frailty of Section 202 residents has led HUD to provide more supportive settings and services. Most projects now include supportive features such as grab bars, ramps, elevators, and emergency call buttons. Approximately 25 percent of projects offer 24-hour on-site personnel. Projects also offer a range of services, such as congregate dining and visiting services (50%), housekeeping services (26%), and staff who offer social work or counseling services (12%) (Heumann, Winter-Nelson, and Anderson 2001).

Federal legislation created several supportive housing programs in Section 202 housing. One of the earliest of these demonstrations, the

Congregate Housing Services Program (CHSP) authorized under Title IV of the Housing and Community Development Act of 1978, provides a service-enriched setting for frail older persons. The program used HUD funds to pay for services such as meals, homemaking, and transportation to select groups of tenants with three ADL or IADL needs. Eligibility for and organization of the services was overseen by a service coordinator and professional assessment team. The program did not expand until the early 1990s (Redfoot and Sloan 1991) with the passage of the National Affordable Housing Act of 1990, and again in 1992 with the passage of the Housing and Community Development Act. The latter expanded operations to almost double the number of original sites. However, instead of HUD paying for most of the basic services, the revised program required a 50 percent match from other sources as well as 10 percent payment from residents, changes that discouraged some potential projects from applying. Currently, a little over 100 facilities still receive extension funding (Golant 2004). Unfortunately, HUD no longer funds new programs, and the first contracts expired in 1998 (HUD 2000). HUD does not consider paying for services its priority or responsibility.

In 1992 the Housing and Community Development Act authorized expenditures for a Service Coordinator program. Service coordination is often described as the "glue" that holds a program together or the linking mechanism between residents of housing complexes and services. It is a less intensive model than the CHSP and relies more on connecting residents with services than on providing them directly. Services coordinated for residents include Meals on Wheels, in-home supportive services, home health care for those that meet Medicare or Medicaid eligibility, transportation services, on-site adult education, and monthly blood pressure checks. In 1999, 37 percent of facilities had a service coordinator on staff and another 35 percent of facilities reported that service coordination was available in the community (Heumann, Winter-Nelson, and Anderson 2001). According to the American Association of Service Coordinators, there were approximately 3,000 service coordinators in Section 202, public housing, and other programs in 2003. More than 37 percent of Section 202 facilities employ professional service coordinators (Heumann, Winter-Nelson, and Anderson 2001). In fiscal year 2003, the HUD budget provided an additional $3 million for the Service Coordinator program, bringing the total to $53 million. In both the CHSP and Service Coordinator programs, the high concentration of elderly persons provided economies of scale in giving comprehensive and coordinated services to residents (Golant 2004).

Assisted Living: A Growing Housing Option for Elderly Persons with Disabilities

During the 1990s assisted living was one of the fastest-growing segments of the senior housing industry, further reflecting the trend toward housing that targets older adults with disabilities. The assisted living industry grew 14.5 percent between 2000 and 2002 (Mollica 2002). Currently, there are 390,730 assisted living units with 528,073 beds in the United States (Promatura Group 2000). Assisted living is a housing option that involves the delivery of professionally managed supportive services and, depending on state regulations, nursing services, in a group setting that is residential in character and appearance. The intent of assisted living is to accommodate physically and mentally frail older adults without imposing a heavily regulated, institutional environment on them (Kane and Wilson 1993). It has the capacity to meet unscheduled needs for assistance with the goal of maximizing the physical and psychological independence of residents. In 2002 the Commission on Affordable Housing and Health Facility Needs for Seniors in the 21st Century, also known as the Seniors Commission, encouraged housing authorities to find innovative new ways to develop assisted living facilities. Specifically, the commissioners recommended the use of HOPE VI modernization funds to build new independent and assisted living facilities for seniors.

Despite the capacity of assisted living to accommodate more frail older adults than other housing options, it is unlikely that it can substitute for nursing home care. In an analysis of six studies of assisted living residents, Golant (2004) found that despite wide variation in impairment level, older residents in assisted living were less physically and cognitively impaired than those in nursing homes. A nationally representative study found that among residents who leave assisted living, most move to a higher level of care; nearly 60 percent end up in nursing homes (Phillips et al. 2003). However, Oregon's affordable assisted living program has lower rates of residents moving to nursing homes (20%) because of the state's liberal skilled nursing care provisions and flexible nurse delegation statutes (Golant 1999). These statistics suggest that even in Oregon, where assisted living facilities accommodate more physically and cognitively impaired residents, a significant number of residents still relocate to nursing homes. Assisted living may only be appropriate for certain frail elderly persons. At some point a threshold may be reached at which relocation to a nursing home may be necessary. The closer that assisted living comes to housing nursing home–eligible residents, the more attention will be paid to regulations that protect residents and ensure quality of care. There is a danger that these regulations could shift assisted living away from a social model to a "medicalized" approach.

The Flexibility of the Housing Stock

Although specific segments of the senior housing industry have expanded rapidly, there is increasing recognition that frail older persons and others with disabilities do not necessarily have to move from one setting to another if they need assistance. Semi-dependent or dependent older persons can live indefinitely in a variety of settings, including their own homes and apartments, if the physical setting is more supportive and affordable services are accessible.

For example, the Assisted Living Conversion Program under the U.S. Department of Housing and Urban Development provides funds for the conversion of Section 202 projects into assisted living to support increasingly frail residents. As of 2000, HUD's budget included $50 million for the conversion into assisted living of entire buildings or floors of Section 202 housing for elderly persons, representing another attempt to make assisted living more affordable. HUD also authorizes the use of housing vouchers in assisted living. Although these programs will facilitate aging in place, they reduce the number of units for more independent older persons and raise concerns about regulating quality of care. The experience of various states with converting Section 202 into assisted living suggests that projects increase residents' access to services and maintain a residential environment. However, projects need more stable sources of funding and face difficulty integrating staff from both housing and services backgrounds (Wilden and Redfoot 2002). If successful, such policies will make assisted living more available to low-and moderate-income older persons.

A similar approach is taking place in single-family housing, where the great majority of older persons reside. Home modifications, which are adaptations to existing residential environments, can make it easier and safer to carry out activities such as bathing, cooking, and climbing stairs. Modifications include grab bars, roll-in showers, handrails, ramps, and wheelchair-accessible kitchens. Increasing evidence suggests that home modifications have an important impact on the ability of chronically ill or disabled persons to live independently. Home modifications are also an important part of multifactorial interventions to prevent falls that include risk assessment, exercise, educational materials and programming, and follow-up (Shekelle et al. 2002). Furthermore, a physically supportive dwelling can facilitate both informal caregiving and formal care services (Newman 1990).

Current approaches emphasize the elasticity of the conventional housing stock in terms of its ability to accommodate a wide spectrum of frail older persons and younger persons with disabilities. This trend has influenced long-term care policy, which is emphasizing community-based care. For example, early in the 1980s Section 2176 of the Omnibus Budget Reconciliation Act allowed states to apply for Medicaid waivers that paid for nonmedical services for older adults who would otherwise face institutionalization (Pynoos and Redfoot 1995). Maintaining older adults in the community is also well aligned with the Olmstead Decision issued by the Supreme Court in 1999 that requires states to administer programs and services to persons with disabilities into the "most integrated setting appropriate" to their needs.

Past court cases further demonstrate that senior housing operators must make accommodations to facilitate aging in place. The practice of relocating or evicting residents to a nursing home because of increasing disability is discriminatory. In *O'Neal v. Alabama Department of Public Health,* the department refused to renew an assisted living center's license until all residents with Alzheimer's disease were evicted. The justification was that residents with Alzheimer's were confused and incapable of exiting the facility in case of fire or other emergencies. The court found this argument to be discriminatory (Ziaja 2001). Senior housing must accommodate residents regardless of their level of physical or mental disability. This case demonstrates that the courts support the rights of elderly persons to age in place and to live in the most integrated setting possible.

Future Directions: Achieving Aging in Place

In the future, housing policy will emphasize aging in place. Achieving this goal requires new approaches to providing suitable housing and to financing long-term care. Several proposals have been promoted to facilitate aging in place, including the creation of more suitable housing and communities, and reverse mortgages. Ultimately, the goal of aging in place will require innovative new approaches and broader conceptualizations of supportive environments.

Visitability and Universal Design

To avoid the necessity of home modification and retrofitting, there is a movement to build newly constructed homes with accessibility features already in place. The relatively new concepts of visitability and universal design involve housing that is beneficial not only for elderly persons but also for persons with disabilities and persons of all ages. It is part of the growing trend that recognizes the elasticity of the housing stock to support increasingly disabled individuals.

Visitability is a small set of basic accessibility features that enable older adults and persons with disabilities to access the main level of single-family homes, duplexes, and triplexes. The concept of visitability does not require a completely accessible house, but rather it is a narrower concept intended to assist residents, friends, and relatives who are functionally impaired, as well as future residents, to enter and get around the home. The three key visitability requirements are: zero-step entrance to home, wide interior doors, and at least a half bath on the main floor. The visitability movement is gaining momentum. As of 2003, at least thirty cities, counties, and states are promoting visitability through voluntary programs, incentives, or mandates. At the national level, a federal visitability bill, the National Inclusive Home Design Act, was introduced in October 2002. The bill would require all newly constructed single-family homes built with federal funds to meet the three key requirements. Advocates view visitability as a "foot in the door" to more fully accessible, universally designed homes in the future.

Universal design is a concept promoting homes that are accessible, adaptable, and usable by persons of all ages and abilities. It is different from visitability because it applies to the entire home by including features such as variable height counters, lever door handles, supportive bars in bathroom and shower, and bathrooms and kitchens designed to accommodate wheelchairs or walkers.

Several barriers limit the spread of accessibility concepts. Developing uniform standards for consumers with diverse health conditions and disabilities is challenging. In addition, advocates have difficulty working together to achieve their goals. Some advocates support visitability, while others view visitability as a limited approach and see universal design as the right approach. This lack of consensus leads to fragmentation among different advocacy groups. Adding to the difficulties facing advocates are disagreements about the actual cost and effectiveness of visitability and universal design. The primary opposition that advocacy groups face is from builders, who oppose regulation because of: (1) concerns that the increased cost of accessibility features negatively impacts the affordability of housing, and (2) resistance toward offering more features to homebuyers who do not request them. Builders prefer voluntary programs or incentives that waive building permit fees. Progress in this area therefore requires an educated group of consumer advocates who are convinced enough about the benefits of universal design to take on the building industry.

Greater Attention to the Broader Environmental Context

In the future, meeting the needs of seniors will require reaching beyond the confines of individual houses or complexes to the larger community. The Americans with Disabilities Act of 1990 brought attention to accessibility in the broader community. While age-specific housing has many benefits associated with security and mutual support among residents, it can be overly insular and isolating. New models of housing need to be developed that incorporate community spaces and provide services to the adjacent neighborhood. More integrative models of elderly housing (e.g., service houses) in some European countries and a few locations in this country are designed to co-locate restaurants, shops, day care, health clinics, and senior centers so that housing for elderly persons is better connected to the community and provides services to older persons and younger persons with disabilities living in the adjacent neighborhood.

The creation of elder-friendly communities has received increasing attention across the nation. Such communities would consider the location of stores, churches, or parks; adequate transportation options; and the legibility of signage as important determinants to maintaining independence. The goal is to help older adults remain mobile and connected to the community. Future planning and policy initiatives must recognize the environmental context as key to healthy aging communities.

Reverse Mortgages

Reverse mortgages are intended to help older Americans on fixed incomes. They allow homeowners over the age of 62 to convert part of the equity in their homes into tax-free income. No repayment of the loan is required until the borrower dies, sells the home, or permanently moves. The market for reverse mortgages may grow significantly as baby boomers enter retirement. Older persons can use cash from these loans for a variety of purposes, including home modifications, home repair, and long-term care services. Approximately 80,000 reverse mortgages exist, and 95 percent of these loans are FHA-insured Home Equity Conversion Mortgage program loans (www.reversemortgage.org).

A recent initiative is to encourage older homeowners to use reverse mortgages to purchase long-term care insurance. The passage of the American Homeownership and Economic Opportunity Act of 2000 is a step in this direction. It waives the up-front fee for the mortgage insurance premium for older Americans who use the money from an FHA Home Equity Conversion Mortgage Program for long-term care insurance. This approach would lessen the reliance on Medicaid, a dominant payer of nursing home care. At the same time, older adults would not have to spend down to qualify for Medicaid coverage of nursing home care. Older adults with long-term care insurance would have more options to remain at home with home health care services or move to an assisted living facility (Scully 2003). This policy initiative represents an emphasis on using one's own resources first to support long-term care before relying on public programs. Nevertheless, the use of reverse mortgages for such purposes can be seen as another form of spending down to receive long-term care.

Conclusion

Senior housing is evolving in the midst of political pressures, competing needs, and dwindling resources. Age is no longer the sole concern of senior housing, which is increasingly focused on the special need of frail seniors. This trend is evidenced by the FHAA, which sanctions senior housing as long as it provides facilities and services specifically designed to meet the physical and social needs of older adults. It recognizes the legitimacy of senior housing that addresses the unique needs of older adults. The fastest growing segments of the senior housing industry, such as assisted living, accommodate frail older adults with disabilities. In addition, policymakers are under increased pressure to address the needs of new family arrangements such as grandparents raising grandchildren. Future approaches to senior housing are likely to emphasize aging in place, using accessibility approaches and innovative funding sources. The focus of senior housing will be to maintain older adults in their homes or in residential settings, despite increasing frailty and disability. This shift will require major changes in both housing and long-term care policy.

References

Carp, F. 1987. The impact of planned housing. Pp. 43–79i In V. Regnier and J. Pynoos, eds., *Housing the Aged*. New York: Elsevier Science Publishing Company.

Commission on Affordable Housing and Health Needs for Seniors in the 21st Century. 2002. *A Quiet Crisis in America*. Washington, D.C.: Author.

Golant, S. M. 1987. In defense of age-segregated housing. Pp. 49–56 in J. A. Hancock, ed., *Housing the Elderly*. New Brunswick, N.J.: Center for Urban Policy Research.

Golant, S. M. 1992. *Housing America's Elderly: Many Possibilities, Few Choices*. Newbury Park, Calif.: Sage.

Golant, S. M. 1999. The promise of assisted living as a shelter and care alternative for frail American elders: A cautionary essay. Pp. 32–59 in B. Schwartz and R. Brent, eds., *Aging, Autonomy, and Architecture: Advances in Assisted Living*. Baltimore: Johns Hopkins University Press.

Golant, S. M. 2004. Do impaired older persons with health care needs occupy U.S. assisted living facilities? An analysis from six national studies. *Journal of Gerontology* 59B(2): S68–S79.

Golant, S. M., and A. J. La Greca. 1995. The relative deprivation of U.S. elderly households as judged by their housing problems. *Journal of Gerontology* 50B(1):S13–23.

Heumann, L. F., K. Winter-Nelson, and J. R. Anderson. 2001. *The 1999 Survey of Section 202 Elderly Housing*. Washington, D.C.: American Association for Retired Persons.

Kane, R.A., and K. B. Wilson. 1993. *Assisted Living in the United States: A New Paradigm for Residential Care for Frail Older Persons?* Washington, D.C.: American Association of Retired Persons.

Khadduri, J., and K. P. Nelson. 1992. Targeting housing assistance. *Journal of Policy Analysis and Management* 11(1):21–41.

Klinenberg, E. 2002. *Heat Wave: A Social Autopsy of Disaster in Chicago.* Chicago: University of Chicago Press.

Minkler, M., and D. Odierna. 2001. *California's Grandparents Raising Children: What the Aging Network Needs to Know as It Implements the National Family Caregiver Support Program.* Berkeley, Calif.: Center for the Advanced Study of Aging Services.

Mollica, R. L. 2002. *State Assisted Living Policy 2002.* Portland, Me.: National Academy for State Health Policy.

Morales, J. 1990. Senior housing as a children's issue: New cases implement Fair Housing Amendments. *Youth Law News* 5 (September/October): 1–9.

Newman, S. J., et al. 1990. Overwhelming odds: Caregiving and the risk of institutionalization. *Journal of Gerontology: Social Sciences* 45(5): S173–83.

Phillips, C. D., Y. Munoz, M. Sherman, M. Rose, W. Spector, and C. Hawes. 2003. Effects of facility characteristics on departures from assisted living: Results from a national study. *Gerontologist* 43:690–96.

Promatura Group, LLC. 2000. *NIC National Supply Estimate of Seniors Housing and Care Properties.* Annapolis, Md.: National Investment Center for the Seniors Housing and Care Industries.

Pynoos, J. 1992. Linking federally assisted housing with services for frail older people. *Journal of Aging and Social Policy* 4(3–4):157–77.

Pynoos, J. 1993. Towards a national policy on home modification. *Technology and Disability* 2(4):1–8.

Pynoos, J., and S. M. Golant. 1995. Housing and living arrangements for the elderly. Pp. 303–24 in R. H. Binstock and L. K. George, eds., *Handbook of Aging and the Social Sciences.* New York: Academic Press.

Pynoos, J., and T. Parrott. 1996. The politics of mixing older persons and younger persons with disabilities in federally assisted housing. *Gerontologist* 36(4):518–29.

Pynoos, J., and D. L. Redfoot. 1995. Housing frail elders in the United States. Pp. 187–210 in J. Pynoos and P. S. Liebig, eds., *Housing Frail Elders: International Policies, Perspectives, and Prospects.* Baltimore: Johns Hopkins University Press.

Pynoos, J., S. Reynolds, E. Salend, and A. Rahman. 1995. *Waiting for Federally Assisted Housing: A Study of the Needs and Experiences of Older Applicants.* Washington, D.C.: American Association of Retired Persons.

Redfoot, D. L., and K. S. Sloan. 1991. Realities of political decision-making on congregate housing. Pp. 99–110 in L. W. Kaye and A. Monk, eds., *Congregate Housing for the Elderly: Theoretical, Policy, and Programmatic Perspectives*. Binghamton, N.Y.: Haworth Press.

Schlesinger, M., and K. Kronebusch. 1994. Sources of intergenerational burdens and tensions. Pp. 185–209 in V. L. Bengtson and R. A. Harootyan, eds., *Intergenerational Linkages: Hidden Connections in American Society*. New York: Springer.

Scully, T. 2003, May. *Perspectives from the Centers for Medicare and Medicaid Services*. A paper presented at the Georgetown University Long-term Care Financing Project: The 21st Century Challenge: Providing and Paying for Long-term Care, Washington, D.C.

Shekelle, P., M. Maglione, J. Chang, W. Mojica, S. C. Morton, S. Y. Wu, and L. Z. Rubenstein. 2002. *Falls Prevention Interventions in the Medicare Population*. Baltimore, Md.: RAND-HCFA Evidence Report Monograph, HCFA Publication #HCFA-500-98-0281.

U.S. Department of Housing and Urban Development, Office of Policy Development and Research. 1999. *The Challenge of Housing Security: Report to Congress on the Housing Conditions and Needs of Older Americans*. Washington, D.C.: U.S. Department of Housing and Urban Development.

U.S. Department of Housing and Urban Development. 2000. *Report to Congress: Evaluation of the HOPE for Elderly Independence Demonstration Program and the New Congregate Housing Services Program*. Washington, D.C.: U.S. Department of Housing and Urban Development.

Wilden, R., and D. Redfoot. 2002. *Adding Assistive Living Services to Subsidized Housing: Serving Frail Older Persons with Low Incomes*. Washington, D.C.: American Association for Retired Persons.

Ziaja, E. 2001. Do independent and assisted living communities violate the Fair Housing Amendments Act and the Americans with Disabilities Act? *Elder Law Journal* 9(2):313–39.

IV. Old Age Politics and Policy

13. The Contemporary Politics of Old Age Policies

Robert H. Binstock

Since 1935, policies to benefit older persons have been prominent on the social policy agenda in the United States. This prominence has been more or less continual regardless of which political party has been in power and despite changing perceptions in public dialogue concerning older people and their worthiness as beneficiaries of government assistance. This chapter explores the politics that have accounted for this persistent attention to old age policies in different eras, including the roles of older voters and age-based interest groups as well broader interests and forces.

Piecemeal Construction of an Old Age Welfare State

In a society where an ideology of individualism and limited government predominated (Hartz 1955; Lipset 1996), the enactment of Social Security was a path-breaking public-sector response to the broad market failure of the Great Depression that resulted in deep impoverishment and unemployment of older people. In turn, the very enactment of this program, providing benefits to a large (and subsequently almost universal) proportion of older Americans, created a subsequent policy-based constituency of older voters and a plethora of interest groups focused on old age issues. As Hudson (1998) observes, the result was both a policy and a political institutionalization of the old (see also Campbell 2003).

The passage of Social Security politically legitimated the status of older persons as a major governmental concern and led to a period of some forty years that witnessed the piecemeal construction of a U.S. old age welfare state. Through Social Security, Medicare (national health insurance for almost all persons aged 65 and older), the Older Americans Act (an omnibus social service program for persons aged

60 and older), income tax deductions, and other measures, the elderly were exempted from income and asset screenings that are applied to welfare applicants in order to determine whether they are worthy of public help.

Moreover, the policy-created constituency of older persons became a useful vehicle for broader agendas. For example, when policy elites during President Lyndon Johnson's Great Society in the mid-1960s wanted to enact Medicare as a first step toward securing national health insurance (Cohen 1985; Ball 1995), the existing legitimization of older people as a deserving group helped make passage of the legislation possible (Marmor 2000).

The incremental creation of an old age welfare state during this period was nourished by compassionate stereotypes of "the aged" in public discourse (Binstock 1983). Elderly persons tended to be stereotyped as poor, frail, socially dependent, objects of discrimination—and above all, "deserving." For some forty years American society accepted this compassionate ageism, the oversimplified notion that all older persons are essentially the same, and all worthy of governmental assistance, without much attention to the substantial variations in economic well-being, health status, and social conditions that prevailed within the elderly population (see Neugarten 1970).

Especially during the 1960s and 1970s, just about every issue or problem that was identified as affecting just some older persons became a governmental responsibility: nutritional, legal, supportive, and leisure services; housing; home repair; energy assistance; transportation; employment assistance; job protection; public insurance for private pensions; special mental health programs; a separate National Institute on Aging; and on and on. By the late 1970s, the proportion of the annual federal budget spent on benefits to older persons had grown to 25 percent (Hudson 1978). A committee of the U.S. House of Representatives (1977), using loose criteria, was able to identify 134 programs benefiting the aging, overseen by 49 committees and subcommittees of Congress.

In addition to expanding the number of and budget for programs on aging, the construction of an old age welfare state had the consequence of creating a latent but large constituency of older voters as well as a number of age-based political interest groups (Binstock 1972; Day 1998; Pratt 1976; Van Tassel and Meyer 1992; Campbell 2003). Both the latent constituency of older voters and the age-based interest groups have helped to keep old age policies prominent on the national agenda in subsequent decades. The political mechanisms through which this prominence is fostered will be considered in detail below.

Intergenerational Constructs

Although the political and policy institutionalization of "the aged" has continued to this day as a major element in keeping old age policies prominent on the national agenda, additional factors have contributed as well in recent decades.

Greedy Geezers

Starting in 1978, the longstanding compassionate stereotype of older persons began to undergo an extraordinary reversal. Older people came to be portrayed as one of the more flourishing and powerful groups in American society and yet attacked as a burdensome responsibility. Throughout the 1980s, the1990s, and into the twenty-first century, the new stereotypes, readily observed in popular culture, have depicted aged persons as a new elite—prosperous, hedonistic, politically powerful, and selfish (e.g., Gibbs 1980).

A dominant theme in such accounts of older Americans is that their selfishness is ruining the nation. The *New Republic* highlighted this motif with an unflattering caricature of aged persons depicted on the cover, accompanied by the caption "greedy geezers." The table of contents "teaser" for the story that followed announced: "The real me generation isn't the yuppies, it's America's growing ranks of prosperous elderly" (Fairlie 1988). This theme was echoed widely, and the epithet "greedy geezers" became a familiar adjective in journalistic accounts of federal budget politics (e.g., Salholz 1990). In the early 1990s *Fortune* magazine claimed that "The Tyranny of America's Old" is "one of the most crucial issues facing U.S. society" (Smith 1992). That these themes concerning seniors persist in public discourse is evidenced by a story entitled "Meet the Greedy Grandparents" (Chapman 2003), commenting on legislation in 2003 that provided some prescription drug coverage under Medicare.

Two elements contributed to this reversal of stereotypes. One was the tremendous growth in the amount and proportion of federal dollars expended on benefits to aging citizens, which had, for the first time, come to be comparable in size to expenditures on national defense (Hudson 1978). Another was the dramatic improvements in the aggregate status of older Americans, in large part due to the impact of Social Security, Medicare, and other federal programs.

Intergenerational Equity: The Contemporary Dimension

In this unsympathetic climate of opinion, the aged emerged as a scapegoat for an impressive list of American problems, and the concept of so-called intergenerational equity—really, intergenerational *inequity*—became prominent in public dialogue. At first, these issues of equity were propounded in a contemporary dimension.

Noting the total and growing proportion of expenditures on benefits to older persons, demographers and advocates for children blamed the political power of elderly Americans for the plight of youngsters who have inadequate nutrition, health care, education, and insufficiently supportive family environments (e.g., Preston 1984). One children's advocate even proposed that parents receive an "extra vote" for each of their children, in order to combat older voters in an intergenerational conflict (Carballo 1981). Former Secretary of Commerce Peter Peterson (1987) suggested that a prerequisite for the United States to regain its stature as a first-class power in the world economy was a sharp reduction in programs benefiting older Americans. Widespread concerns about spiraling U.S. health care costs were redirected, in part, from health care providers, suppliers, administrators, and insurers—the parties that were responsible for setting the prices of care—to elderly persons for whom health care is provided. A number of academicians and public figures expressed concern that health care expenditures on older persons would soon absorb an unlimited amount of our national resources and crowd out health care for others as well as various worthy social causes. Some of them even proposed that age-based health care rationing would be necessary, desirable, and just (e.g., Callahan 1987; Smeeding et al. 1987; Daniels 1988).

By the end of the 1980s, the themes of intergenerational equity and conflict had been adopted by the media and academics as routine perspectives for describing many social policy issues (see Cook et al. 1994) and had also gained currency in elite sectors of American society and on Capitol Hill. For instance, the president of the prestigious American Association of Universities asserted, "The shape of the domestic federal budget inescapably pits programs for the retired against every other social purpose dependent on federal funds" (Rosenzweig 1990).

Indeed, the construct of intergenerational inequity had gained such a strong foothold in the thinking of many policy elites that they took it for granted as they analyzed American domestic policy issues. For example, in 1989 a distinguished "executive panel" of American leaders convened by the Ford Foundation designated older persons as the only group of citizens that should be responsible for financing a broad range of social programs for persons of all ages. In a report entitled *The Common Good: Social Welfare and the American Future,* the panel recommended a series of policies costing a total of $29 billion (Ford Foundation 1989). The panel proposed that this $29 billion be financed solely by taxing Social Security benefits. In fact, every financing alternative considered in the report assumed that elderly people should be the exclusive financiers of the panel's package of recommendations for improving social welfare in our nation. The Ford panel apparently felt that the reasons for this assumption were self-evident; it did not even bother to justify its selections of these financing options as opposed to others (also see, e.g., Beatty 1990).

The Aging of the Baby Boom: Older People versus Society

The construct of intergenerational equity also had a future dimension, focusing on impending changes in the age structure of American society that would be brought about by the aging of the baby boom cohort, the 76 million persons born between 1946 and 1964 (Hobbs 1996). One aspect of this issue was highlighted by the "generational accounting" analyses of economist Laurence Kotlikoff (1992), which, though controversial (see Haveman 1994), have continued to receive considerable attention. He suggested that future generations of older people will do less well than contemporary older people in terms of the taxes they pay for income security purposes and the subsequent lifetime payments they will receive through public programs.

Concern about the consequences for society of sustaining the old age welfare state in the twenty-first century was initially highlighted by the efforts of Americans for Generational Equity (AGE). Formed as an interest group in 1985 with backing from the corporate sector as well as a handful of Congressmen who led it, AGE recruited some of the prominent "scapegoaters" of older people to its board and as its spokespersons. According to its annual reports, most of AGE's funding came from insurance companies, health care corporations, banks, and other private sector businesses and organizations that are in financial competition with Medicare and Social Security (Quadagno 1989).

Since the mid-1980s, anxieties about the societal consequences of an aged baby boom have been expressed in an apocalyptic fashion. For instance, biomedical ethicist Daniel Callahan, concerned about future health care expenditures for older people, characterized the elderly population as "a new social threat" and a "demographic, economic, and medical avalanche . . . one that could ultimately (and perhaps already) do [sic] great harm" (Callahan 1987, p. 20). Accordingly, he proposed that Medicare reimbursement for life-saving care be categorically denied to anyone aged 80 and older. Economist Lester Thurow (1996) saw baby boomers and their self-interested pursuit of government benefits as a fundamental threat to the American political system.

Even in this political climate there were new initiatives in policies on aging; however, they took on features that reflected some of the changes in political discourse regarding older persons that had taken place since the mid-1970s. No longer were the policies blind to variations in the income and asset situations of older persons. No longer was it essential that benefits be simply age categorical. No longer was it assumed that earmarked payroll taxes or general revenues would finance old age benefit programs.

For one thing, a number of policy changes were made to reflect the diverse economic situations of elderly individuals (although the redistributive aspect of Social Security's benefit formulas had been recognizing such diversity for many years). Some of them took benefits away from "greedy geezers." Others directed benefits toward poor older persons.

The Social Security Reform Act of 1983 began this trend by making Social Security benefits subject to taxation for the first time for beneficiaries at higher income levels. The Older Americans Act programs of supportive and social services, for which all persons aged 60 and older are eligible, became gradually targeted by Congress to the low-income and minority elderly. The Qualified Medicare Beneficiary and the Specified Low-Income Medicare Beneficiary programs, established

by the Medicare Catastrophic Coverage Act (MCCA) of 1988, required Medicaid to pay Part B premiums, deductibles, and co-payments
for older persons with very low incomes and assets. And the Omnibus
Budget Reconciliation Act of 1993 continued this trend by adding to
taxation of Social Security benefits for wealthier older Americans.
These policy changes clearly established the principle that the diverse
economic circumstances of older people can be addressed through legislative reforms. Consequently, they gave the lie to the frequently asserted shibboleth that old age programs would only be politically viable if they made no distinctions based on economic status.

The MCCA also introduced the notion that old age benefits could
be directly financed solely by program beneficiaries with no support
from a payroll tax or general revenues. A portion of the bill (later repealed) provided that coverage for catastrophic hospital expenses be
financed by surtaxes on the income of Medicare participants, cali-
brated on a sliding scale in relation to income. This portion of the
MCCA was repealed after a minority of older persons, scattered in
congressional districts throughout the country, vociferously protested
this provision because they thought they already had such coverage
and they regarded the surtax as too expensive (see Himmelfarb 1995).

A New Era: Conservatism Meets Policies on Aging

Even as attention to the projected future costs and societal consequences of the aging of the baby boom characterized the politics of
aging in the late 1980s and the 1990s, the broader political arena
began to turn much more conservative than it had been since the New
Deal. Bill Clinton, supported by the somewhat centrist Democratic
Leadership Council, adopted the theme of "end big government as we
know it." His most notable step in that direction was to sign the
Republican-inspired Personal Responsibility and Work Opportunity
Reconciliation Act (1996), aka Welfare Reform.

Before the Republicans gained control of Congress in 1995, the U.S.
old age welfare state was widely assumed to be a permanent feature of
American society, especially the entitlement programs, Social Security
and Medicare. Changes in these programs might take place, but their
general contours would remain the same, and their revenues and expenditures would probably continue to grow.

However, the escalation of conservatism as the Republicans took control of Congress in 1995, combined with growing concerns about the impact of an aging baby boom on future entitlement obligations, began to undermine that assumption. Another ingredient in the mix was the bipartisan belief at the time that growing budget deficits had to be brought under control, Social Security and Medicare being the two largest single items.

Conservatism and Medicare

Toward this end, Congress submitted to President Clinton a budget bill for fiscal year 1996 that included a $452 billion reduction in projected Medicare and Medicaid spending over seven years. Although the president was willing to approve smaller reductions in Medicare and Medicaid spending, he vetoed the bill, citing the size of the reduction and some structural changes proposed for the programs as among his reasons for doing so. The following year Congress developed a budget resolution for more modest reductions in projected expenditures for the two programs, but no legislative action was taken as the 1996 election approached.

Meanwhile, Congress and the Clinton administration were shifting some measure of Medicare's financial risk to the private sector by encouraging the proliferation of Medicare managed care organizations (MCOs). In 1990, 3 percent of Medicare beneficiaries were enrolled in MCOs; by the end of 1997, the proportion had climbed to 14 percent (Medicare Payment Advisory Commission 1998). In contrast to the traditional fee-for-service (FFS) reimbursement system under Medicare, MCOs limit the federal government's financial risk in that Medicare makes a fixed per capita payment to these organizations for each Medicare participant they enroll; in turn, the MCOs are responsible for providing all needed services that are covered by Medicare.

The strategy of shifting financial risk from the government to the private sector was amplified by the Balanced Budget Act (BBA) of 1997 that established a Medicare+Choice program offering beneficiaries a panoply of private sector options for receiving their health care. However, the strategy proved to be less than a success. The percentage of Medicare enrollees opting for these private sector options reached a peak of 16 percent in 1999 before dropping to 11 percent in 2003 (Pear 2003a).

The BBA also created a Bipartisan Commission on the Future of

Medicare. A majority of the Commission members wanted to complete the transition from the FFS system by proposing that each Medicare enrollee be given a voucher by the government to shop for insurance in the private sector. Two members who were sympathetic to the voucher proposal also demanded that adequate outpatient prescription drug coverage under Medicare be included in return for their votes supporting vouchers. When they did not win this concession, they did not join the majority, and the Commission was unable to make an official recommendations when it concluded its work in 1998 (Pear 1999; Vladeck 1999). Yet these dynamics of the Commission set the stage for further efforts to cover prescription drugs and to privatize Medicare.

During the 2000 presidential election campaign, both candidates pledged to secure Medicare prescription drug coverage. Then, when Republicans took control of both houses of Congress in 2003, they joined President Bush in viewing legislation to cover drugs as an opportunity to curry favor with older voters, perhaps displacing Democrats as the traditional champions of Medicare. However, by the time a final bill—formally named the Medicare Prescription Drug, Improvement, and Modernization of Medicare Act (MMA) of 2003—was enacted, it also contained many features to lure Medicare participants into private sector health plans and to subsidize private Medicare plans to make them more attractive to both providers and potential enrollees (Freudenheim 2004). According to the actuary of the Centers for Medicare and Medicaid Services, an estimated increase of $46 billion in Medicare payments would be provided to the private plans over the ten years following the legislation (Pear 2004a).

In addition, the legislation and subsequent administrative actions involved a considerable amount of spin-doctoring to present private plans as better choices for Medicare enrollees. The MMA changed the name of Medicare+Choice to Medicare Advantage, and a March 2004 letter to Medicare beneficiaries from the secretary of the U.S. Department of Health and Human services touted Medicare Advantage as "among the most common and popular plans right now for working Americans" and giving persons eligible for Medicare "better benefits" (Thompson 2004). Ultimately, of course, a strategic goal of expanding Medicare enrollments in private plans is to shift the financial risk of paying doctors, hospitals, and other health care providers from the government to the private sector and to beneficiaries.

Conservatism and Social Security

Privatizing Social Security has been on the agenda of conservatives and libertarian think tanks since the 1970s (Williamson 1997) but did not reach the mainstream political agenda until the late 1990s. A key event was a 1997 report of an Advisory Council on Social Security that addressed long-term financing issues facing the Old-Age and Survivors Insurance (OASI) program. It presented three plans for partially privatizing OASI as a means of improving the long-range financial status of the traditional program and/or providing retired workers with a greater probability of sufficient income in retirement (1994–1996 Advisory Council on Social Security 1997). Each called for investing tens to hundreds of billions of additional dollars in the private sector.

These and subsequent proposals for partial privatization from Democratic and Republican members of Congress as well as other sources transformed the politics of Social Security reform. The rapidity with which this notion gained political acceptability was underscored in the spring of 1998 when the Senate passed a resolution calling for private investment accounts to be part of any Social Security reform package (Stevenson 1998a). By that summer, the president was seriously considering some form of equity investment as part of Social Security reform (Stevenson 1998b).

George Bush picked up this theme during his 2000 election campaign, and in his first year in office he appointed a special commission on Social Security reform that only included members who were in favor of privatization ideas. Events related to 9/11 pushed these ideas into the background, but key members of the Bush administration continued to make clear that they intended to eventually move forward on the agenda of privatizing Social Security. And in his State of the Union speech in 2004, President Bush once again indicated that he wanted to make it possible for workers to save "part of their taxes in a personal retirement account" (Andrews 2004).

The Roles of Older Voters and Age-Based Interest Groups

As this overview of various eras in the politics of aging indicates, a number of different factors have accounted for the continuing prominence of old age policies on the national legislative agenda, including the political and policy institutionalization of the aged, the emergence of arguments around intergenerational inequity, and the advent of a resurgent conservatism in American politics. Throughout these different eras, older voters and a number of age-based organizations or interest groups have played a variety of roles.

Older Voters

The role of older voters with respect to old age policies has been indirect and complex. On the one hand, election exit polls over the past several decades show little evidence that old age issues have been a dominant factor in influencing the votes of the elderly. Indeed, older persons have distributed their votes among candidates in roughly the same proportions as younger age groups (although the very youngest age group does tend to vote differently from the others) (see Connelly 2000). Indeed, the differences *within* age groups are much sharper than differences *between* age groups. The votes of older persons divide along the same partisan, economic, social, gender, and other lines as those of the electorate at large.

There are many reasons to expect that old age policy issues would not critically influence the choices of older voters. Age is only one of the many personal characteristics of aged people, and only one of the issues with which they may identify themselves and their self-interests. Even if some older voters primarily identify themselves in terms of their age status, this does not mean that their self-interests in old age policies are the most important factors in their electoral decisions. Other policy issues, strong and longstanding partisan attachments, and other electoral stimuli in an electoral campaign can be of equal or greater importance. Moreover, as Jacobson (1992) has shown, voters rarely know much about candidates' positions on the issues, and few elections are determined by them.

On the other hand, older voters do have an indirect latent group power that affects political elites, a power that does not necessarily require a behavioral reality of electoral cohesion. Members of Congress are characteristically concerned with how the next legislative vote they cast might become a defining issue—negative or positive—in their next electoral campaigns (see Arnold 1992). Politicians at all levels know that older persons vote at a higher rate than other age groups and that they are a steadily increasing percentage of voters (Binstock 2000). So they look for opportunities to curry favor with older voters, as exemplified by the success of President Bush and congressional Republicans to enact a Medicare prescription drug bill in 2003 (Toner 2003a). Alternatively, they are wary of being cast as villains with respect to old age policies, thereby giving rise to the journalistic cliché: Social Security is the third rail of politics—touch it and you're dead! And in fact, when proposals arise for cutting back Social Security and other old age benefits, older people are generally quite active in making their views known to members of Congress (Campbell 2003).

In electoral campaigns, candidates seek to ensure that their opponents will not outdo them in courting older voters. This can take the form of promises to champion the expansion of old age benefits, as in the case of the 2000 presidential election when both candidates promised to secure prescription drug benefits for the Medicare program. Or it can manifest itself in candidates' portraying themselves as preservers or defenders of existing old age policies, as was the case in 1996, when both Bob Dole and Bill Clinton portrayed themselves as saviors of Medicare (*New York Times* 1996a, 1996b), despite the fact that Dole had led a legislative effort in Congress to cut the program and Clinton had vetoed that bill.

Old Age Interest Groups

Age-based political organizations have been in existence for most of the twentieth century. However, those founded in the early decades were primarily amorphous and transient social movements guided by charismatic leaders (Messinger 1955; Pinner, Jacobs, and Selznick 1959; Holtzman 1963), and those of the middle decades were more service-oriented than politically oriented. Since the 1960s, however, the number of stable old age advocacy groups has proliferated, and those that existed before the 1960s have become more politically active (Pratt 1976, 1993; Powell, Branco, and Williamson 1996; Day 1998). Today dozens of old age interest groups are more or less exclusively preoccupied with national policy issues related to aging, and they are reputed to be among the most powerful lobbies in Washington (Cook and Barrett 1992; Birnbaum 1997; Day 1998), particularly AARP (formerly the American Association of Retired Persons), which is by far the largest mass-membership organization of older persons (Morris 1996).

Numerous factors account for the proliferation and stability of political organizations focused on aging concerns. Government expansion in the aging policy arena generates organizational activity not only because millions of older persons have a stake in old age programs but also because politicians and bureaucrats working in the aging field mobilize political support for their own legislation and programs. The patronage of government agencies as well as of foundations and service provider associations in the private sector propels the growth and politicization of existing interest groups and the emergence of new ones (Estes 1979; Walker 1983).

It is important to note, however, that the enactment and amendment of major policies on aging from 1935 through the late 1970s can largely be attributed to policy elites rather than to pressures from old-age interest groups (e.g., on Social Security, see Derthick 1979; on Medicare, see Ball 1995 and Cohen 1985). The impact of these groups was largely confined to promoting relatively minor policies of the latter half of the twentieth century involving the distribution of benefits to professionals and practitioners in the field of aging rather than directly to older persons themselves (Binstock 1972; Estes 1979; Lockett 1983). But more recently these groups have been active in opposing cutbacks in Social Security and Medicare (see Day 1998; Campbell 2003), and, as discussed below, AARP played a critical role in the passage of a Medicare amendment in 2003.

Forms of Power. Although old age political organizations have had not initiated or shaped the major old age policies over the years, their professed role as representatives of and advocates for "the elderly" has given them some entrée into the policy process. Public officials often find it useful to invite such organizations to participate in policy activities, demonstrating in this way that they been "in touch" symbolically with tens of millions of older persons. A brief meeting with the leaders of AARP and other old age organizations enables an official to claim that he or she has obtained the views of older people.

The symbolic legitimacy of old age organizations affords them several types of power. First, they have easy informal access to public officials. Second, their legitimacy enables them to obtain public platforms in the national media, in congressional hearings, and in other age-related policy forums. And third, old age interest groups can mobilize their members when changes are being contemplated in old age programs.

Perhaps the most important form of power available to the old age interest groups might be termed "the electoral bluff." Although these organizations have not demonstrated a capacity to swing a decisive bloc of older voters, incumbent members of Congress are hardly inclined to risk upsetting the existing distribution of votes that puts them and keeps them in office. The perception of being powerful is, in itself, a source of political influence (see Banfield 1951). Hence, when congressional offices are flooded with letters, faxes, and phone calls expressing the (not necessarily representative) views of older persons, members of Congress take heed.

Many old age interest groups have attempted to enhance their power by banding together in a 51-member Leadership Council of Aging Organizations (LCAO), a self-defined coalition of "national non-profit organizations concerned with the well-being of America's older population and committed to representing their interests in the policy-making arena" (Leadership Council of Aging Organizations 2004a). The coalition sends letters to members of Congress and the current administration on policy issues, conducts issue briefings and forums, holds press conferences, and comments on presidential and congressional budgets affecting older persons (although not all members sign on to any given statement or letter). Members of LCAO have tended to be liberal in their political orientation, for example, being squarely opposed to Social Security privatization (Leadership Council of Aging Organizations 2004b). There have been occasions over the years, however, when these organizations have been divided on such aging policy issues as catastrophic hospital coverage (Himmelfarb 1995), mandatory retirement (Day 1990; Pratt 1993), and elimination of the Social Security "earnings test" (Dumas 1992). Such divisions limit the effectiveness of the coalition.

Types of Interest Groups. In addition to the organizations that participate in the LCAO coalition, there are a number of old age interest groups that represent for-profit as well as not-for-profit nursing homes and other business and service interests in the field of aging, such as the American Health Care Association and the American Federation of Home Care Agencies. There are also some conservative direct-mail organizations that do not publicize the size of the membership, such as the United Seniors Association and the Seniors Coalition, initially founded by conservative fund-raisers to oppose tax hikes on Social Security benefits (Kosterlitz 1993). The Seniors Coalition bills itself as "*the* responsible alternative to the AARP" (Seniors Coalition 2004).

Even among the fifty-one organizations in the LCAO, however, there is considerable diversity in types of organizations. The missions of some of them involve concern for a wide range of health and welfare issues. They include such organizations as the American Public Health Association, Families USA, the American Foundation for the Blind, Volunteers of America, the Catholic Health Association of America, United Jewish Communities, and the Gray Panthers. Because older people are but one of their many constituencies, the depth of their commitment to lobbying in the old age policy arena is diluted by the totality of their interests.

In contrast to these is a grouping of old age political organizations that are focused on causes that affect selected categories of older persons, including older women (e.g., the Older Women's League); various ethnic and racial subgroups of older people (e.g., the National Caucus and Center on Black Aged, the National Asian Pacific Center on Aging, Associacion Nacional pro Personas Mayores, and the National Indian Council on Aging); and older persons afflicted by specific illnesses (e.g., the Alzheimer's Association and the National Osteoporosis Foundation). These groups tend to lobby Congress armed with policy analyses highlighting their concerns for their respective subgroups. Perhaps the most effective of these has been the Alzheimer's Association, which has a substantial public policy operation (see Binstock 1998) and has managed to have a significant portion of the budget of the National Institute on Aging earmarked for research on Alzheimer's disease (Adelman 1995).

Another grouping of organizations in the LCAO coalition is trade associations involved in providing programs and services to older persons as clients and customers, such as the American Association of Homes and Services for the Aging, the National Association of Area Agencies on Aging, the National Association of State Units on Aging, the National Association of Nutrition and Aging Services Programs, the National Association of Foster Grandparent Program Directors, and the National Adult Day Services Association, among others. Such trade associations tend to focus on the likely impact of policies on their respective industries, with a more secondary concern about policy effects on older people themselves. These organizations draw on state and local political connections as well as on their clients to protest possible cutbacks in the programs that sustain their operations. In 1995, for instance, such protests led Congress to scrap its plan to enfold funds that were earmarked for congregate and home-delivered meals for the elderly into a broad nutrition block grant to the states (*Newsweek* 1995).

There is also a cluster of professional organizations especially attuned in their public policy efforts to promoting aging-related research, education, and favorable conditions for professional practice in the field of aging (e.g., geriatric medicine). This group includes the American Geriatrics Society, the Gerontological Society of America, the Alliance for Aging Research, the American Society on Aging, and the National Council on the Aging. The public policy operations of these organizations are comparatively small when compared, say, with that of the Alzheimer's Association. Yet on occasion some of them have effectively lobbied Congress to fund programs to promote their professional activities, including a five-year effort by the Gerontological Society of America that established a separate National Institute on Aging at the National Institutes of Health (Lockett 1983).

The old age interest groups that have the greatest potential for political power are, of course, those that have mass memberships of older persons, because their members are part of the latent constituency of older voters who might, in principle, be influenced by their parent organizations in upcoming elections. Among these are the National Association of Retired Federal Employees (NARFE), the National Committee to Preserve Social Security and Medicare (NCPSSM), the Alliance for Retired Americans (ARA), and AARP.

NARFE is the smallest of the mass-membership organizations in the LCAO that are primarily focused on issues of old age and retirement directly affecting its members. It has about 400,000 members, and its mission has remained the same since it was founded in 1921: "to protect and improve the retirement benefits of federal retirees, employees and their families" (National Association of Retired Federal Employees 2004).

NCPSSM was founded in 1982 in the midst of a funding crisis in Social Security (see Light 1985) "to serve as an advocate for the landmark federal programs of Social Security and Medicare" (National Committee to Preserve Social Security and Medicare 2004a). Although it has only 1.2 million dues-paying members (Richtman 2004), its Web site claims "millions of members and supporters" (National Committee to Preserve Social Security 2004b).

The Alliance for Retired Americans (ARA), with a membership of about 3 million retirees (Alliance for Retired Americans 2004) was created in 2001 as an organization in which all AFL-CIO union members automatically become members as they retire and to which all other retirees are welcome (Greenhouse 2001). It is a successor to the liberal National Council of Senior Citizens, also an AFL-CIO creation, which was formed explicitly to promote public health insurance for older people. The union movement in the 1960s saw the enactment of Medicare as a means of eliminating retiree health benefits as a troublesome part of the overall compensation packages for which it bargained (Quadagno, in press). As might be expected given ARA's origins in the AFL-CIO, immediately after its creation it began lobbying for Medicare low-cost prescription drug coverage (Greenhouse 2001).

The Unique Position of AARP. Although AARP is also a mass-membership organization, it deserves special mention because of its huge membership, vastly superior financial and staff resources, and reputation in Washington as the most politically powerful of the age-based groups (Morris 1996; Birnbaum 1997). The latest annual report and financial accounting statements posted on its Web site place its membership at "more than 35 million members" and portray a large business operation (AARP 2003a, 2003b). AARP had assets of $178 million at the end of 2002 and annual operating revenues of $636 million. The largest portion of this revenue—34.3 percent ($218 million)—came from "royalties" on the insurance programs and other products it markets to its members. In 2002, for instance, AARP processed $4.2 billion in insurance premium payments from members; from this it retained $123.3 million for the use of its brand name and logo, $10.8 million for member list access fees, $.9 million for quality control services, as well as $26.7 million earned by investing insurance premiums from members until the date when the premiums must be forwarded to the insurance companies (AARP 2003b). The other sources of revenue in 2002 were: membership dues, $186 million; advertising in its publications, $76 million; federal and other grants, $61 million; investments and "other," $56 million; and member service and programs, $39 million. In addition to insurance, AARP offers a prescription drug service, mutual funds, credit cards, travel services (including hotel and automobile discounts), and other programs and services. It maintains offices in all fifty states, the District of Columbia, Puerto Rico, and the U.S. Virgin Islands.

Although more than 90 percent of AARP's $613 million in annual expenditures in 2002 was for membership development, management, member programs and field services, publications, and other revenue-generating activities, the organization also spent $57 million on public policy research and legislative lobbying. This level of expenditure, together with a membership of approximately 35 million, makes it dominant among old age interest groups in framing age-related policy issues.

The political positions of AARP over the years, however, have tended to be restrained. Essentially, its activities in the public policy arena have been membership marketing strategies and avenues through which AARP's staff and national volunteer leaders could be "players" in the Washington national scene. Its approach to lobbying has always been constrained by the overriding consideration that its political views and tactics should not alienate substantial portions of its dues-paying and product-and-services-buying membership. In short, AARP's incentive system has long dictated that it should clearly establish a record that it is "fighting the good fight" with respect to policy proposals affecting old-age programs. But the fight, win or lose, should *not* include positions and tactics that threaten to jeopardize the stability of the organization's membership and financial resources.

From 1994 until 2003, AARP assumed a noticeably withdrawn public posture due to two episodes that noticeably antagonized some of its members and eroded some of its standing in Washington. One was its endorsement of the Medicare Catastrophic Coverage Act that increased Part B premiums paid by Medicare enrollees and levied a progressive income surtax on relatively well-off older people to pay for new hospital insurance benefits—legislation that was unpopular and was repealed the next year (Himmelfarb 1995). The other episode was support for the Democratic leadership's 1994 health care reform bills in the Senate and the House (*New York Times* 1994a, 1994b). On both occasions it was rumored that a small minority of AARP members resigned. Following the ineffectual endorsement of the health bills, the president of AARP publicly acknowledged that his membership had widely divergent and strongly held views and that representing a diverse membership in public policy affairs is an ongoing struggle for the organization (Lehrman 1995).

AARP's legitimacy as an advocate for older people was further tarnished in two 1995 Senate hearings where various witnesses criticized AARP's organizational practices and its tax-exempt status. Senator

Alan Simpson of Wyoming charged that AARP had "drifted considerably from any reasonable description of a nonprofit organization that should enjoy a tax exemption and unlimited lobbying privileges," and he also asserted that the organization "imposes a policy agenda on an unwilling membership" (Pear 1995). These hearings and media coverage of them also raised questions about the propriety of AARP lobbying the federal government when in one year alone it received $86 million in federal grants, and it opened up a wider discussion of lobbying by tax-exempt organizations in general (e.g., *New York Times* 1995). In 1994 AARP had settled a dispute regarding its business income by agreeing to pay $135 million to the Internal Revenue Service. In 1996 the organization was fined $5.6 million by the U.S. Postal Service for illegally using cheaper nonprofit mailing rates to send out millions of solicitations for commercial insurance (Holmes 2001). Subsequently, AARP became sufficiently cautious in its policy stances that, as a staff member for a Democrat in the House of Representatives perceived the situation in 2001, "I've almost stopped thinking of them as a lobby. They have all kinds of valuable member services and do really good research work. But in terms of being a tough lobby, they're not what they used to be" (Holmes 2001, p. D1)

AARP and the Medicare Modernization Act. The public affairs posture of AARP became markedly more prominent during the legislative process that resulted in the enactment of the MMA of 2003. In fact, its impact on this process may have been the most influential that any old age interest group has had in U.S. politics.

Given that the most widely publicized feature of the House and Senate MMA bills was to provide $400 billion over ten years for Medicare coverage of outpatient prescription drugs—a critical gap in the program—it would have been difficult for AARP to continue its relatively low visibility of the preceding years. Indeed, as an organization purporting to represent the needs of older Americans, how could AARP do anything but support such an expansion of Medicare, and do so prominently?

Yet, as indicated above, the MMA legislation also contained a number of provisions to further the privatization of Medicare. These included incentives to lead program participants to abandon the program's traditional FFS system for managed care organizations and preferred provider organizations and arrangements to set up direct competition between FFS and private sector Medicare that would favor the latter. These provisions concerned AARP as well as other members of the LCAO and substantial segments of the social policy community on the grounds that they would undermine the Medicare program and achieve little in the way of program efficiency or savings (Hacker and Marmor 2003; White 2003; Iglehart 2004). In July, AARP sent an eight-page letter to members of Congress in which it outlined its objections to various features of the legislation (including some inadequacies in drug coverage) and threatened to oppose the legislation unless there was an adequate response to these concerns (*USA Today* 2003). When the House and Senate versions of the legislation emerged from a congressional conference committee in November as a unified bill, NCPSSM and the Alliance for Aging Research were opposed to it. At a rally sponsored by the Alliance, attendees denounced it as a "lemon" constructed by Republicans committed to destroying Medicare (Pear and Toner 2003a).

A clear but little-noticed signal as to what would be AARP's eventual response emerged two weeks before the MMA achieved final passage in the Senate. AARP sponsored rallies in five major cities to which were transmitted a televised speech by President Bush calling for passage of the MMA. Five high-level White House surrogates—the administrator of the Centers for Medicare and Medicaid Services, the surgeon general, the director of National Institutes of Health, the commissioner of the Food and Drug Administration, and the commissioner of the Centers for Disease Control—were present at the five sites to introduce the president's speech and to answer questions following it (America's Future 2003).

Four days later AARP endorsed the bill and announced that it would spend $7 million worth of newspaper and television advertising during the week to support passage of the legislation (Pear and Toner 2003b)—a promise on which it delivered. Two additional members of the liberal LCAO—the National Council on the Aging and the Alzheimer's Association—also supported the legislation, but other mass membership liberal organizations in the coalition such as NCPSSM were "surprised" and "disappointed" by AARP's actions (Budge and Marini 2003).

By all accounts (Pear 2003b; Toner 2003b; Iglehart 2004), AARP's endorsement was decisive in enabling the bill to pass the Senate. Some Democratic senators who might have been prepared to sustain a filibuster against the bill were clearly concerned that it would be difficult for them to explain to their constituents in subsequent campaigns how they could be against this legislation which the "800-pound gorilla" representing the interests of older people had strongly supported (see Stolberg 2003).

Democrats were particularly disappointed and angry with AARP because many of them—as had Republicans—had come to view AARP as basically in harmony, politically, with their party. In 2002 Republican Senator Trent Lott had characterized AARP as a "wholly owned subsidiary of the Democratic party" (Stolberg 2003). In contrast, following AARP's endorsement and the passage of MMA, Democratic Representative Pete Stark, a leading health policy spokesman, sent a letter to House Democrats in which he said, "AARP—what does it stand for? Always Advocating for the Republican Party" (Pear 2004b). Eighty-five House Democrats proclaimed that they "would either resign from AARP or refuse to join it," and Democrat Nancy Pelosi, minority leader in the House, complained that AARP was "in the pocket of Republicans" (Stolberg 2003). In addition, congressional Democrats and many other commentators charged AARP with a conflict of interest in supporting the MMA because about one-third of the organization's income is derived from selling insurance, and the new legislation provides tens of billions in subsidies to insurance companies (Drinkard and Welch 2003; Krugman 2003).

Although the conflict-of-interest accusations suggested that AARP endorsed the MMA in order to increase its income (an accusation that the organization strongly denied), its decision probably turned on other factors. One obvious explanation for the organization's decision is that the new drug coverage, though far from perfect, would be of some assistance to most older Americans, of great assistance to many of them, and a good first step toward better coverage. This was, in fact, an argument that AARP made at the time in newspaper advertisements throughout the country and in other venues as well.

Another explanation is that the endorsement made sense from an organizational maintenance perspective. For AARP, maintaining and growing its membership is a prime directive, because all of its activities—marketing and providing products and services, and "representing" older people in public policy affairs—are dependent on the size of its mass membership. In making a choice on whether to endorse or oppose the MMA—a choice it could not avoid—a paramount consideration had to be which choice would be likely to alienate the fewest members. A rationale for endorsing the bill could be readily conveyed to AARP members and the larger community: There is no drug coverage now, and this bill provides an opportunity to have some that cannot be passed up; we can work to improve things later. Most of the rationales for opposing the bill would be much more impersonal and difficult to convey, centered on arguments regarding erosion of traditional Medicare FFS in the future, probable ineffectiveness of private competition in holding down program costs, and overly generous subsidies to private plan providers and insurers.

AARP's endorsement of the MMA did create some backlash within its membership. According to William Novelli, AARP's CEO, by about eight weeks after the endorsement at least 45,000 members had resigned in anger (Pear 2004b). Yet one wonders how many resignations there would have been if AARP had opposed a bill that provided prescription drug coverage under Medicare for the first time. It is probably safe to say that the number would have been far, far more than 45,000. Perhaps millions of members would have been at stake.

In any event, AARP moved swiftly to contain whatever damage had been done to its image. Novelli, a former public relations executive, immediately disseminated defensive "op eds" to major newspapers (e.g., Novelli 2003). In the next issue of the AARP's newsletter to members, he explained the organization's decision (Novelli 2004). And the following issue of the newsletter outlined AARP's agenda for reforming the Medicare law it had endorsed just three months earlier (Barry 2004).

Looking Ahead

Regardless of how its members or others may judge AARP's actions in relation to the MMA of 2003, the organization certainly emerged as a much more influential force in the politics of old age policies than it had been before. It is also far more influential than the other age-based organizations—most of which opposed the MMA but were ignored by Congress.

It is clear that under Novelli's leadership AARP will continue to draw on its standing as a massive membership organization of older persons to undertake a visible and active role in the old age policy arena. Since he took charge of the organization in early 2002, "social change" has become an explicitly avowed priority of the organization

(AARP 2003a). Moreover, his intention for the organization to be a major "player" in Washington politics is unambiguous. In response to Democratic complaints that his organization had cooperated with the Republicans on the MMA, he acknowledged that these actions had re-aligned AARP politically. Shortly after the legislation passed, he opined that "AARP was taken for granted" by Democratic leaders in the past, and he observed that "the best thing we can do is not be aligned with either party" (Cook 2003).

But even as AARP steps forward aggressively, it is important to note that forces other than old age interest groups and the latent con-stituency of older voters play a powerful role in the old age policy arena. In the legislative process of the MMA, interests other than age-based ones, representing powerful economic and professional con-stituencies, played active roles. Also endorsing the bill, for instance, were the American Association of Health Plans (which includes both HMOs and health insurers), the American Hospital Association, the American Medical Association, and a coalition of employers, includ-ing General Motors and Dow Chemical, who hoped that prescription drug coverage would enable them to reduce their retiree health insur-ance commitments or receive subsidies for not doing so (Pear and Toner 2003a). In addition, the footprints of the pharmaceutical in-dustry were all over the MMA in such provisions as a ban on reim-portation of relatively low-cost drugs from Canada and other coun-tries and a measure that prohibited Medicare from directly negotiating drug prices with manufacturers (see Weissert 2003; Iglehart 2004).

The strongest factor in shaping old age policies in the foreseeable fu-ture, however, will be the broader political milieu of American society. Certainly, old age policies will remain prominent on the policy agenda throughout the first half of the twenty-first century because of the sheer size of the aging baby boom cohort. If neoconservatism remains in the ascendance, then the old age welfare state may be partially disassem-bled through privatization measures. If a more liberal milieu emerges, a range of new measures manifesting government involvement and control will be more likely to shape old age policies.

References

1994–1996 Advisory Council on Social Security. 1997. *Report of the 1994–1996 Advisory Council on Social Security, Volume I: Findings and Recommendations.* Washington, D.C.: Government Printing Office.

AARP. 2003a. *Annual Report 2002.* Retrieved March 27, 2004 from http://assets.aarp.org/www.aarp.org-articles/aboutaarp/annualreports2002-f.pdf.

AARP. 2003b. *Consolidated Financial Statements as of December 31, 2002 Together with Independent Auditor's Report.* Retrieved March 26, 2004, from http://assets.aarp.org/www.aarp.org_/articles/aboutaarp/financia12002.pdf.

Adelman, R. C. 1995. The Alzheimerization of aging. *Gerontologist* 35:526–32.

Alliance for Retired Americans. 2004. *About Us.* Retrieved March 27, 2004, from www.retired americans.org/indes.php?tg=topusn&cat=2.

America's Future. 2003. *Coordinated Events by Bush, Trade Association, and AARP.* Retrieved November 12, 2003, from action@action.ourfuture.org.

Andrews, E. L. 2004. Bush promotes earlier proposals for tax-advantaged savings accounts. *New York Times,* January 21, A12.

Arnold, R. D. 1992. *The Logic of Congressional Action.* New Haven, Conn.: Yale University Press.

Ball, R. M. 1995. What Medicare's architects had in mind. *Health Affairs* 14(4):62–72.

Banfield, E. C. 1951. *Political Influence: A New Theory of Urban Politics.* New York: Free Press.

Barry, P. 2004. Pushing down drug costs: AARP opens drive to lower drug prices with a range of fixes to new Medicare law. *AARP Bulletin, 45*(2):8.

Beatty, J. 1990. A post–cold war budget. *Atlantic Monthly* 256(2):74–82.

Binstock, R. H. 1972. Interest-group liberalism and the politics of aging. *Gerontologist* 12:265–80.

Binstock, R. H. 1983. The aged as scapegoat. *Gerontologist* 23:136–43.

Binstock, R. H. 1998. *Public Policy and Voluntary Health Agencies.* Washington, D.C.: National Health Council.

Binstock, R. 2000. Older people and voting participation: Past and future. *Gerontologist* 40:18–31.

Bipartisan Commission on Entitlement and Tax Reform. 1995. *Final Report.* Washington, D.C.: Government Printing Office.

Birnbaum, J. H. 1997. Washington's power 25. *Fortune,* December 8. www.pathfinder.com/fortune/1997/971208/was 1.htm.

Budge, R. M., and R. Marini. 2003. AARP still getting whacked over backing of bill. *San Antonio Express/News,* December 26. Retrieved December 29, 2003, from http://news.mysanantonio.com/story.cfm?xla=saen&xlc=1104697.

Callahan, D. 1987. *Setting Limits: Medical Goals in an Aging Society.* New York: Simon and Schuster.

Campbell, A. L. 2003. *How Policies Make Citizens: Senior Political Activism and the American Welfare State.* Princeton, N.J.: Princeton University Press.

Carballo, M. 1981. Extra votes for parents? *Boston Globe,* December 17, 35.

Chapman, S. 2003. Meet the greedy grandparents. *Slate,* December 10. Retrieved December 17 from http://slate.msn.com/id/2092302/%20.

Cohen, W. J. 1985. Reflections on the enactment of Medicare and Medicaid. *Health Care Financing Review, Annual Supplement,* 3–11.

Connelly, M. 2000. Who voted: A portrait of American politics, 1976–2000. *New York Times,* November 12, wk4.

Cook, D. 2003. The point man on AARP's controversial move. *Christian Science Monitor.* December 11. Retrieved December 29, 2003, from www.christiansciencemonitor.com/2003/12/11/p03s01-supo.hmtl

Cook, F. L., and E. J. Barrett. 1992. *Support for the American Welfare State.* New York: Columbia University Press.

Cook, F. L., V. M. Marshall, J. E. Marshall, and J. E. Kaufman. 1994. The salience of intergenerational equity in Canada and the United States. Pp. 91–129 in T. R. Marmor, T. M. Smeeding, and V. L. Greene, eds., *Economic Security and Intergenerational Justice: A Look at North America.* Washington, D.C.: Urban Institute Press.

Daniels, N. 1988. *Am I My Parents' Keeper? An Essay on Justice between the Young and the Old.* New York: Oxford University Press.

Day, C. L. 1990. *What Older Americans Think.* Princeton, N.J.: Princeton University Press.

Day, C. L. 1998. Old-age interest groups in the 1990s: Coalition, competition, strategy. Pp. 131–50 in J. S. Steckenrider and T. M. Parrott, eds., *New Directions in Old-Age Policies.* Albany: State University of New York.

Derthick, M. 1979. *Policymaking for Social Security.* Washington, D.C.: Brookings Institution.

Drinkard, J., and W. M. Welch. 2003. AARP accused of conflict of interest. *USA Today,* November 24, 11A.

Dumas, K. 1992. Budget buster hot potato: The earnings test. *Congressional Quarterly Weekly Report,* January 11, 52–55.

Estes, C. L. 1979. *The Aging Enterprise.* San Francisco: Jossey-Bass.

Fairlie, H. 1988. Talkin' 'bout my generation. *New Republic* 198:19–22.

Ford Foundation, Project on Social Welfare and the American Future, Executive Panel. 1989. *The Common Good: Social Welfare and the American Future.* New York: Ford Foundation.

Freudenheim, M. 2004. Using new Medicare billions, H.M.O.s again court elderly. *New York Times,* March 9, A1.

Gibbs, N. R. 1980. Grays on the go. *Time* 131(8):66–75.

290   Robert H. Binstock

Greenhouse, S. 2001. A.F.L.-C.I.O. forms retiree advocacy Group. *New York Times,* May 24, A14.

Hacker, J. S., and T. Marmor. 2003. Medicare reform: Fact, fiction and foolishness. *Public Policy and Aging Report* 13(4):1, 20–23.

Hartz, L. 1955. *The Liberal Tradition in America.* New York: Harcourt Brace.

Haveman, R. 1994. Should generational accounts replace public budgets and deficits? *Journal of Economic Perspectives* 8 (Winter): 95–111.

Himmelfarb, R. 1995. *Catastrophic Politics: The Rise and Fall of the Medicare Catastrophic Coverage Act of 1988.* University Park: Pennsylvania State University Press.

Hobbs, F. B. 1996. *65+ in the United States.* U.S. Bureau of the Census, Current Population Reports, Special Studies, P23-190. Washington, D.C.: Government Printing Office.

Holmes, S. A. 2001. The world according to AARP. *New York Times,* March 21, D1.

Holtzman, A. 1963. *The Townsend Movement: A Political Study.* New York: Bookman Associates.

Hudson, R. B. 1978. The "graying" of the federal budget and its consequences for old age policy. *Gerontologist* 18:428–40.

Hudson, R. B. 1998. Privatizing old-age benefits: Re-emergent ideology encounters organized interest. Pp. 11–19 in J. G. Gonyea, ed., *Re-Securing Social Security and Medicare: Understanding Privatization and Risk.* Washington, D.C.: Gerontological Society of America.

Iglehart, J. K. 2004. The new Medicare prescription-drug benefit—a pure power play. *New England Journal of Medicine* 350:826–33.

Jacobson, G. C. 1992. *The Politics of Congressional Elections,* third edition. New York: Harper Collins.

Kosterlitz, J. 1993. Golden silence? *National Journal,* April 3, 800–804.

Kotlikoff, L. J. 1992. *Generational Accounting: Knowing Who Pays, and When, for What We Spend.* New York: Free Press.

Krugman, P. 2003. AARP gone astray. *New York Times,* November 21, A31.

Leadership Council of Aging Organizations. 2004a. LCAO Mission and Purpose. Retrieved March 26, 2004, from http://lcao.org/himssion.htm.

Leadership Council of Aging Organizations. 2004b. Social Security privatization. Retrieved March 26, 2004, from http://lcao.org/legagenda/ss_private.htm.

Lehrman, E. I. 1995. Health-care reform at the crossroads. *Modern Maturity,* January–February, 12.

Light, P. C. 1985. *Artful Work: The Politics of Social Security Reform.* New York: Random House.

Lipset, S. M. 1996. *American Exceptionalism: A Double-Edged Sword.* New York: Norton.

Lockett, B. A. 1983. *Aging, Politics, and Research: Setting the Federal Agenda for Research on Aging.* New York: Springer Publishing Company.

Marmor, T. R. 2000. *The Politics of Medicare.* Hawthorne, N.Y.: Aldine de Gruyter.

Medicare Payment Advisory Commission. 1998. *Report to the Congress: Medicare Payment Policy, Volume I: Recommendations.* Washington, D.C.: Government Printing Office.

Messinger, S. L. 1955. Organizational transformation: A case study of a declining social movement. *American Sociological Review* 20:3–10.

Morris, C. R. 1996. *The AARP: America's Most Powerful Lobby and the Clash of Generations.* New York: Times Books

National Association of Retired Federal Employees. 2004a. About NARFE. Retrieved March 28, 2004, from www.narfe.org/guest/about_narfe _guest.cfm.

National Committee to Preserve Social Security and Medicare. 2004a. Message from the President. Retrieved March 27, 2004, from www .ncpssm.org/about/index.html.

National Committee to Preserve Social Security and Medicare. 2004b. Join Us. Retrieved March 27, 2004, from www.ncpssm.org/join/indes/html.

Neugarten, B. L. 1970. The old and the young in modern societies. *American Behavioral Scientist* 14:13–24.

Newsweek. 1995. Senior power rides again. February 20, 31.

New York Times. 1994a. Endorsement riles members of retiree group. August 12, A10.

New York Times. 1994b. Not all in A.A.R.P. are behind health plan. August 13, A7.

New York Times. 1995. G.O.P. senator investigates finances of retirees' group. April 9, Y13.

New York Times. 1996a. A transcript of the first televised debate between Clinton and Dole. October 8, A14–17.

New York Times. 1996b. Excerpts from the second televised debate between Clinton and Dole. October 18, C22–23.

Novelli, W. D. 2003. AARP stays sharp. *Wall Street Journal,* December 4, A16.

Novelli, W. D. 2004. Now, the next phase. *AARP Bulletin* 45(1):28.

Pear, R. 1995. Senator challenges the practices of a retirees association. *New York Times,* June 14, A14.

Pear, R. 1999. Medicare panel, sharply divided, submits no plan. *New York Times,* March 17, A1.

Pear, R. 2003a. Fewer people on Medicare are dropped by H.M.O.s. *New York Times*, September 9, A21.

Pear, R. 2003b. Sweeping Medicare change wins approval in congress; President claims a victory. *New York Times*, November 26, A1.

Pear, R. 2004a. Medicare actuary gives wanted data to Congress. *New York Times*, March 20, A8.

Pear, R. 2004b. AARP, eye on drug costs, urges change in new law. *New York Times*, January 17, A12.

Pear, R., and R. Toner. 2003a. Counting votes and attacks in final push for Medicare bill. *New York Times*, November 20, A21.

Pear, R., and R. Toner. 2003b. Medicare plan covering drugs backed by AARP. *New York Times*, November 18, A21.

Personal Responsibility and Work Opportunity Reconciliation Act. 1996. Public Law No. 104-93.

Peterson, P. G. 1987. The morning after. *Atlantic Monthly* 260(4):43–49.

Pinner, F. A., P. Jacobs, and P. Selznick. 1959. *Old Age and Political Behavior*. Berkeley, Calif.: University of California Press.

Powell, L. A., K. J. Branco, and J. B. Williamson. 1996. *The Senior Rights Movement: Framing the Policy Debate in America*. New York: Twayne Publishers.

Pratt, H. J. 1976. *The Gray Lobby*. Chicago: University of Chicago Press.

Pratt, H. J. 1993. *Gray Agendas: Interest Groups and Public Pensions in Canada, Britain, and the United States*. Ann Arbor: University of Michigan Press.

Preston, S. H. 1984. Children and the elderly in the U.S. *Scientific American* 251(6):44–49.

Quadagno, J. 1989. Generational equity and the politics of the welfare state. *Politics and Society* 17:353–76.

Quadagno, J. In press. Why the United States has no national health insurance: Stakeholder mobilization against the welfare state, 1945–1996. *Journal of Health and Social Behavior*.

Richtman, M. 2004. Personal communication to the author from the executive director of the National Committee to Preserve Social Security and Medicare, February, 5.

Rosenzweig, R. M. 1990. Address to the president's opening session, 43rd Annual Meeting of the Gerontological Society of America, Boston, November 16.

Salholz, E. 1990. Blaming the voters: Hapless budgeteers single out "greedy geezers." *Newsweek*, October 29, 36.

Seniors Coalition. 2004. About TSC. Retrieved March 26, 2004, from www.senior.org/bin/view.fpl/10142/article/327/cms_article/327.html.

Smeeding, T. M., M. P. Battin, L. P. Francis, and B. M. Landesman, eds.

1987. *Should Medical Care Be Rationed by Age?* Totowa, N.J.: Rowman & Littlefield.

Smith, L. 1992. The tyranny of America's old. *Fortune* 125(1):68–72.

Stevenson, R. W. 1998a. Privatization of Social Security is gaining ground. *New York Times*, April 6, A1.

Stevenson, R. W. 1998b. Clinton may use Wall Street to ease Social Security ills. *New York Times*, July 28, A9.

Stolberg. S. G. 2003. An 800-pound gorilla changes partners over Medicare. *New York Times*, November 23, wk5.

Thompson, T. G. 2004. The Facts about Upcoming New Benefits in Medicare. Undated letter received by Medicare enrollees in March.

Thurow, L. C. 1996. The birth of a revolutionary class. *New York Times Magazine*, May 19, 46–47.

Toner, R. 2003a. G.O.P. steals thunder. *New York Times*, June 28, A1.

Toner, R. 2003b. An imperfect compromise. *New York Times*, November 25, A1.

U.S. House of Representatives. 1977. *Federal Responsibility to the Elderly: Executive Programs and Legislative Jurisdiction.* Report of the Select Committee on Aging. Washington, D.C.: Government Printing Office.

USA Today. 2003. AARP balks at drug plan. July 17. Retrieved July 21, 2003, from www.aarp.org/bulletin/departments/2001/news/article.html.

Van Tassel, D. D., and J. E. W. Meyer. 1992. *U.S. Aging Policy Interest Groups: Institutional Profiles.* New York: Greenwood Press.

Vladeck, B. C. 1999. Plenty of nothing—a report from the Medicare Commission. *New England Journal of Medicine* 340:1503–6.

Walker, J. L. 1983. The origins and maintenance of interest groups in America. *American Political Science Review* 77:390–406.

Weissert, W. G. 2003. Medicare Rx: Just a few of the reasons why it was so difficult to pass. *Public Policy and Aging Report* 13(4):1, 3–6.

White, J. 2003. The Social Security and Medicare debate three years after the 2000 election. *Public Policy and Aging Report* 13(4):15–19.

Williamson, J. B. 1997. A critique of the case for privatizing Social Security. *Gerontologist* 37:561–71.

14. Using Local Tax Levies to Fund Programs for Older People
Good Politics and Good Policy?

Robert Applebaum, Sarah Poff Roman,
Marc Molea, and Alan Burnett

In the late 1970s a retiree named Lois Brown Dale was looking for financial support to build and operate a senior center in a small county in southwest Ohio. She believed the public would support such an effort through local taxes but was informed that placing such a referendum on the ballot would require special legislation. Undeterred, she successfully lobbied the Ohio legislature to allow counties to earmark local funds for elder services. It is safe to say that neither Ms. Dale nor the members of the legislature envisioned that twenty-five years later 58 of Ohio's 88 counties would have property tax levies raising nearly $85 million for services for older people.

In some metropolitan counties, such as Hamilton (Cincinnati) and Franklin (Columbus), the property tax revenues are large, generating more than $18 million per year for community and in-home services. In nonmetropolitan counties, funds generated by levies range from $9,000 to $860,000, with more than half generating less than $250,000 annually. Levy funds in these counties are typically used to fund services provided by a local senior center. Regardless of the size, each levy has in common that local voters determine the ultimate fate of the program. In several urban counties, umbrella human services property tax levies support multiple community needs, including but not limited to mental retardation/developmental disabilities, health, mental health, children services, and senior services. Several municipalities and townships, most notably where there is no countywide levy, have used property tax levies to support senior services and facilities in their jurisdictions.

In addition to the extensive effort in Ohio, other states, including Michigan, Kansas, Louisiana, and North Dakota, have local levies in place. It seems likely that such efforts will continue and expand as we age as a nation. The growth of this approach, while praised by some as a major innovation, is also accompanied by a series of critical policy questions. Does such an approach represent good public policy? Do such efforts create intergenerational conflict? Are older citizens getting too large a share of societal resources? Are levies designed for older people successful at the expense of other age- and need-based levies such as children's services, mental health, or health programs? Although answers to such questions are difficult to assess, a review of the Ohio experience in the context of national studies on support for local tax initiatives provides some insight into this issue.

Levy Support for Aging Service Programs in Ohio

As noted, the use of local tax levies to support programs for older people has become a core element of the aging network funding base in Ohio. Because of variations in local politics, economic conditions, and aging service organizational structures, the levies vary dramatically in size, scope, host agency, and nature of support (see Table 14.1). For example, about one-third of Ohio levies are relatively small, generating less than $300,000 annually in financial support. Another third are moderate in size, drawing between $300,000 and $900,000 annually. The final group consists of levies with revenues over $1 million, with one at $8 million and two over $18 million annually. Regional differences also exist, with southwestern Ohio accounting for more than one-third of the levy dollars generated for the entire state.

There are also trends in how levy dollars are spent, depending on the size of the levy. The predominant services funded with levy dollars include transportation, senior center operations and maintenance, home-delivered and congregate meals, information and referral, homemaker services, and recreation activities. Levies generating $300,000 per year or less are typically used to fund services provided by a local senior center. The moderate group ($300,000–$900,000) often funds senior centers and an array of social services provided through a combination of local providers and the senior centers themselves. The larger levies (more than $1 million) have been used to set up extensive in-home care programs, using care management and a variety of providers to deliver a range of community-based services to older people in their communities. Twenty-three (59%) of Ohio's 39 metropolitan counties and 33 (67%) of Ohio's 49 nonmetropolitan counties have levies that exclusively support senior services.

Table 14.1 Summary of aging services levies in Ohio, by revenue, duration, and services funded

Annual Revenue Amount	Number of Levies in Ohio	Duration of Levies		Types of Services and Host Agencies Typically Funded
		3 Years	5 Years	
Less than $300,000	23	2 (8.7%)	21 (91.3%)	Senior center services
$300,00–$900,000	20	0 (0.0 %)	20 (100%)	Senior center/local providers services
$1,000,000+	15	1 (6.7%)	14 (93.3%)	Local AAA's (HCBS programs)
State total: $82,452,687	58	3 (5.2%)	55 (94.8%)	

Source: Ohio Department of Aging 2003

The senior services levies are county based and can be placed on the ballot through citizen petition ("initiative") or by local elected officials ("resolution"). The host agency is determined through the political process by those placing the issue on the ballot. In some instances the local senior center serves as the catalyst for the effort and is the named levy recipient. In many counties, a local council on aging serves as the host agency for the levy. In some communities, the regional entity (the area agency on aging) serves as the host agency for the administration of levy funds.

How Other States Compare

As previously mentioned, levy programs also exist in Kansas, Louisiana, Michigan, and North Dakota. While these programs tend to generate smaller revenues than those in Ohio, they have become reliable sources of funding for aging services at the county level (see Table 14.2 for a comparison of state levy programs). In Kansas, 64 out of 104 counties (62%) had levy programs in 2001, generating a total of $8,025,080 to fund senior services. Annual revenues among these counties ranged from $5,668 to $1,918,887, with 49 of them (77%) under $100,000. Consistent with smaller levy programs in Ohio, levy funds in Kansas are typically used to fund senior center programs and support services such as transportation and nutrition programs.

Levy programs are less common in Louisiana, where 13 out of 46 counties (28%) have a local millage (property tax levy) for aging serv-

Table 14.2 State comparison of aging services levies, 2001

State	Number of Counties with Levies	Total Revenues ($)	Low ($)	High ($)
Kansas	64 of 104 (62%)	8,025,080	5,668	1,918,887
Louisiana	13 of 46 (28%)	6,055,147	50,000	2,700,000
Michigan	59 of 85 (69%)	25,441,562	25,000	3,250,000
North Dakota	50 of 53 (94%)	1,538,141	4,020	278,991
Ohio	58 of 88 (66%)	82,452,687	9,000	18,200,000

Source: Data from 2001, except for North Dakota (2002).

ices administered by area agencies on aging. In 2002 Louisiana levies generated a total of $6,055,147 for senior services programs. Annual county revenues ranged from $50,000 to $2,700,000, with nearly half below the $200,000 mark. In Michigan, 59 out of 85 counties (69%) had levies in 2001, contributing a total of $25,441,562 to senior services. Among these programs, revenues ranged from $25,000 to $3,250,000, with 7 counties over $1 million and 9 under $100,000. Mill levies in North Dakota are common, with 50 out of 53 counties participating in such programs. These levies generated $1,538,141 for senior services in North Dakota in 2002. The size of these levies ranged from $4,020 to $278,991, with 47 (94%) generating less than $100,000 in revenues.

Why Seek Levy Funding?

Our analysis suggests several major reasons why Ohio counties have embraced this strategy: the limitations of the state's long-term care system, the lack of a comprehensive approach to serving older people with chronic disability at the federal level, and the failure of the Older Americans Act to keep pace with inflation and with the rising number of older people. At the state level, Ohio has relied primarily on the home and community-based Medicaid waiver program to support in-home services. State funds are used to provide the required match to Medicaid. Dollars from a state-funded community services block grant and a state Alzheimer's Respite Program supplement aging network services. Ohio does not have the general revenue dollar support that is available in many states to supplement the limitations associated with the Medicaid program. Two major criticisms of the federal Medicaid waiver programs are that they are designed for very low-income people, and that those participating must be severely disabled, meeting the nursing home level of care criteria for the state. This is problematic because many low-income older people are ineligible for Medicaid assistance because of Ohio's stringent $1,500 asset limitation. Also, many individuals may need in-home assistance in such areas as bathing, shopping, and meal preparation, but would not meet the criteria for nursing home entry, making them ineligible for the federal program. With these major limitations in the existing system, and with little or no action expected at the state or federal levels, local counties have decided to act on their own to develop a more comprehensive long-term care service delivery system in their communities.

In the communities that have large levies, these dollars have typically been used to actually create a community-based system. Used in conjunction with Medicaid waiver dollars, programs established in these counties have tried to develop a comprehensive service system. With a centralized intake and assessment process, older residents in these communities can call a well-publicized telephone number to receive detailed information on available services and an assessment or referral, depending on client circumstances. This approach has generated a larger volume of telephone calls and applications for long-term care assistance. Because most state home care programs rely heavily on Medicaid and restrict access to home care based on income and disability, a centralized information and intake process does not typically exist across the state or the country.

In some communities, local tax dollars supplement funding from the Older Americans Act, which has been considerably underfunded over the past two decades. The Act has remained at essentially the same level of federal funding for the past twenty-five years. Given inflation and the growth in the older population, the program faces serious limitations in its ability to make services available to older people. Although it remains important as a foundation for the aging network, the Older Americans Act has never achieved an adequate level of support to operate even basic programs for all older adults.

Engaging local levies by local constituencies receives both praise and criticism. On the positive side, such efforts provide an example of communities stepping up to meet the needs of the local citizenry. Program sponsors often discuss the fact that if they waited for the state and federal government to develop a comprehensive long-term care policy, most of the consumers and families that they are helping would be long gone. With a federal or state program unlikely any time soon, advocates argue that the local approach is the only alternative. The local strategy also provides considerable recognition and support at the community level, something that does not always occur in state and federal efforts. Interestingly, the levy renewals in Ohio have drawn even more positive support than the initial levy votes, typically winning between 60 and 80 percent of the votes. These margins are rarely seen in other tax issues placed on the ballot. In communities that have implemented such levies, local citizens and politicians are well aware of the programs and tend to be proud of their community's investment. Levies earmarked for older people do indeed appear to be good politics.

While this approach has garnered widespread support in Ohio and other states, there are some that contend that such initiatives do not represent a good public policy strategy. They argue that such a system has many of the same limitations as experienced in local funding of schools. One argument is that it creates a class system across the state, with wealthy counties having a greater ability to raise funds than poorer counties. In other words, a two-tiered long-term care system is being created, depending on which county one resides in. Critics also argue that because the property tax is not based on income, it places a proportionally higher burden on older people who are likely to own their homes but be on fixed incomes. Some have also argued that the expansion of local strategies allows and even encourages the state or federal government to ignore the policy issue because the problem is being addressed at the local level. Finally, it is suggested that this approach represents one more incremental step in the creation of a fragmented system, with different funding levels, eligibility criteria, host agencies, and services provided.

Good Politics versus Good Policy

Perhaps the most controversial issue about the property tax levies targeted for older people is the question of intergenerational equity and fairness. Are levies receiving support at the expense of other groups in need? What role does the older voter play in supporting local tax levies? Do individuals support only those levies that will benefit themselves? Although policy analysts have speculated about the effects of such initiatives, there is limited empirical data from which to draw conclusions. Because of the relative newness of levy-supported programs for older adults, there is a dearth of information about the effects on local politics and social policies.

Review of Existing Data

Whether supporting levies for older people hurts other populations in need of services, and how older voters affect passage of such initiatives is a difficult question to answer empirically. We identified a series of articles on this topic, with somewhat mixed results. For the past two decades, policy analysts have raised questions about intergenerational equity and the distribution of societal resources (Preston 1984; Heclo 1988; Van Parijs 1999; Silverstein et al. 2000). Two main points of dissension are debated in this body of work: whether older people are getting too big a share of societal resources, and whether older people are supportive of other age and need groups. Exploring both sides of these debates offers insight into the viability of property tax levy initiatives. As will be presented, this approach to funding could potentially be criticized in both of these areas.

Distribution of Societal Resources

Questions about the distribution of social resources are ultimately answered subjectively, depending on one's values and beliefs of societal equity. The contention that increased local spending on older adults will come at the expense of other need groups (especially children) is based on the assumption that these populations are in direct competition for resources. Although there has been considerable publicity about the graying of the federal budget, an argument largely driven by the funds allocated by beneficiaries themselves to the Social Security and Medicare trust funds, such expenditure patterns do not exist at the state and local levels. For example, the three leading expenditure categories in Ohio's budget are education, corrections, and Medicaid. Even the Medicaid program, which represents about one-fifth of the entire state budget, spends only about one-third of its revenues on older people. Education and corrections are clearly not targeted toward older people, as is the case for other major expenditure categories such as transportation, welfare and employment assistance, public safety, and emergency assistance. At the local level, schools, libraries, and public services such as water, sewer, and refuse disposal dominate budget allocations. Service levies designed for special populations such as mental health, children with special needs, and older people round out the local funding but are small in comparison to the primary expenditure group. Funding for senior services is not in direct competition with any one need group, suggesting that high spending for seniors does not necessitate low spending on children. Studies have shown that in many states an increase in the proportion of older people and a subsequent decrease in the proportion of younger people often translates into higher spending per child (Adams and Dominick 1995). Based on this analysis of state and local budget allocations, it is difficult to make the argument that older people are receiving an excessive share of state and local resources in comparison to other age groups.

Support for Other Need Groups

The other side of the equity debate is whether older people are supportive of other groups at the polls. Because of their growing numbers and high voter turn-out, questions have been raised about the effect older people will have on the passage of funding for other interest groups. Relative to local taxation, critics have argued that increasing support for aging services might be catastrophic for education and other programs for children.

A body of work does indicate that a high proportion of older voters in a community may result in resistance to supporting local initiatives (Button 1992; Poterba 1997). Panel data from a national study over a thirty-year period concluded that an increase in the proportion of older people in a state resulted in a decrease in per child student expenditures (Poterba 1997). This argument suggests that local taxes for schools might be viewed as resources that do not offer the same benefit for older residents as for the rest of the population. It has also been argued that older people who migrate may have less commitment to their new community and are thus less likely to support initiatives that do not directly benefit them (Button 1992).

Some studies, however, have found that there might be other variables at play, and that these trends are not related entirely to an aging population. These data reveal distinct trends in support for educational spending, depending on the ethnic background and socioeconomic status of the voting public. For example, studies have found that older voters are less likely to support spending on education and children's programs when the majority of the younger population is of a different racial background (Poterba 1997; Ladd and Murray 2001). Additionally, analysts have reported the majority of "selfish" voting patterns among older people with low incomes (Button and Rosenbaum 1990).

An equal number of articles found that an increased aging population has little to no effect on the ability of a local community to raise revenue for education or other locally supported programs (Button and Rosenbaum 1990; Ladd and Murray ; Harris, 2001Evans, and Schwab 2001). A range of reasons were identified to explain this outcome. Primarily, these analysts argue that the economic and social diversity of the older population makes it unlikely that they will vote as a block on any political issue (Button 1992; Adams and Dominick 1995). Additionally, older people who migrate to a new area can choose their new location based on the local tax structure, thus choosing to live in communities that best meet their needs (Button 1992; Adams and Dominick 1995; Poterba 1998). If these migratory elders elect to live in communities where there is minimal taxation for education or children's programs, they should have little effect on the tax structure in the community (Poterba 1998).

Ohio's Experience

With some of the largest, longest-running, and most successful property tax initiatives to fund services for older people, Ohio should provide experience that sheds light on the applicability of this approach. Although data are not available state-wide on the effect of the Ohio tax levies, the experience of the two largest counties shows that existing community levies continue to receive support and that new funding initiatives are not jeopardized. For example, Hamilton County (Cincinnati) continues to support such diverse efforts as the zoo and the children's hospital, while levies for new football and baseball stadiums were passed, along with a new levy for the largest school district. Also noteworthy is the huge success and public support that these levies have had. To illustrate, the levy in Hamilton County has received an increasing majority of the vote since its inception in 1992 and has grown from $12 million to $18 million today.

Local Levies as Good Public Policy:
Policy Directions for an Aging Society

While the implications of using property tax levies to fund programs for older people raise some interesting policy questions, it is clear that new policy directions to support an aging society are critical. Given the current economic climate and the political focus on reduced domestic spending and federal taxes, it seems unlikely that major federal initiatives to support services for older people outside of the current Social Security and Medicare frameworks will occur. With the incredible demographic shifts to be experienced, the pressure on states to provide supportive services for older people with chronic disability will continue to mount. In many states the response to these pressures is primarily through the Medicaid program, allowing states to focus on the most disabled and lowest income population while at the same time receiving federal match. This excludes the majority of older people residing in the community who are not eligible for Medicaid because of the stringent income and asset requirements and the strict disability requirements and leaves local communities to address the problem.

As evidenced through this review, the feasibility of implementing a local approach depends on the community in question and its unique sociodemographic characteristics. In the case of Ohio, property tax levies have become a viable alternative, and these programs are an essential backbone to the aging network. Such efforts have certainly proven to be good politics. It appears that the lack of federal and state policy may mean that such efforts represent sound future policy as well.

References

Adams, P., and Dominick, G. L. 1995. The old, the young, and the welfare state. *Generations* 19(3):38–42.

Button, J. W. 1992. A sign of generational conflict: The impact of Florida's aging voters on local school and tax referenda. *Social Science Quarterly* 73(4):786–97.

Button, J. W., and W. Rosenbaum. 1990. Gray power, gray peril, or gray myth? The political impact of the aging in local sunbelt politics. *Social Science Quarterly* 71(1):25–37.

Harris, A. R., W. N. Evans, and R. M. Schwab. 2001. Education spending in an aging America. *Journal of Public Economics* 81:449–72.

Heclo, H. 1988. Generational politics. Pp. 381–411 in J. Palmer, T. Smeeding, and B. B. Torrey, eds., *The Vulnerable*. Washington, D.C.: Urban Institute Press.

Ladd, H. F., and S. E. Murray. 2001. Intergenerational conflict reconsidered: County demographic structure and the demand for public education. *Economics of Education Review* 20:343–57.

Poterba, J. M. 1997. Demographic structure and the political economy of public education. *Journal of Policy Analysis and Management* 16(1):48–66.

Poterba, J. M. 1998. Demographic change, intergenerational linkages, and public education. *American Economic Review Papers and Proceedings* (May):315–20.

Preston, S. H. 1984. Children and the elderly: Divergent paths for America's dependents. *Demography* 21(4):435–57.

Silverstein, M., T. M. Parrott, J. J. Angelelli, and F. L. Cook. 2000. Solidarity and tension between age-groups in the United States: Challenge for an aging America in the 21st century. *International Journal of Social Welfare* 2000(9):270–84.

Van Parijs, P. 1999. The disenfranchisement of the elderly, and other attempts to secure intergenerational justice. *Philosophy and Public Affairs* 27(4):292–333.

Index

AARP, 237–38, 277, 281–86, 287
activities of daily living (ADLs), 134, 142, 166, 253
African Americans, 76; disability and, 112; economic status of, 10, 165; health care costs of, 72–73; labor force participation of, 121, 122; as old-old, 164–66; retirement and, 118–20, 122, 129–30, 135–53; Social Security and, 31, 78–82 passim, 195–98
age-based benefits: critique of, 8–11, 123–24, 152; development of, 3, 4–7; Medicare and, 206–10, 217; oldest-old and, 168–70; rationale for, 8, 14–16, 23–24, 109–10, 157; risk and, 209–10
Age Discrimination in Employment Act (ADEA), 4
Alliance for Retired Americans, 280–81
Alzheimer's Association, 238, 279, 280
Americans for Generational Equity (AGE), 269–70
Americans with Disabilities Act (1990), 258
assisted living, 254–56, 260
Assisted Living Conversion Program, 255

baby boom generation, 11; disability and, 172; intergenerational equity and, 269–70; long-term care and, 176; Medicaid and, 74; Medicare

and, 207; oldest-old and, 159–61; Social Security and, 81
Balanced Budget Act (1997), 70, 97, 271–72
Berenson, R., 72
Beveridge Plan, 94–96
Binstock, R., 159
Bipartisan Commission on the Future of Medicare, 272–73
blacks. *See* African Americans
Blahous, C., 199
Bonelli, G., 58, 59
Bongaarts, J., 111
bridge jobs, 9, 143
Bush, G. W., 193

Callahan, D., 270
Camacho, T., 164
Canada, pension policy in, 54–55
care work, 32, 77–78
children, 38, 301, 302; elderly and, 23, 38, 42–43, 158; ratio to older people, 188–89
Clinton, B., 7, 237, 271
Congregate Housing Services Program (CHSP), 253
conservatism, 36, 85, 92–93, 99–101; interest groups and, 278; Medicaid and, 226, 236; Medicare and, 85, 272–73; Social Security and, 100, 186, 188–89, 192–93, 274; welfare state and, 5, 49, 92, 174

Dale, L., 294
Diamond, P., 12, 198

dignity, 27–30
disability, 2, 110–12; housing and, 256; oldest-old and, 166–68; retirement and, 117–18; self-assessment of, 165; trends in, 172
Dole, B., 276

earnings test (Social Security), 9, 79
Employee Benefits Research Institute, 121
Employee Retirement Income Security Act (ERISA, 1974), 45
employment-based benefits, 68, 85, 210
employment of aged. *See* labor force participation
entitlement programs, 23–24, 34, 36, 96

Fair Housing Amendments Act (FHAA, 1988), 248, 260
Federal Employee Retirement System (FERS), 103
Federal Interagency Forum on Aging-Related Statistics, 110, 160, 170, 210
Feeney, G., 11
Foner, A., 175
Ford Foundation, 269

general revenue financing, 58–59
"generational accounting," 13, 269
generations, 11–12, 42–60 passim
Gokhale, J., 12, 13
Goldwater, B., 186
Goodin, R., 28
Great Britain, pension reform in, 94–97, 101–3, 194, 198–99
Great Society, 4, 266
"greedy geezers," 14, 267–68
Greenspan, A., 6

Haber, C., 2
Health and Retirement Study (HRS), 118, 130, 132–34
health insurance, private, 26, 67–68, 73–74, 85, 116, 121, 123, 207–10, 215

health maintenance organizations (HMOs), 33, 71, 72, 208, 215, 271
Hispanics, 11, 92; disability and, 112; health and, 72–73; 165–66; labor force participation of, 121, 122; life expectancy of, 161; retirement of, 118–20, 122, 129–52 passim; Social Security and, 78–82 passim, 195–98
Hohaus, R., 184
home and community care programs, 69–70, 295, 297–98
housing: aging in place in, 257; development of senior, 244–46, 256; elderly and handicapped, 249; elderly and younger persons, 250; grandparents in, 250–51; Section 202, 245–47, 253–55
Housing and Community Development Act (1992), 250, 253

ideology, 2–3, 13–14, 38, 85–86, 92–93, 99–100, 102–4, 105n. 4
Institute of Medicine, 115, 116
intergenerational equity, 11, 42–51 passim, 59–60, 61n. 7, 178, 231, 247, 268–69, 300
intragenerational justice, 51–59

Jacoby, J., 188

Kahn, R., 175
Kennelly, B., 234–35, 238
Kerr-Mills program, 222–23
Kohli, M., 42
Kotlikoff, L., 12, 269
Krugman, P., 192

labor force participation, 8, 9, 117–21, 130–53; African Americans and, 66, 78, 119; Hispanics and, 66, 78, 119; medical benefits and, 121–23; Social Security and, 9, 129, 196–97; women and, 9, 66
Landon, A., 186
Leadership Council of Aging Organizations (LCAO), 278–79